Practical Periodontics

Practical Periodontics

Second Edition

Edited by

Kenneth Eaton

PhD, MSc, BDS, MGDSRCS, FFGDP(UK) Hon.,
FCGDent, FFPH, FHEA, FICD, FNCUP, DHC
Specialist in Periodontics and Dental Public Health,
Visiting Professor University College London; Honorary
Professor University of Kent, Advisor to the Council of
European Chief Dental Officers

Philip Ower

MSc, BDS, FFGDP(UK) Hon., MGDSRCS (Eng & Ed)
Formerly Specialist in Periodontics and Director,
PerioCourses Ltd, UK

For additional online content visit Elsevier eBooks+

ELSEVIER

Notices

Practitioners and researchers must always rely on their own experience and knowledge in evaluating and using any information, methods, compounds or experiments described herein. Because of rapid advances in the medical sciences, in particular, independent verification of diagnoses and drug dosages should be made. To the fullest extent of the law, no responsibility is assumed by Elsevier, authors, editors or contributors for any injury and/or damage to persons or property as a matter of product liability, negligence or otherwise, or from any use or operation of any methods, products, instructions or ideas contained in the material herein.

ISBN: 978-0-3238-7845-6

Content Strategist: Alex Mortimer
Content Development Specialist: Supriya Barua Kumar
Design: Ryan Cook
Illustration Manager: Akshaya Mohan
Marketing Manager: Deborah Watkins

Printed in Scotland

Last digit is the print number: 9   8   7   6   5   4   3   2   1

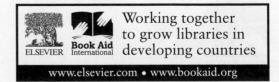

Contents

Foreword

After the success of the first edition, *Practical Periodontics* is now released as a second edition with fully updated chapters. This new edition maintains its scientific rigour, combining the introduction of new knowledge with a detailed description of current therapeutic concepts and the advent of new technologies. This work continues to focus on educating students with evidence-based concepts and acquisition of relevant professional competences. The information provided is clear, well organized and very practical, but at the same time it has been rigorously reviewed and is updated with current knowledge, comprehensively covering modern periodontology from the basic knowledge necessary to understand aetiology and pathogenesis to the most relevant aspects of the prevention and therapy of periodontal diseases.

The authors, led by Professor Kenneth Eaton and Dr Philip C. Ower, together with many contributors, are not only well respected in the United Kingdom but also throughout Europe and beyond. Their contribution to this work clearly demonstrates not only excellent preparation but also the academic spirit and the teaching abilities that are needed to produce a book such as this with scientific rigour and practical relevance for students and professionals.

In summary, this book continues to provide useful and relevant content in line with contemporary educational concepts and with a practical approach to modern periodontology.

Mariano Sanz
Professor and Chairman of Periodontology
Faculty of Odontology, University Complutense of
Madrid (Spain)

Preface

We were honoured when Elsevier approached us with an invitation to edit a second edition of *Practical Periodontics*. We were tasked with producing a textbook for dental hygiene and therapy undergraduates and general dentists that is in the same style as other recent textbooks published by Elsevier. We chose the title to reflect the fact that we wanted this text not only to be a useful learning resource but also to have practical application. As a result this new book contains numerous figures and tables to illustrate the text and also the key points, highlighted in every chapter. It is hoped that this layout will help dental, hygiene and therapy undergraduates when they are preparing for examinations, as well as provide a resource for qualified clinicians.

We have also provided additional aids for revision and understanding in the form of questions, cases and videos. These resources can be found on the following website using the pin code in the front of this book for access: http://ebooks.health.elsevier.com/.

The sections of the new edition follow a logical progression starting with the aetiology of periodontal diseases. In the first section, the chapters cover the basic sciences relevant to periodontology and are on the anatomy of the periodontal tissues, periodontal pathogenesis, the epidemiology of periodontal diseases, host response and susceptibility, the role of bacterial biofilm and systemic and local risk factors for periodontitis. In the second section, the chapters cover classification of periodontal diseases, periodontal assessment of patients, gingival overgrowth, periodontal/systemic disease relationships and determining prognosis. The chapter on assessment is supplemented with an extensive video on the subject. The third section on treatment planning covers treatment planning for gingivitis and periodontitis, gingival recession, periodontal problems in children and young adults and specialist referrals. The fourth section deals with patient education and self-performed biofilm control. Its chapters are on the role of self-care and oral hygiene methods, clinical imaging and patient adherence. At a simplistic level this is perhaps the key section, as without excellent communication with patients and total cooperation on their part to control their biofilm, the efforts of a clinician are likely to be doomed to failure. The fifth section details non-surgical periodontal management and includes chapters on the nature of root surface contamination, periodontal instrumentation, the use of antimicrobials, the assessment of treatment outcomes and supportive therapy. The sixth section covers surgical periodontal therapy and the rationale for a surgical approach. The seventh and final section explains the interaction of periodontology with other dental disciplines, and there is a new chapter on dental implants – monitoring, maintenance and management of complications.

There is increasing emphasis nowadays on the role of evidence-based healthcare. It is therefore essential that from the outset undergraduate clinicians are prepared to question everything they read or are told. The questions "Who says so?", "Is it true?" and "Where is the evidence?" are key. For this reason all chapters contain several citations to lead the reader to the source texts for the statements made, and as a result there is an extensive reference list for most chapters. It is hoped that the reader will refer to the source papers when wanting to challenge any statement in the textbook, as deeper understanding comes from challenge and debate and not from rote learning.

We are deeply indebted to our colleagues who have either written or contributed to chapters in the textbook or who have made video or case reports available for the online part of this publication. They come from academia, specialist practice, general practice and industry. All have a passion for periodontology that we hope shines through in their chapters. Our sincere thanks to all of them. In addition we would like to thank Professors Peter Heasman and Philip Preshaw for permission to use the Newcastle University online material on assessing the periodontium and Dr Anastasiya Orishko and Professor Francesco D'Auito for permission to use the radiographs and periodontal charts for four cases. We would also like to thank the team at Elsevier for their support and for guiding us through the publication process, in particular Alexandra Mortimer and Supriya Barua Kumar.

We dedicate this book to the late Graham Smart and to the late Bernie Kieser, who was such an inspiration to us and Graham during our postgraduate training and subsequent careers in periodontology.

Kenneth Eaton and Philip Ower

Contributors

Paul Baker, MSc, BDS, MClinDent, FDSRCS(Eng), MRDRCS
Specialist in Periodontics, PerioLondon, UK

Leo Briggs, MSc, BDS
Specialist in Periodontics and Deputy Head, Dental Defence Union, UK

Iain Chapple, PhD, BDS, FDSRCS, FDSRCPS, CCST (Rest Dent)
Professor of Periodontology, Consultant in Restorative Dentistry and Director of Research, Institute of Clinical Sciences, University of Birmingham, UK

Marilou Ciantar, PhD(Hons), MSc, BChD(Hons), ILTM, MFDSRCS, MFDRCSI, FFDRCSI
Senior Clinical Lecturer in Periodontology, University of Edinburgh, UK

Valerie Clerehugh, PhD, BDS, FDSRCS, FHEA
Emeritus Professor of Periodontology, School of Dentistry, University of Leeds, UK

Paul Cooper, PhD, BSc
John Arnaud Bell Professor of Oral Biology, University of Otago, Dunedin, New Zealand

Ulpee Darbar, MSc, BDS, FDSRCS (Rest Dent) Ed, FDSRCS Eng, FHEA
Consultant in Restorative Dentistry & Honorary Associate Professor, Eastman Dental Hospital & Institute, University College, London

Ian Dunn, MSc, BChD, MCGDent
Specialist in Periodontics, UK

Kenneth Eaton, PhD, MSc, BDS, MGDSRCS, FFGDP(UK) Hon., FCGDent, FFPH, FHEA, FICD, FNCUP, DHC
Specialist in Periodontics and Dental Public Health, Visiting Professor University College London, Honorary Professor University of Kent, Advisor to the Council of European Chief Dental Officers

David Gillam, BA, BDS, MSc, DDS, FRSPH, MICR
Clinical Reader in Oral Bioengineering, Institute of Dentistry, Barts and the London School of Medicine and Dentistry, Queen Mary University London

Monica Lee, MSc, BDS, MFDSRCPS (Glas), MClinDent, MRDRCPS (Glas)
Specialist in Periodontics, Cambridge, UK

Martin Ling, BDS, MFDS, MFGDP, FHEA
Lecturer in Periodontology, University of Birmingham, UK

Philip D. Marsh PhD, BSc
Professor Emeritus in Oral Microbiology, Department of Oral Microbiology, School of Dentistry, University of Leeds, UK

John Matthews, PhD
Professor and Honorary Consultant in Periodontology, University of Birmingham, UK

Ewen McColl, BSc(Hons), BDS, MFDS, FDSRCPS, MCGDent, MRDRCS Ed, MClinDent, FDSRCS, FHEA, FDTF(Ed)
Director of Clinical Dentistry, Peninsula Dental School, University of Plymouth, UK

Neil Meredith, PhD, MSc, BDS, FDSRCS, LDSRCS, FICD
Professor in Prosthodontics and Head of Dental School, James Cook University, Queensland, Australia

Mike Milward, PhD, BDS, MFGDPRCS, MFDSRCPS, FHEA (UK)
Professor and Honorary Consultant in Periodontology, University of Birmingham, UK

Philip Ower, MSc, BDS, FFGDP(UK) Hon., MGDSRCS (Eng & Ed)
Formerly Specialist in Periodontics and Director, PerioCourses Ltd, UK

Colin Priestland, MSc, BDS, MGDSRCS
Private Practice, Townsville, Queensland, Australia

Elaine Tilling, MSc, RDH, DMS MIPHE
Education and Projects Manager, TePe Oral Hygiene Projects, UK

Aradhna Tugnait, PhD, MDEntSci, BChD, FDSRCS (Ed), FHEA
Associate Professor in Restorative Dentistry, School of Dentistry, University of Leeds, UK

Wendy Turner, BDS, FDS

Clinical Professor, Centre for Dentistry, School of
Medicine, Dentistry and Biomedical Science, Queen's
University Belfast

Andrew Walker, BDS, MFDS (Edin), MClinDent (Perio), DLM

Specialist in Periodontics, Dentolegal Consultant, Dental
Protection, Tutor, University of Liverpool Dental
School, UK

Alan Woodman, MSc, BDS, DGDP(UK), MRDRCS(Eng)

Formerly Specialist in Periodontics and Tutor, University
of Portsmouth Dental Academy, UK

José Zurdo, MBBS, BDS, Cert.Perio MSc

Specialist in Periodontics

Aetiology of Periodontal Diseases

1.1

THE MACRO- AND MICROANATOMY OF PERIODONTAL TISSUES

IAIN CHAPPLE AND MIKE MILWARD

CHAPTER OUTLINE

Introduction

Embryological Origins of the Periodontal Tissues

Microanatomy of the Gingival Tissues

Microanatomy of the Periodontal Ligament and Cementum

Periodontal Ligament
Cementum

Microanatomy of the Alveolar Bone

Acknowledgement

OVERVIEW OF THE CHAPTER

This chapter provides a description of basic periodontal anatomy and outlines the functions of the periodontal tissues.

By the end of the chapter the reader should be able to:

- Describe the macroscopic anatomy of the periodontal tissues and their embryological origins
- Identify key features of applied periodontal anatomy, visible during clinical examination
- Recognize how anatomical landmarks are related to definitions of health, gingivitis and periodontitis
- Recognize the changes in anatomical relationships that occur during disease processes

- Describe the microscopic features of normal anatomy and understand how they are related to normal structure and function, as well as how they change during disease.

The chapter covers the following topics:

- The embryological origins of the periodontium
- The tissues comprising the periodontium
- The microanatomy of the gingival tissues
- The microanatomy of the periodontal ligament and cementum
- The microanatomy of alveolar bone.

Introduction

Inflammatory periodontal diseases are among the most prevalent chronic diseases of humans and are a major cause of tooth loss.

They can also be risk factors (see Chapter 1.6 for definition) for other systemic inflammatory diseases such as atherogenic cardiovascular disease, type 2 diabetes, rheumatoid arthritis, chronic obstructive pulmonary disease, chronic kidney disease, neurodegenerative diseases and certain other inflammatory conditions.

In addition, many systemic conditions can present in and around the periodontal tissues, and their diagnosis and/or symptomatic management is aided by a detailed knowledge

of periodontal anatomy at both macroscopic and microscopic levels. The latter is complex, being of mixed ectodermal and mesodermal origins. Periodontal anatomy includes the gingival, alveolar bone and dental tissues.

Embryological Origins of the Periodontal Tissues

The gingival epithelium is of ectodermal origin.

The periodontal ligament and cementum are of neural crest (ectomesenchymal) origin.

The alveolar bone is of mesodermal origin (Figure 1.1.1).

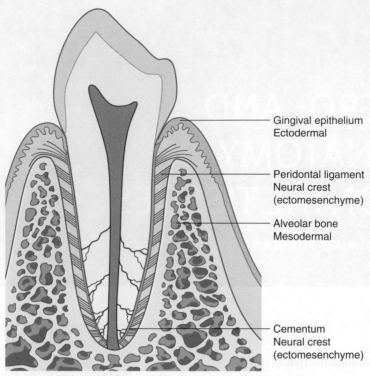

Gingival epithelium
Ectodermal

Peridontal ligament
Neural crest
(ectomesenchyme)

Alveolar bone
Mesodermal

Cementum
Neural crest
(ectomesenchyme)

• **Figure 1.1.1** The embryological origins of the periodontal tissues.

Microanatomy of the Gingival Tissues

The microanatomy of the gingival tissues is shown in Figure 1.1.2, and the appearance of healthy gingival tissues is shown in Figure 1.1.3.

The key elements of the normal gingival tissues are:

1. Outer gingival epithelium: the outer gingival epithelium is an orthokeratinised, stratified squamous epithelium. The keratinisation makes it resistant to abrasion from rough and hard food particles. A histological section of the outer gingival epithelium is shown in Figure 1.1.4. The gingival epithelium covers a core of fibrous connective tissue, which was defined in the 2017 world workshop classification system as the "supracrestal connective tissue attachment", replacing the term "biological width". Like all stratified squamous epithelia, the gingival epithelium undergoes constant renewal with shedding of the surface cells as they are replaced by cell proliferation from the deeper layers. Keratinocytes make up the majority of the cells of the gingival epithelium, which comprises basal cells (stratum basale), prickle cells (stratum spinosum), granular cells (stratum granulosum) and keratinised cells (stratum corneum). The cells at the surface lose their nuclei and form a solid layer of protective keratin. Cell division takes place in the basal layer, and the cells produced travel through the gingival epithelium where they are eventually shed. During this process, the cells increase in size and become flattened, producing more and more keratin as they do so. It is the keratin that results in the mechanical toughness of the most superficial epithelium. The rates of cell division and shedding are balanced so that the thickness of the epithelium is constant. The epithelium is attached to the underlying connective tissue by a basal lamina consisting of two layers of a protein/polysaccharide complex, the lamina lucida and the lamina densa.

2. Gingival connective tissue: the gingival connective tissues consist of a mesh of collagen fibres in an extracellular matrix made up of noncellular ground substance of glycosaminoglycans (such as hyaluronic acid), proteoglycans, and glycoproteins (such as fibronectin), all of which are synthesized by the principal cell type in the gingival connective tissues, the fibroblast. The matrix contains blood vessels, nerves and cells, most of which are fibroblasts (which also synthesize collagen), but immune system cells are also found, including neutrophils, lymphocytes, tissue macrophages (called Langerhans cells) and plasma cells. The gingival connective tissue is highly vascular, allowing for the entry of circulating inflammatory cells that perform "immune surveillance". The collagen fibres run in different directions in groups (Figures 1.1.5 and 1.1.6), and the groups are interlinked, giving the gingival tissues both strength and resilience. The collagen is initially secreted in the form of inactive procollagen, which is converted into tropocollagen. This is polymerized into collagen fibrils that are then combined into collagen bundles by the formation of cross linkages. The collagen in gingival connective tissue is mostly type I but types III and V are also found.

3. The dentogingival, circular and transeptal fibres form a physical barrier to the spread of gingival inflammation

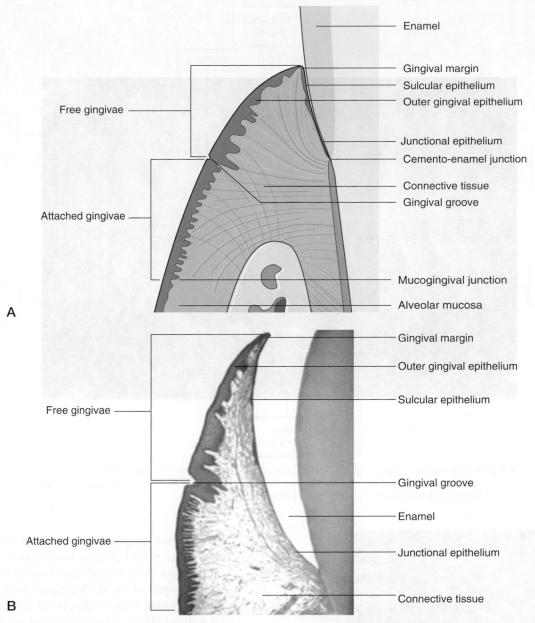

Enamel

Gingival margin

Sulcular epithelium

Outer gingival epithelium

Junctional epithelium

Cemento-enamel junction

Connective tissue

Gingival groove

Mucogingival junction

Alveolar mucosa

Free gingivae

Attached gingivae

A

Gingival margin

Outer gingival epithelium

Sulcular epithelium

Free gingivae

Gingival groove

Enamel

Attached gingivae

Junctional epithelium

Connective tissue

B

• **Figure 1.1.2** Microanatomy of normal gingival tissues.

toward the alveolar crest, thus affording some protection from alveolar bone loss around teeth: these fibres are absent in peri-implant mucosa, and peri-implant bone loss thus progresses in a more rapid concentric manner.

4. The gingival margin: the visible edge of the gingivae, 1.5–2 mm coronal to the cemento-enamel junction (CEJ).

5. The gingival groove: in health, this line separates the free from the attached gingiva at the level of the CEJ. It is only present in 30–40% of adults.

6. The sulcular epithelium: this lies between the oral and junctional epithelium. It has rete ridges. This tissue displays rapid turnover and para-keratinisation (cell nuclei still present). It is thinner and less keratinised than the outer gingival epithelium.

7. The free gingiva: this is a mobile cuff of keratinised gingival tissue lying above the alveolar crest. It extends from the gingival margin to the gingival groove (when present), which is at the level of the CEJ. The free gingiva forms a cuff around the neck of the tooth, and its surface is smooth. It is separated from the attached gingiva by the free gingival groove. Between the teeth, the free gingiva forms the cone-shaped interdental papilla, and it forms the interdental "col" beneath the contact points of the abutting teeth. The col area has very thin, nonkeratinised epithelium that makes this area more vulnerable. This is often a site of bacterial accumulation, which explains why periodontal diseases (gingivitis or periodontitis) usually start in this area.

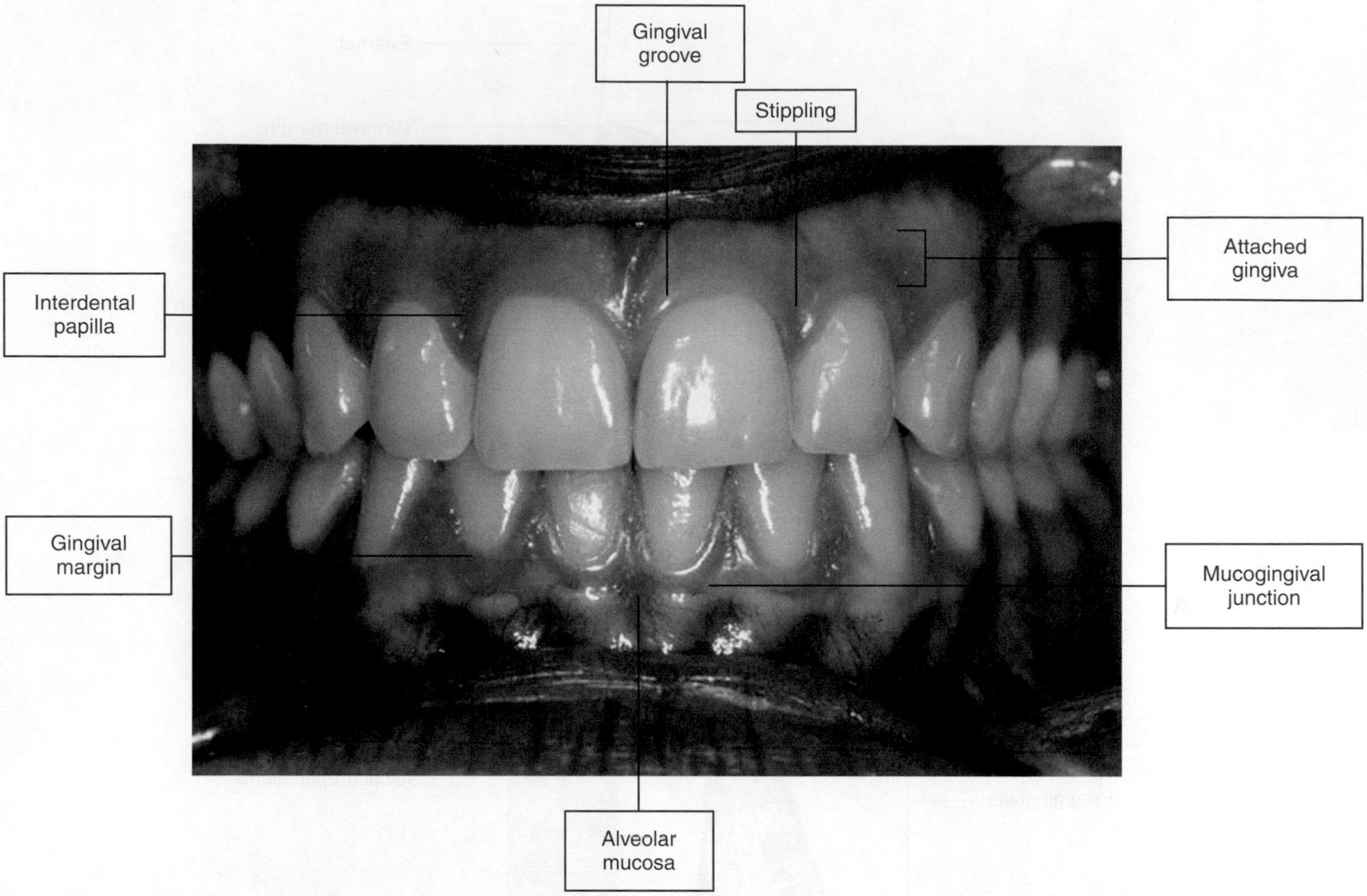

Gingival
groove

Stippling

Attached
gingiva

Interdental
papilla

Gingival
margin

Mucogingival
junction

Alveolar
mucosa

• **Figure 1.1.3** Healthy gingival tissues (Reproduced with kind permission by Quintessence from Chapple, I.L.C., Gilbert A.D., 2002. *Understanding Periodontal Diseases: Assessment and Diagnostic Procedures in Dental Practice.* Quintessence, London. ISBN: 1-85097-053-X).

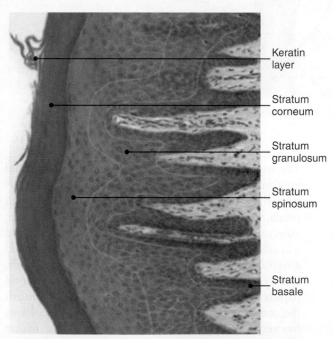

Keratin
layer

Stratum
corneum

Stratum
granulosum

Stratum
spinosum

Stratum
basale

• **Figure 1.1.4** The histology of the outer gingival epithelium.

8. The attached gingiva: this is a band of between 1 and 9 mm of keratinised gingival tissue that is tightly bound down to the underlying alveolar bone/periosteum by the collagen fibres of the dentogingival complex. It is pale pink compared with the deeper red colour of the alveolar mucosa. These differences in colour are due to the alveolar mucosa being more vascular and the overlying epithelium being thinner and nonkeratinised. It extends from the free gingival groove apically to the mucogingival junction (MGJ) where it becomes continuous with the nonkeratinised and mobile alveolar mucosa. The attached gingiva has a "stippled" appearance (depressions on the surface) because of epithelial rete ridges.

9. The mucogingival junction: the MGJ is a well delineated line that marks the boundary between the pink keratinised attached gingiva, which is tightly bound down to the alveolar bone, and the darker red, nonkeratinised alveolar mucosa, which is only loosely bound down to alveolar bone.

10. The enamel space: this is a demineralised section (as a result of histological preparation) in which the enamel is absent and indistinguishable from the gingival crevice.

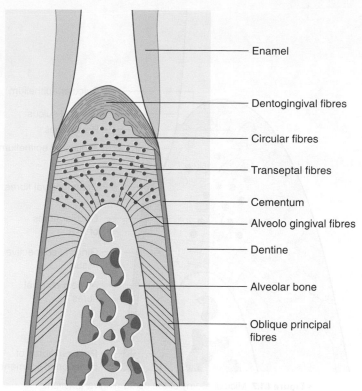

• **Figure 1.1.5** The interdental periodontal tissues in health.

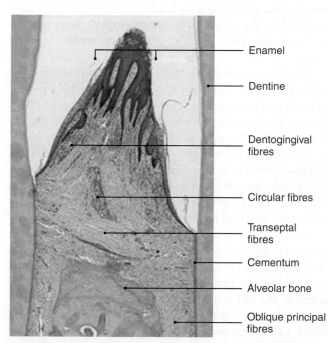

• **Figure 1.1.6** Histological longitudinal section of the interdental periodontal tissues in health.

11. The junctional epithelium (JE): the JE provides the contact between the gingiva and the tooth and attaches to enamel via hemidesmosomes, forming a tight attachment to the tooth surface. A thin basement lamina lies between the JE and connective tissue and also between the JE and the tooth surface. This attachment to the tooth is also known as the "epithelial attachment". Unlike the sulcular epithelium the JE has no rete ridges. It is fragile and is 20 to 30 cells thick with the most apical cells positioned at the CEJ (unless there has been recession, in which case the JE lies on cementum). The length of the JE is about 40 cells, or about 1 mm. The cells of the JE are larger than other oral epithelial cells and oriented parallel to the tooth surface. They also have wider intercellular spaces resulting in increased permeability of the JE to bacteria (and their products), gingival crevicular fluid (GCF) and inflammatory cells. Neutrophils are often seen in the JE, even in health. These cells pass through the JE into the gingival crevice where they form part of the host's immune defence against bacteria in the biofilm. Cell turnover in the JE is rapid. When the most apical cell of the JE migrates apically below the CEJ, this defines periodontal true pocket formation.

Figure 1.1.7 shows the microanatomy of the dento-gingival junction.

Microanatomy of the Periodontal Ligament and Cementum

Periodontal Ligament

The periodontal ligament forms the fibrous attachment between the tooth and bone. It is mostly made up of collagen fibres that insert into the root cementum and also into the alveolar bone in an acellular matrix that is similar to that

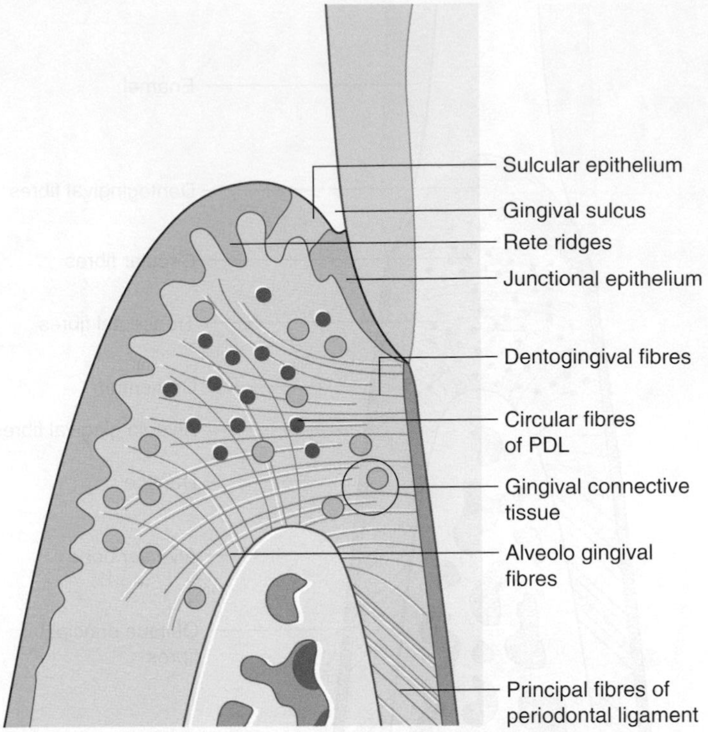
Sulcular epithelium
Gingival sulcus
Rete ridges
Junctional epithelium
Dentogingival fibres
Circular fibres of PDL
Gingival connective tissue
Alveolo gingival fibres
Principal fibres of periodontal ligament

• **Figure 1.1.7** Microanatomy of the dento-gingival junction.

found in the gingival connective tissues. The ligament has the following functions:

- Maintains the tooth in a functional position
- Resists occlusal loading
- Protects dental tissues from excessive loading
- Maintains and repairs alveolar bone and cementum (contains stem cells)
- Controls the neurological functions of mastication via mechanoreceptors.

The ligament varies in thickness (0.3–0.1 mm), being wider coronally and apically, and is at its narrowest at the axis of rotation of the tooth. Its main collagen fibres (the "principal fibres") run obliquely from bone to tooth in an apical direction (Figure 1.1.8).

The fibres are not straight but follow a wavy course, which allows for tooth movement during mastication. The fibres that are embedded in bone and cementum are known as Sharpey's fibres. The main types of collagen are types I, III and V, but there is more type III than in the gingival connective tissue. Type III collagen is more extensible than other types of collagen and may be important in maintaining the integrity of the periodontal ligament during tooth movements in mastication. The ligament also contains oxytalan fibres that are not found elsewhere in the body; these are elastic fibres that insert into cementum and run more longitudinally. They are more numerous in teeth that are subject to high loading, such as bridge abutments.

The periodontal ligament matrix also plays an important role in the absorption of functional stress during tooth movements, providing a hydraulic "cushion" effect. This is provided by the ability of the matrix components (glycosaminoglycans, proteoglycans and glycoproteins) to bind water.

Fibroblasts are the main cell type of the periodontal ligament, producing and degrading collagen through a process of repair and regeneration. They have phagocytic capabilities that enable them to remove damaged collagen and replace it with new collagen, thus maintaining the integrity of the periodontal ligament. The ligament also contains stem (mesenchymal) cells that can differentiate into osteoblasts (bone-forming cells) and cementoblasts (cementum-forming cells). This allows the periodontal ligament to maintain and repair itself and its insertions into bone and cementum. Osteoblasts, osteoclasts, cementoblasts and cementoclasts are found lining the bone and cementum surfaces within the ligament, all these cell types being derived from stem cells within the periodontal ligament. The ligament also contains the cell rests of Malassez, which are the odontogenic remnants of the epithelial root sheath of Hertwig, and which can differentiate into cementoblasts during guided tissue regeneration.

The periodontal ligament has a rich blood and nerve supply that is derived from the neural supplies to the pulp (which branch off before entering the tooth's apical foramina) and also from the blood supply to the alveolar bone. The ligament's nerve supply, which has both sensory and autonomic fibres, permits the monitoring of loading during mastication through proprioceptive fibres and mechanoreceptors.

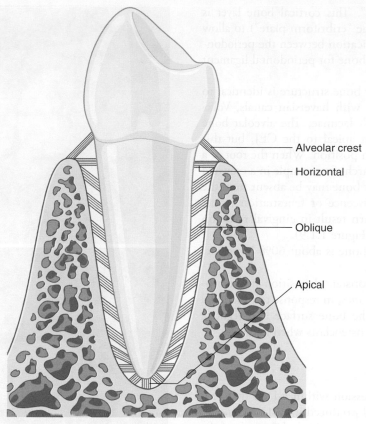

• Figure 1.1.8 Periodontal ligament fibres.

Alveolar crest

Horizontal

Oblique

Apical

Cementum

The cemental layer of the root provides an anchorage site for the collagen fibres of the periodontal ligament. It is a calcified connective tissue, which is a highly mineralised tissue, similar to bone, and it is tightly bound to the underlying dentine. It comprises collagen fibres in a calcified organic matrix and is about 65% inorganic (mostly hydroxyapatite), 23% organic (mostly type I collagen) and 12% water. Unlike bone, cementum is less readily resorbed. This may be because a layer of uncalcified matrix (precementum) is laid down by cementoblasts before calcification and remains on the surface of the mature cementum. As cementum formation occurs throughout life, there is always a layer of precementum present on the cementum surface.

At the cementoenamel junction, the cementum usually abuts onto enamel but, occasionally, it may either overlap enamel or stop short, leaving a band of exposed dentine. There is no direct blood or nerve supply to cementum. Cementum formation is continuous throughout life to accommodate changes within the periodontal ligament. The thickness of cementum coronally is 16 to 60 μm and, if exposed (for example, in recession), it can be easily removed by a toothbrush, resulting in dentinal sensitivity (see Chapter 3.2). In the apical third of the root, the cementum can be up to 200 μm thick. The thickness of cementum increases throughout life.

There are two types of cementum: cellular and acellular.

Cellular cementum is found near the apex of the root. It contains cementocytes in lacunae that communicate through a network of canaliculi (channels).

Acellular cementum covers most of the root surface of the tooth and contains no cementocytes, but its surface is populated with cementoblasts.

Cementoblasts are similar to osteoblasts and are responsible for the synthesis of the organic components of the matrix and for their calcification. As cementum formation occurs, the cementoblasts become trapped in the calcifying matrix and become cementocytes.

The inserting Sharpey's fibres are arranged at right angles to the cementum surface. In acellular cementum, the fibres are closely packed and mostly calcified; in cellular cementum, they are only partially calcified and are more loosely arranged.

Microanatomy of the Alveolar Bone

Alveolar bone is part of the mandible and maxilla, but its existence depends on the presence of teeth and, in the absence of teeth, it gradually resorbs. There is, however, no identifiable boundary between the alveolar bone and the bones of the jaws.

Alveolar bone comprises cancellous bone covered by a thin layer of cortical bone. The Sharpey's fibres of the periodontal ligament insert into the alveolar bone in what is referred to as "bundle bone". This cortical bone layer is perforated (it is also called the "cribriform plate") to allow vascular and neural communication between the periodontal ligament and the alveolar bone for periodontal ligament remodelling.

Anatomically, the alveolar bone structure is identical to other bones of the skeleton with haversian canals, Volkmann's canals and Howship's lacunae. The alveolar bone crest usually lies 1 to 2 mm apical to the CEJ, but this may vary depending on tooth position. When the root of a tooth is displaced out of the arch, for example in a crowded mouth, the overlying alveolar bone may be absent from the root surface, creating a dehiscence or fenestration in the alveolar bone that may in turn result in gingival recession defects (see Chapter 3.2 and Figure 1.1.9).

Like cementum, alveolar bone is about 60% inorganic, 25% organic and 15% water.

Alveolar bone undergoes constant deposition and resorption, just like other skeletal bones, in response to functional demands. Osteoblasts line the bone surface and regulate bone remodelling, recruiting osteoclasts when necessary.

Acknowledgement

This chapter is based on a session within e-Den that Professors Chapple and Milward produced in 2011. Acknowledgement is given to the Faculty of Dental Surgery of the Royal College of Surgeons of England for giving permission for material from the e-Den session to be used in this chapter.

Multiple Choice Questions on the contents of this chapter are available online at Elsevier eBooks+.

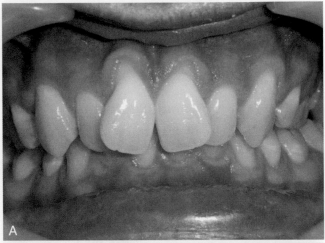

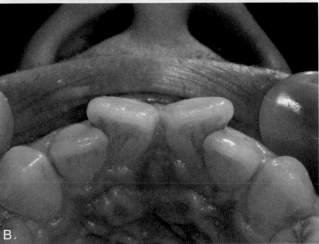

• **Figure 1.1.9** Upper incisors showing localized recession as a result of underlying bone dehiscences that have developed as a result of overcrowding during tooth eruption. (A) Labial view; (B) incisal view.

1.2

THE PATHOGENESIS OF PERIODONTAL DISEASES

MIKE MILWARD, JOHN MATTHEWS, AND IAIN CHAPPLE

CHAPTER OUTLINE

OVERVIEW OF THE CHAPTER

Inflammatory periodontal diseases are among the most prevalent of human chronic diseases and are a major cause of tooth loss. Much research has been directed at unravelling the complex processes underpinning their aetiology and pathogenesis.

This chapter will provide key information on the pathogenesis of chronic periodontal diseases, including the bacteria involved, host/bacterial interactions, and the role of host responses, with particular emphasis on hyper-responsive neutrophils and the role of antioxidants.

By the end of the chapter the reader should understand:

- The concept of disease pathogenesis
- Inflammatory and immune responses to biofilm bacteria and their products
- The role of periodontal bacteria in provoking damaging host responses
- The potential for reactive oxygen species–mediated tissue damage and the role of antioxidants
- The critical factors in the pathogenesis of periodontal diseases.

This chapter covers the following topics:

- Periodontal disease or diseases?
- Introduction
- Bacterial factors
- Host factors
- Inflammatory response to biofilm bacteria
- Immune responses to biofilm antigens
- Bacteria versus host
- Does gingivitis inevitably lead to periodontitis?

Periodontal Disease or Diseases?

There are many forms of disease that can affect the periodontal tissues, including gingivitis, necrotising periodontal diseases and periodontitis. All manifest as an inflammatory and an immune response to bacterial biofilm (also known as plaque). Therefore the term "periodontal disease" does not describe a single disease entity but is a general term encompassing all diseases of the periodontal tissues. Although widely used, this term causes much confusion. It (periodontal disease in the singular) will therefore not be used in this book; instead, throughout the book the terms gingivitis and periodontitis will be used. The former implies that the disease process is limited to the gingiva and that there has been no destruction of the periodontal ligament or alveolar bone. The latter implies that there has been destruction of the periodontal ligament and alveolar bone and that this process is generally concurrent with the presence of gingivitis.

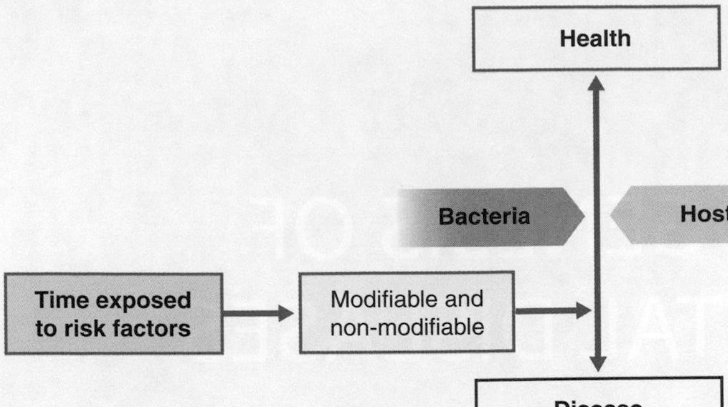

Health

Bacteria ← → Host

Time exposed to risk factors → Modifiable and non-modifiable →

Disease

• **Figure 1.2.1** Interactions that are responsible for disease.

Introduction

Pathogenesis describes how a disease develops. It includes the origin of the disease and the events that take place leading to that disease. Whether periodontitis develops in a patient depends on the interaction between biofilm bacteria and the host's inflammatory and immune responses. This interaction can be modified by a variety of complex factors, collectively called "risk factors" (Figure 1.2.1 and see Chapter 1.6).

> ### KEY POINT 1
> Periodontitis is the result of complex interactions between plaque bacteria and the host response.

In many mouths and at many sites in a mouth, the long-term presence of bacterial biofilm results in gingivitis but does not progress to periodontitis. Periodontitis is in part due to direct damage of the periodontal tissues by certain bacteria in the biofilm and also by bacterial activation of the host's immune/inflammatory responses. Grossi et al. (1994) have suggested that, on average, the relative direct effect from biofilm bacteria contributes to 20% of the tissue damage seen in periodontitis and the other 80% comes from an aberrant host response (Figure 1.2.2).

Periodontitis is regarded as a condition that is seen in susceptible patients who have an exaggerated inflammatory/immune response to bacterial biofilm and/or reduced levels of antioxidant defence (intracellular molecules present in cells that offer protection from excess inflammatory response). This leads to chronic collateral damage of the periodontal tissues because the host response is unable to successfully remove the biofilm, resulting in propagation of the periodontal lesion. Over the years there has been much debate over whether the change to a pathogenic microbial biofilm comes before or after the inflammatory response. A review by Van Dyke et al. (2020) has proposed that the inflammatory response is the key factor that modulates the change to a pathogenic biofilm, and it is only in the latter stages that the microbial pathogenicity becomes important. These findings offer the potential that management of inflammation can result in a shift to a healthy microbial balance.

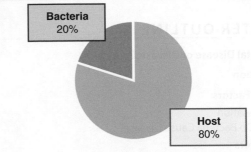

• **Figure 1.2.2** Most of the damage seen in periodontitis is host mediated.

Bacterial Factors

Colonisation

Bacteria need to colonise (become established) in the gingival sulcus/periodontal pocket for periodontitis to develop. The stages in this process are:

- Acquisition—occurs predominantly at birth from parental or environmental sources and on tooth eruption (i.e., appearance of new habitats such as enamel surfaces and the gingival crevice)
- Adherence/retention—the ability of bacteria to attach to a surface or occupy a site not affected by saliva flow, essential for bacterial survival
- Initial survival—after adherence/retention the bacteria have to acquire essential nutrients to survive
- Prosperity—the ability of bacteria to be able to survive in a biofilm with other microorganisms in the long term
- Avoidance of elimination—bacterial strategies to help bacteria evade host defence mechanisms
- Multiplication—division to ensure a critical mass for survival
- Virulence factors—factors expressed by certain bacteria for their benefit that concurrently cause tissue damage and disease
- Maturation of biofilm—as the biofilm develops the flora will change and, in disease, Gram-negative anaerobic motile bacilli will predominate
- Invasion—to cause tissue damage and elicit an inflammatory/immune response.

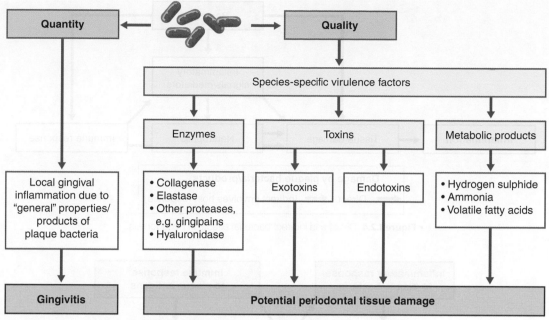

• **Figure 1.2.3** Overview of periodontitis pathogenesis.

How Do Bacteria Cause Disease?

Both the quantity and the quality of bacteria that have coloniscd thc gingival sulcus/periodontal pocket can contribute to disease. The quantity causes local gingival inflammation (gingivitis). The quality (species of bacteria) can produce specific virulence factors, especially enzymes, toxins and other metabolic products, all of which have the potential to damage the periodontal tissues (and activate the host's inflammatory/immune response).

Specific enzymes, toxins and metabolic products that are involved in the pathogenesis of periodontal diseases are shown in Figure 1.2.3.

The bacterial flora changes from health to disease. Thus Gram-positive, aerobic, nonmotile species of bacteria such as *Streptococcus sanguis*, *Actinomyces viscosus* and *Streptococcus oralis* are associated with health, and Gram-negative, anaerobic, motile bacteria such as *Porphyromonas gingivalis* are associated with disease.

Because there are frequently more than 400 species of microorganisms present in the mouth, it is often difficult to know exactly which species or combinations of species are responsible for periodontitis. However, in the flora for acute necrotising ulcerative gingivitis (ANUG), a fusospirochetal complex can be seen with a predominance of *Treponema vincenti*, *Fusobacterium nucleatum* and *P. gingivalis*, and, in patients with periodontitis Grade C in the absence of risk factors (previously termed aggressive periodontitis), *Aggregatibacter actinomycetemcomitans* is strongly associated.

Host Factors

Damage to the periodontal tissues from the products of the bacterial biofilm may be direct (via bacterial toxicity) or indirect (by stimulation of the host response). Figure 1.2.4 summarises possible direct and indirect damage mechanisms that may be operating.

A summary of how the host response can cause plaque-induced disease is shown in Figure 1.2.5.

Inflammatory Response to the Bacterial Biofilm

The host's innate inflammatory response is the first line of defence against bacterial challenge; it is rapid and nonspecific. If this response is excessive, it can cause collateral tissue damage. It involves the epithelial barrier, the complement cascade, cytokines, neutrophils and mast cells. These features will now be considered in further detail.

The Epithelial Barrier

The epithelial barrier provides an interface between the external environment of the gingival crevice or the pocket and the underlying connective tissues. It is not an inert barrier, and both cells and fluids pass across it. Evidence suggests that it has a role in initiating and propagating the inflammatory response via cytokine release after stimulation by bacterial products such as lipopolysaccharides (LPS). In addition, stimulated epithelium also releases antibacterial peptides such as beta-defensins, which help maintain its integrity to bacterial attack.

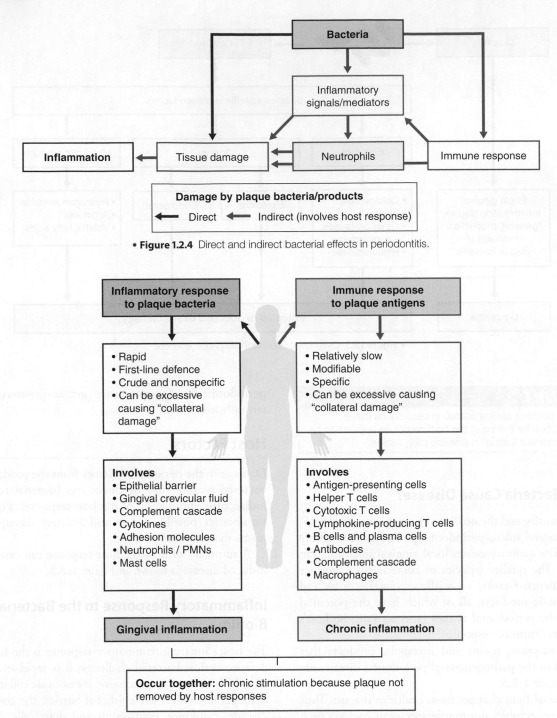

• **Figure 1.2.4** Direct and indirect bacterial effects in periodontitis.

• **Figure 1.2.5** Host response mechanisms in biofilm-induced periodontitis.

Complement

Complement consists of 20 serum glycoproteins that are inactive in circulating blood/tissue fluid. They can be activated via two pathways—the alternate pathway (activated by bacterial endotoxin/proteases) or the classical pathway (activated by antibody–antigen interaction).

When activated, these glycoproteins initiate a range of proinflammatory effects (a "cascade") that ultimately cause:
• Neutrophil recruitment (movement of neutrophils to the damaged site)
• Phagocyte binding to bacteria

• Cell lysis (both of the host's cells and bacteria)
• Mast cell degranulation with the release of vasoactive amines, resulting in increased vascular permeability
The "cascade" is shown in Figure 1.2.6.

Cytokines

Cytokines are signalling molecules released by a variety of cells that have a range of actions that include proinflammatory activity, for example, neutrophil chemotaxis.

The types of cytokine and their effects are shown in Table 1.2.1.

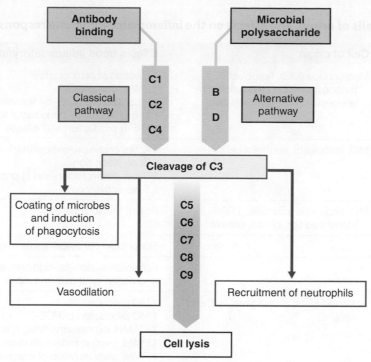

• **Figure 1.2.6** The complement cascade.

Inflammasomes

One of the key cytokines in the periodontitis is interleukin 1 (IL-1), which causes a proinflammatory response including activation of osteoclasts and neutrophil recruitment (see Table 1.2.1). IL-1 expression is controlled via central regulators of innate immunity called inflammasomes. A number of these multiprotein complexes have been identified that trigger the host's response after detection of bacteria or tissue damage (Lamkanfi & Dixit, 2017). Research has identified dysregulation of this system in periodontitis, which may contribute to the aberrant host response characteristic of periodontitis.

Neutrophils (Polymorphonuclear Leucocytes [Pmnls])

Neutrophils:

- are the most commonly occurring white blood cells and the most abundant and important inflammatory cell in periodontitis,
- play a key role in the first-line defence of these tissues,
- move toward the site of infection through the process of chemotaxis,
- kill bacteria either through intra- or extracellular methods,
- kill by means of enzymes and free radicals as well as neutrophil extracellular traps (NETS) and
- may produce an exaggerated response that can lead to collateral local tissue damage (periodontitis).

A diagrammatic example of how neutrophils kill bacteria is shown in Figure 1.2.7.

Mast Cells

Mast cells:

- are resident in all connective tissues, including gingiva and periodontal ligament;
- contain numerous granules that are released after mild mechanical or chemical stimulation;
- have granules that include neutrophil chemotactic factor, histamine, and heparin;
- can be activated and caused to degranulate by mild chemical or physical trauma, complement activation, and cross-linking IgE receptors; and
- degranulate and cause a local increase in vascular permeability with dilation of blood capillaries, which aids neutrophil migration from blood into the tissues.

Table 1.2.2 shows the chemicals that are released from an activated mast cell, together with the actions.

Immune Responses to Biofilm Antigens

Immune responses have three basic characteristics:
- specificity to particular antigens
- the ability to distinguish between self and nonself
- a memory to produce a modified response (faster and bigger) on secondary exposure to a specific antigen.

The immune response involves T lymphocytes, B lymphocytes, and antigen-presenting cells.

These cells will now be discussed in more detail.

T Lymphocytes (T Cells)

1. Make up the so-called cell-mediated immune response, as the antigen-specific molecule is not secreted (like an antibody) and remains bound to the cell surface (the T-cell antigen receptor).
2. Direct contact between the T cell and its associated antigen is required to initiate an immune response and to destroy the antigen.

TABLE 1.2.1 Cytokines, their cells of origin, and effects on the inflammatory/immune response

Cytokine	Cell of origin	Effects upon inflammatory/immune response
Interleukin 1 (IL-1)	Macrophage (MØ), fibroblast, monocytes upon stimulation by endo/exotoxins, epithelial cells	Activation of osteoclasts ↑ PMNL margination ↑ Prostaglandin PGE_2 by fibroblasts ↑ IL-6 synthesis by periodontal fibroblasts ↑ TNF-α production and release
Interleukin 6 (IL-6)	MØ, fibroblasts, epithelial cells	↑ Acute phase protein synthesis by liver ↑ Bone resorption ↑ B-cell differentiation and Ig production ↑ T-cell activation
Interleukin 8 (IL-8)	MØ, endo/epithelial cells, LPS-stimulated fibroblasts, platelets	Potent PMNL chemotaxin
Interleukin 10 (IL-10)		Suppression of cytokines (anti-inflammatory)
Transforming growth factor beta (TGF-β)		Anti-inflammatory (at high concentrations) stimulates collagen synthesis and repair
Tumour necrosis factor alpha (TNF-α)	Activated MØs, monocytes, epithelial cells	↑ MØ production IL-1 ↑ MØ production of PGE-2 ↑ ICAM-1 expression/PMNL margination ↑ PMNL oxygen radical production ↑ PMNL degranulation of enzymes
Prostaglandin E2 (PGE_2)	Activated MØs, monocytes, PMNLs, mast cells, epithelial cells	↑ Vascular permeability ↑ Vasodilation ↑ PMNL chemotaxis Stimulates bone resorption
Granulocyte–macrophage colony stimulating factor (GM-CSF)	Epithelial cells, monocytes, endothelial cells, fibroblasts	↑ Release of PMNLs from bone marrow ↑ PMNL chemotaxis ↑ Apoptosis ↑ Degranulation ↑ Oxygen radical formation

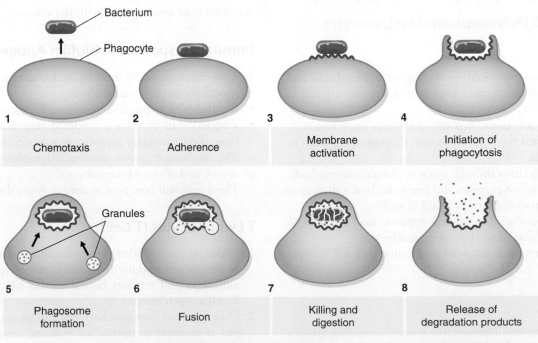

• **Figure 1.2.7** Diagram of a neutrophil phagocytosing a bacterium and the subsequent degranulation.

TABLE 1.2.2	Substances released from an activated mast cell and their actions		
		Preformed	**Effect**
Granule release	▸	Histamine	Vasodilation, increased capillary permeability chemokinesis, bronchoconstriction
		Proteoglycan	Binds granule proteases
		Neutral proteases β-Glucosaminidase	Activates C3 Splits off glucosamine
		ECF NCF	Eosinophil chemotaxis Neutrophil chemotaxis
		Platelet-activating factor	Mediator release
		Interleukins 3,4, 5, & 6 GM-CSF, TNF	Multiple, including macrophage activation, trigger acute phase proteins, etc.
		Newly synthesized	**Effect**
Lipoxygenase pathway	▸	Leukotriene C_4, D_4 (SRS-A) Leukotriene B_4	Vasoactive, bronchoconstriction, chemotaxis, and/or chemokinesis
Cyclo-oxygenase pathway	▸	Prostaglandins Thromboxanes	Affect bronchial muscle, platelet aggregation, and vasodilation

3. Antigen-specific T cells can only interact with antigens when present on a host cell surface.
4. Helper T cells start immune responses by interacting with specific antigens displayed on the surface of an antigen-presenting cell.
5. Effector T cells interact with specific antigens displayed on host cell surfaces and either lyse the cell (cytotoxic T cells) or release soluble mediators (lymphokines) that attract macrophages and/or other inflammatory cells to the area.
6. A diagrammatic representation of the T-cell response is shown in Figure 1.2.8.

B Lymphocytes

7. Form part of the so-called humoral immune response.
8. When activated by its associated antigen, the B cell proliferates and differentiates into antibody-secreting cells (plasmablasts and plasma cells).
9. B-cell responses to most antigens will not occur without the help of T cells and the mediators they produce (e.g. IL-2, IL-4).
10. Antibodies are released into the tissue/circulation where they can bind soluble and insoluble antigens that do not have to be associated with host cells.
11. Antibody–antigen binding, with or without complement activation, allows removal and destruction of the antigen via phagocytosis.
The B-cell response is shown in Figure 1.2.9.

Antibodies/Immunoglobulins

In humans, there are five main classes of antibody (immunoglobulin): IgG, IgA, IgM, IgD, and IgE. These differ in their secondary (non–antigen binding) biological functions such that only IgG and IgM antibodies can activate complement.

Normally, a B-cell response to antigen will result in the production of specific antibodies including all five classes. However, the IgG class usually predominates.

Dimeric IgA is predominant in responses to antigen that is swallowed (not via the gingival sulcus) and is present in saliva where it aggregates antigens/bacteria/viruses, preventing them from harming the body.

In terms of periodontal diseases, IgG class antibodies to plaque antigens are of most importance. They are within periodontal tissues and present within gingival crevicular fluid.

The mechanism for the removal or destruction of antigen by an antibody is shown in Figure 1.2.10.

Antibody–bacteria aggregation is shown in Figure 1.2.11.

Bacteria Versus Host

If there is an ongoing imbalance between the host's inflammatory/immune response and biofilm bacteria then disease will occur. This is demonstrated in patients with periodontitis by an aberrant inflammatory/immune response with excess nonresolving inflammation, resulting in collateral tissue damage. Although the aberrant host response is the major cause of tissue damage, bacteria are required to initiate and propagate the host response and have the ability to cause some tissue damage directly. The quantity of the bacteria in the biofilm and the specific species present are the two most important bacterial factors that can lead to periodontal destruction. Both the host and plaque factors are modulated by risk factors (Figure 1.2.12).

An excessive host response can cause periodontal breakdown. The mechanism for this is thought to be due to

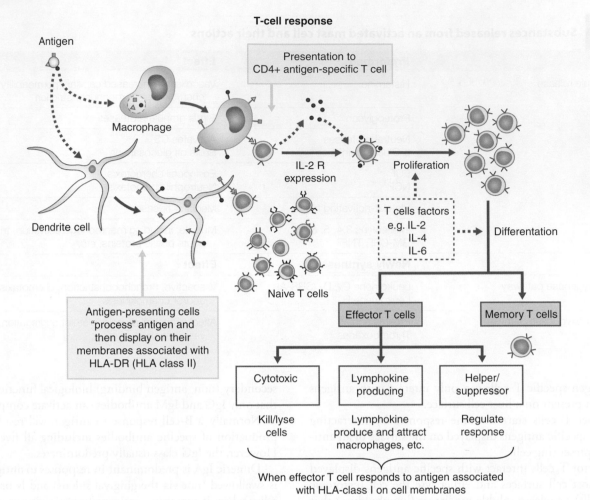

T-cell response

Antigen

Presentation to
CD4+ antigen-specific T cell

Macrophage

Dendrite cell

IL-2 R
expression

Proliferation

T cells factors
e.g. IL-2
IL-4
IL-6

Differentation

Naive T cells

Antigen-presenting cells
"process" antigen and
then display on their
membranes associated with
HLA-DR (HLA class II)

Effector T cells

Memory T cells

Cytotoxic

Lymphokine
producing

Helper/
suppressor

Kill/lyse
cells

Lymphokine
produce and attract
macrophages, etc.

Regulate
response

When effector T cell responds to antigen associated
with HLA-class I on cell membranes

• **Figure 1.2.8** The T-cell response.

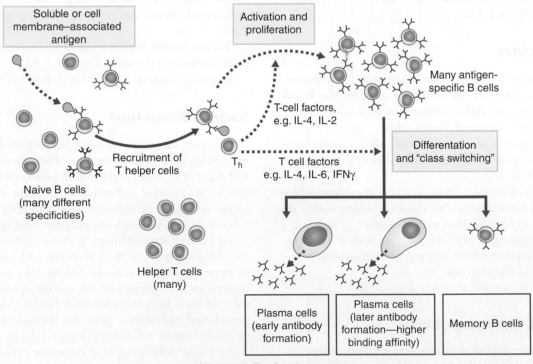

Soluble or cell
membrane–associated
antigen

Activation and
proliferation

Many antigen-
specific B cells

T-cell factors,
e.g. IL-4, IL-2

Recruitment of
T helper cells

T_h

T cell factors
e.g. IL-4, IL-6, IFNγ

Differentiation
and "class switching"

Naive B cells
(many different
specificities)

Helper T cells
(many)

Plasma cells
(early antibody
formation)

Plasma cells
(later antibody
formation—higher
binding affinity)

Memory B cells

• **Figure 1.2.9** The B-cell response.

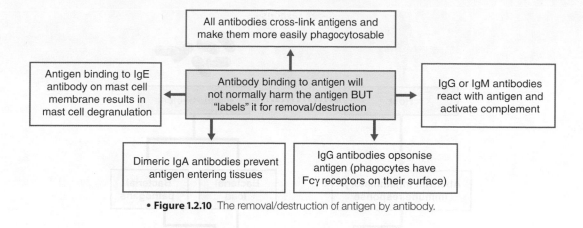

• **Figure 1.2.10** The removal/destruction of antigen by antibody.

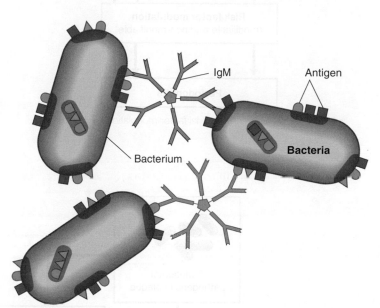

• **Figure 1.2.11** Antibody–bacteria aggregation (mainly a function of polymeric antibodies—IgM and dimeric secretory IgA).

periodontal pathogens in the biofilm stimulating a proinflammatory response, resulting in neutrophil recruitment leading to the local release of reactive oxygen species (free radicals) and enzymes capable of damaging host tissue. Although host tissue antioxidants can neutralize reactive oxygen species, if the latter predominate (due to either low local levels of antioxidants and/or excess reactive oxygen species production), oxidative stress can result in an excessive and aberrant response leading to tissue damage (Figure 1.2.13).

The action of the excess free radicals and enzymes on the periodontal tissues is summarised in Figure 1.2.14.

The critical role that oxidative stress and reactive oxygen species play in local tissue damage is shown in Figure 1.2.15.

Does Gingivitis Inevitably Lead to Periodontitis?

In the past, it was thought that gingivitis inevitably led to periodontitis. However, it is now accepted that this is not the case. The risk for the progression to periodontitis is greatest in individuals who are susceptible, representing between 5% and 15% of the population. At the other end of the scale, about 10% of the population are resistant to periodontal breakdown, despite persistent long-term plaque accumulation, and disease progression in these individuals is rare.

Clinically, there are some shared signs of disease between gingivitis and periodontitis: biofilm accumulation, bleeding, inflamed gingivae, loss of stippling and loss of a knife-edge gingival margin.

In addition to these signs, in periodontitis the following signs may be seen: pocket formation, suppuration, attachment loss, bone loss and furcation exposure. Furthermore when periodontitis is present, teeth may become mobile and drift and diastemas (spaces between the teeth) may develop. However, these last three signs can also be due to aberrant occlusal forces or a combination of periodontitis and aberrant occlusal forces.

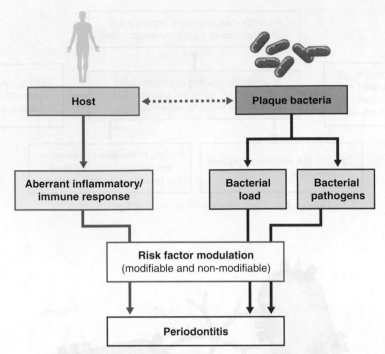

• **Figure 1.2.12** Host and bacterial factor modulation by risk factors.

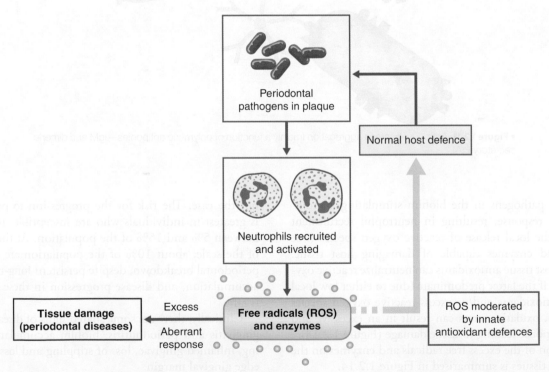

• **Figure 1.2.13** How an excessive host response can contribute to disease.

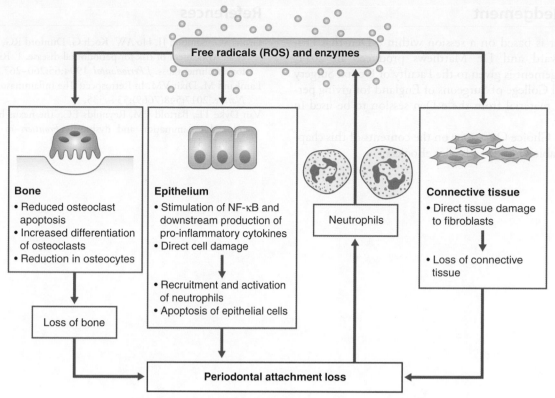

• **Figure 1.2.14** Tissue damage caused by free radicals and enzymes.

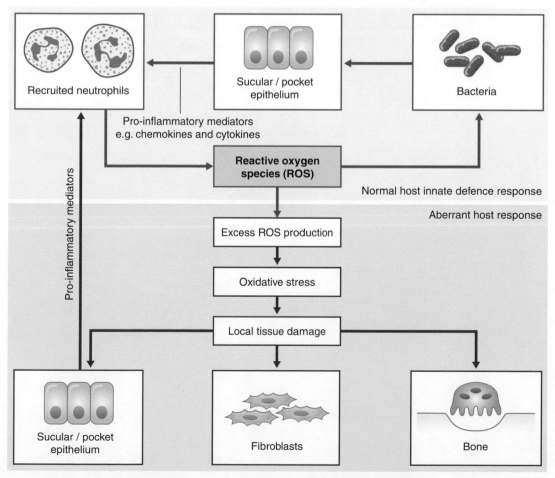

• **Figure 1.2.15** The role of oxidative stress in local tissue damage.

Acknowledgement

This chapter is based on a session within e-Den that Professor Milward and Dr. Matthews produced in 2011. Acknowledgement is given to the Faculty of Dental Surgery of the Royal College of Surgeons of England for giving permission for material from the e-Den session to be used in this chapter.

Multiple Choice Questions on the contents of this chapter are available online at Elsevier eBooks+.

References

Grossi SG, Zambon JJ, Ho AW, Koch G, Dunford RG, Machtei EE, et al. Assessment of risk for periodontal disease. 1. Risk indicators for attachment loss. *J Periodontol.* 1994;65:260–267.

Lamkanfi M, Dixit VM. In Retrospect: The inflammasome turns 15. *Nature.* 2017;548(7669):534–535.

Van Dyke TE, Bartold PM, Reynolds EC. The nexus between periodontal inflammation and dysbiosis. *Frontiers in immunology.* 2020;11:511.

1.3

EPIDEMIOLOGY OF PERIODONTAL DISEASES

KENNETH EATON

CHAPTER OUTLINE

OVERVIEW OF THE CHAPTER

This chapter explains the principles of epidemiology and why clinicians need to be aware of the epidemiology of diseases and conditions that they treat. It then outlines the current deficiencies in periodontal epidemiology and gives brief details of two national studies and a positive development.

By the end of the chapter the reader should:

- Understand the principles of epidemiology and periodontal epidemiology
- Be able to describe indices that have been used in periodontal epidemiology
- Recognise the problems in periodontal epidemiology relating to: what to measure, how to measure, examiner training and consistency
- Describe the major findings of the periodontal aspects of the National Health and Nutrition Examination Survey (2002/2013) and the Adult Dental Health Survey (2009).

The chapter covers the following topics:

- Introduction
- The principles of descriptive epidemiology
- Why is there a need for data on periodontal diseases?
- Indices that have commonly been used in periodontal epidemiology
- Problems with periodontal epidemiology – what to measure, how to measure, examiner consistency
- National surveys
- A positive development
- Possible future developments.

Introduction

Porta and Last (2008) have defined epidemiology as the study of the distribution and determinants of health-related states or events in specified populations and the application of the study to control health problems. Epidemiology can also be defined as the science of epidemics.

In healthcare, epidemiological techniques are used to investigate, at a specific time, the proportion of people in a population that is affected by a disease. The principles of epidemiology are therefore based on the need to find information about a population, which may be the entire population of a town, region or country or a subset with problems of interest.

KEY POINT 1

In practical terms, where commonly occurring diseases such as dental caries or periodontal diseases are concerned, it is not possible to investigate/examine the entire population, so only a sample is examined. The selection of a representative sample is therefore of paramount importance.

MacMahon et al. (1960) suggested that epidemiology should be more than just counting numbers of people within the population with disease but should also try to clarify the factors contributing to, or causing, the disease in question. They therefore suggested that there are four stages:

- **Descriptive epidemiology**: in which the distribution of the disease under investigation is described, with a comparison of its frequency in different populations and different subsets of the population. The description is based on prevalence, incidence and severity.
- **Formulation of hypotheses**: which sought to explain specific factors relating to the disease in question.
- **Analytical epidemiology**: in which observational studies were designed and performed to examine these hypotheses.
- **Experimental epidemiology**: in which experimental studies were performed in human populations to test the hypotheses that had been proved in observational and analytical studies.

In practice, oral epidemiology, including periodontal epidemiology, has been largely descriptive.

Principles of Descriptive Epidemiology

As mentioned in the introduction, descriptive epidemiology is based on prevalence, incidence and severity.

KEY POINT 2
Descriptive epidemiology is based on prevalence, incidence and severity.

Prevalence is the amount of disease present in a population at a given time (measured as a percentage) and depends on the duration of a disease and its previous incidence.

Incidence is the number of new cases or events that occur during a specified time period.

Severity has been defined as the quality of being severe in the disease, or in the extent and severity index (Carlos et al. 1986), as "the stage of advancement of periodontal destruction".

The basic principles for a descriptive epidemiological study are that:

- The methods should be described clearly with a detailed explanation and should be easily reproducible by any clinician or scientist who works in the same discipline.
- The assessment of the variables should be performed in an objective manner and follow the documented methods for data collection precisely and consistently.
- The environment in which the data are collected should be controlled and standardised.
- The examiners should be well trained and calibrated so that they are consistent in their assessments.
- The size of the sample should be determined using a power calculation, be of adequate size and be representative.
- The data should be collected in such a manner that they can easily be analysed.

Why is There a Need for Data on Periodontal Health/Disease?

Leroy et al. (2010) suggested that accurate epidemiological data on periodontal health/disease are needed to:

- identify people at risk of periodontal diseases in the population
- assess the efficacy of preventive strategies and curative therapies at a population level
- inform workforce planning
- evaluate the interplay with risk factors for periodontitis
- assess the interaction between periodontal health/disease and systemic diseases
- assess the effect of periodontal diseases on the quality of life.

Periodontal Epidemiology

Techniques for periodontal epidemiology have evolved over the last 60 years. As will be seen later in this chapter, there have been problems deciding exactly which variables to measure and how to measure them.

Until the 1950s, both clinically and in epidemiological surveys, periodontal health was frequently classified as good, moderate or poor. These were very subjective assessments, which were not based on any specific criteria and, as a result, were frequently interpreted differently by different examiners or by the same examiner from 1 day to another. As a result, a series of periodontal indices were developed to achieve greater consistency of assessment, both during the clinical examination of patients and in epidemiological surveys. The indices used in clinical practice for assessing and monitoring patients are described in Chapter 2.2. Additional ones have been used in epidemiological surveys.

Indices used in Epidemiological Surveys

The first was *Russell's Periodontal Index (PI)* (Russell 1956). This involved assessing the periodontal tissues around each tooth and awarding a score to the tooth. The scores used in "field" studies (where no radiographs were available) were:

0 Neither overt inflammation in the investing tissues, nor loss of function due to destruction of supporting tissue

1 Mild gingivitis: an overt area of inflammation in the free gingiva but the area does not circumscribe the tooth

2 Gingivitis: inflammation completely circumscribes the tooth but there is no apparent break in the epithelial attachment

4 There is early, notch-like resorption of the alveolar crest. Not used in field studies

6 Gingivitis with pocket formation: the epithelial attachment has been broken and there is a pocket (not merely a deepened gingival crevice due to swelling of the free gingivae). There is no interference with normal masticatory function, the tooth is firm in its socket and not drifted

8 Advanced destruction with loss of masticatory function: the tooth may be loose, may have drifted, may sound dull on percussion with a metallic instrument and may be depressed in its socket.

All the resulting scores were added together and divided by the number of teeth to give an overall score.

The next index to be devised for periodontal epidemiology was *Ramfjord's Periodontal Disease Index (PDI)* (Ramfjord 1959). Ramfjord highlighted two significant weaknesses of the Russell's Periodontal Index: it did not involve probing to assess periodontal pocket depth and did not "orientate pockets to the cemento-enamel junction". He claimed that, as a result, it underestimated the true extent of periodontitis. The Ramfjord PDI was based on the assessment of six teeth which were: the upper right first molar, the upper left central incisor, the upper left first premolar, the lower left first molar, the lower right central incisor and the lower right first premolar. The following assessments took place at each tooth:

- Four-point pocket probing (mid-buccal, mid-palatal/lingual, mesio-buccal, disto-buccal) relating the crest of the gingiva and the bottom of the pocket to the cemento-enamel junction (CEJ)
- Recording of gingivitis, calculus, plaque, attrition, mobility and lack of contact using a four-point scale (0–3) for each of these variables
- If the gingival crevice had migrated apically from the CEJ by no more than 3 mm at any of the probing sites, the score for the tooth was 4. If this migration was between 3 mm and 6 mm, it was 5, and if it was more than 6 mm, it was 6. The six scores were added together and divided by 6 to give an overall score for periodontitis. The other scores were treated individually to give scores for gingivitis, plaque, etc., but not amalgamated with the score for pocket depth/attachment loss.

KEY POINT 3

Ramfjord highlighted two significant weaknesses of the Russell's Periodontal Index which were that it did not involve probing to assess periodontal pocket depth and did not "orientate pockets to the cemento-enamel junction". He claimed that, as a result, it underestimated the true extent of periodontitis.

The advantage of the Ramfjord index was that it did measure pocket depth and loss of attachment. However, it was complicated to record and did not assess all teeth. There was therefore a need for a simpler index.

KEY POINT 4

The advantage of the Ramfjord index was that it did measure pocket depth and loss of attachment. However, it was complicated to record and did not assess all teeth.

To address this need, the *Community Periodontal Index of Treatment Need (CPITN)* was devised for the World Health Organization (WHO) (Ainamo et al. 1982). As its name implies, it was designed to assess treatment needs

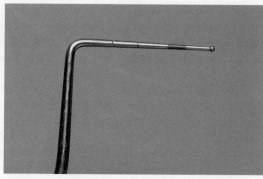

• **Figure 1.3.1** Picture of WHO epidemiological probe. Note the round tip, first band (silver) from 0 to 3.5 mm, second band (black) from 3.5 to 5.5 mm.

rather than periodontal status and not specifically as an epidemiological index. However, it has been used (or misused) for this purpose for the last 30 years. A simplified periodontal probe was designed to be used with the index (Figure 1.3.1).

For adults, 10 teeth (all upper and lower first and second molars and the upper right and lower left central incisors) are assessed for:

- Gingival bleeding after probing
- Supragingival calculus
- Subgingival calculus
- Pocket depths of 4 or 5 mm
- Pocket depths of 6 mm or more.

The following scores are given:

0 = periodontal health (no bleeding, calculus or pockets)
1 = gingival bleeding but no calculus or pockets
2 = supra- or subgingival calculus present
3 = a 4 or 5 mm pocket
4 = a 6 mm or deeper pocket present.

The worst score for each sextant (Figure 1.3.2) is recorded, and the overall score is taken as the worst score from the sextants.

After a few years, CPITN was redesignated as CPI to denote its use as an epidemiological tool rather than to assess treatment need. Its use in epidemiological surveys has been recommended by WHO in both the third (1989) and fourth (1997) editions of *Oral Health Surveys: Basic Methods*.

However, in the light of growing evidence that CPITN underestimates the extent of periodontal breakdown in a mouth and that from an epidemiological standpoint, calculus is an irrelevance (Leroy et al. 2010), WHO has revised their recommendations in the fifth edition of *Oral Health Surveys: Basic Methods*, as will be described later in this chapter.

KEY POINT 5

However, in the light of growing evidence that CPITN underestimates the extent of periodontal breakdown in a mouth and that from an epidemiological standpoint, calculus is an irrelevance (Leroy et al. 2010), WHO has revised their recommendations in the fifth edition of *Oral Health Surveys: Basic Methods*.

A modified version of CPITN, known as the basic periodontal examination (BPE), has been developed as a screening tool by the British Society of Periodontology and Implant Dentistry. It is widely used in the UK and is described in Chapter 2.2.

The Extent and Severity Index (ESI) was proposed by Carlos et al. (1986). It involves assessing half the mouth – the upper right and lower left quadrants. Mid-buccal and mesio-buccal sites and all the teeth other than third molars are assessed for attachment loss (Figure 1.3.3). Attachment loss is thought to be a more reliable indicator of past periodontal breakdown than pocket depth.

In the ESI, attachment loss is considered to be due to disease if it is greater than 1 mm.

Extent is measured by the percentage of sites where such a measurement was found, e.g. if it was found at 7 of the 28 sites assessed in a half mouth, then the extent would be 25%. The severity is calculated as the mean loss of attachment at all the sites. Thus if the total attachment loss for the half mouth was 56 mm, the severity score would be 2.0 and the extent and severity score would be 25, 2.0. The advantage of the ESI is that it is simple to use and can provide a measurement against which to compare when it is repeated

3	0	3
1	2	1

Overall score = 3

• **Figure 1.3.2** Example of CPITN scores for each sextant and the overall score.

subsequently. However, like the PDI and CPITN, it does not assess all teeth in a mouth.

Problems with Periodontal Epidemiology

The problems with periodontal epidemiology arise from three main areas. These are:

- What to measure
- How to measure
- How to ensure that examiners measure consistently.

What to Measure

As explained in Chapter 1.2, it is currently recognised that the presence of gingivitis at a site does not necessarily mean that it will progress to periodontitis. A number of studies have also shown that the presence of calculus does not necessarily lead to either gingivitis or periodontitis. This is not to say that patients with gingivitis or calculus do not need advice on oral hygiene and professional cleaning. From a periodontal epidemiological point of view, the most important consideration is the life expectancy of a tooth; if periodontal attachment (periodontal ligament and alveolar bone) has been lost, then a tooth is at a greater risk than if the attachment level is normal. Historically, a

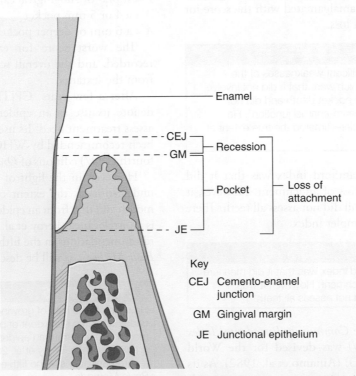

• **Figure 1.3.3** Diagram showing loss of attachment (LOA) which is the sum of recession plus pocket depth.

Key

CEJ Cemento-enamel junction

GM Gingival margin

JE Junctional epithelium

TABLE 1.3.1 American Academy of Periodontology and Centre for Disease Control case definitions for periodontitis

Disease category	Attachment loss (AL)	Pocket depth (PD)
Severe periodontitis	At 2 or more interproximal (IP) sites with AL ≥6 mm (not on the same tooth)	And 1 or more IP site(s) with PD ≥5 mm
Moderate periodontitis	At 2 IP sites with AL ≥4 mm (not on same tooth)	Or 2 or more IP sites with PD ≥5 mm (not on same tooth)
No or mild periodontitis	Neither "moderate" nor "severe"	

Reprinted from *Journal of Periodontology*, 78(7S):13, Page & Eke (2007), with permission from John Wiley & Sons.

healthy attachment level has been taken to be when the base of the gingival sulcus is no more than 1 mm apical to the cemento-enamel junction. However, this is a rather simplistic assumption because, with age, teeth erupt, and as long as the teeth are not mobile and there is no ongoing periodontitis, an 80-year-old can happily live with a generalised 25% attachment loss, whereas this would be a cause for concern in an 18-year-old. Nevertheless, the measurement of attachment loss is taken to be the gold standard for periodontal epidemiology. Pocket probing depth is also an important variable to assess but in combination with attachment loss.

KEY POINT 7

If its periodontal attachment (periodontal ligament and alveolar bone) has been lost, then a tooth is at a greater risk than if the attachment level is normal.

KEY POINT 8

The measurement of attachment loss is the gold standard for periodontal epidemiology. Pocket probing depth is also an important variable to assess but in combination with attachment loss.

Unfortunately, there is no consensus on a "case" definition for periodontitis in epidemiological studies (Savage et al. 2009), i.e. the threshold at which loss of attachment and pocket depth should be considered a threat to the teeth and the number of sites where this threshold has been crossed. This makes meaningful comparisons between studies impossible. Two case definitions have been suggested by Page and Eke (2007) for the American Academy of Periodontology/Centre for Disease Control (AAP/CDC) (Table 1.3.1) and Tonetti and Claffey (2005) for the European Federation of Periodontology (EFP) (Table 1.3.2).

How to Measure

Probes

Both attachment loss and pocket depth are measured with a periodontal probe. Ideally, a probe with 1 mm markings, such as the North Carolina 15 (Figure 1.3.4), should be used.

TABLE 1.3.2 European Federation of Periodontology case definitions for periodontitis

Incipient periodontitis	IP attachment loss of ≥3 mm in ≥2 non-adjacent teeth
Periodontitis with substantial extent and severity	IP attachment loss of ≥5 mm in ≥30% of teeth

Reprinted from *Journal of Clinical Periodontology*, 32(S6):4, Tonetti and Claffey (2005), with permission from John Wiley & Sons.

KEY POINT 9

There are a number of potential inaccuracies which can occur when measuring pocket depth. These may be due to:
- The extent to which a probe penetrates into a pocket, which can vary depending on the degree of inflammation at the base of the pocket. If the tissues are very inflamed, then there will be less resistance to pressure and the probe tip will penetrate further than in a pocket without an inflamed base.
- The diameter of the probe tip. The smaller the tip the greater its potential to penetrate.
- The thickness (width) of the tine (the part of the probe with markings).
- The probing force used.
- The angulation of the probe to the pocket wall.
- The accuracy of the markings on the probe.
- Presence of overhanging restorations or calculus.

Apart from measuring attachment loss and pocket probing depth, the exposure of furcations, tooth mobility, gingival bleeding, gingival recession, plaque and calculus have frequently been recorded. Details of the techniques for recording these variables are in Chapter 2.2. Finally, nonclinical details such as frequency of toothbrushing and use of oral hygiene aids, such as interdental brushes and dental floss, may be recorded.

Use of radiographs in epidemiological surveys

It is considered unethical to take oral radiographs for the population en masse. The needs of the individual must be

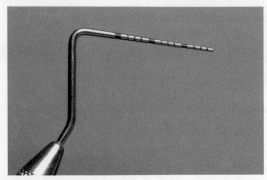

• **Figure 1.3.4** A picture of a North Carolina (NC) 15 periodontal probe. Note the 1 mm markings.

assessed prior to taking a radiograph, and there must be a good clinical indication to do so. For this reason and for reasons of time and cost, radiographs are not usually taken during epidemiological surveys.

What to Measure – Full Versus Part Mouth Assessment

Because a periodontal assessment is usually part of a larger oral or other epidemiological survey, there are often constraints on the time available to perform this assessment. As a result, historically, part mouth rather than full mouth assessments have been performed, and indices such as those described earlier in this chapter have been employed. However, the publication of the results of the periodontal section of the National Health and Nutrition Examination Survey (NHANES) (2009/2010) has reinforced the fact that part mouth assessment underestimates the true level of disease (Eke et al. 2012, Papapanou 2012).

Examiner Consistency

The potential difficulties in assessing pocket depth accurately were discussed earlier in this chapter.

> ### KEY POINT 10
> There are also difficulties in assessing and scoring variables such as plaque and gingivitis accurately and consistently. These difficulties may be due to variation between examiners (inter-examiner variability) or variation by one examiner (intra-examiner variability) such that he/she scores the same site with the same amount of plaque or gingivitis inconsistently.

To try to overcome lack of consistency, examiners for epidemiological surveys undergo training and calibration prior to performing the survey and perform repeat scores on a proportion of subjects each day during the survey. *Oral Health Surveys: Basic Methods, 4th Edition* (1997) recommended that after 4 or 5 days of training inter- and intra-examiner agreement on assessments should be in the 85–95% range.

> ### KEY POINT 11
> Examiners who are persistently inconsistent during training and calibration should not take part in the survey concerned.

National Surveys

The results of two national surveys, NHANES 2009/2010 in the United States and the UK Adult Dental Health Survey (ADHS) 2009, have raised some interesting issues which will need to be addressed in the future.

In previous NHANES surveys, part mouth assessments were performed. The results of NHANES III, which was performed in the late 1990s and used a part mouth assessment, indicated that 53.1% of Americans aged 30 years or older who were examined had attachment loss of ≥3 mm and 23.1% pocket depth of ≥4 mm. When full mouth assessment was used in the 2009/2010 survey, these figures increased to 85.9% and 40.9% respectively (Eke et al. 2012). The survey confirmed previous findings that the periodontal health of those with lower socio-economic status was worse than that of those with higher socio-economic status.

> ### KEY POINT 12
> Eke et al. (2012) concluded that the higher burden of periodontitis in the adult US population and the prevailing disparities among socio-demographic segments detected from this survey, coupled with the potential economic cost for prevention and treatment, suggest periodontitis as an important dental public health problem, especially among our ageing population.

In the ADHS (2009), pocket depth, gingival bleeding, calculus and plaque were recorded at two teeth in each sextant. However, in the South Central area of England, the BPE was used. Loss of attachment was only recorded for those over 55 years of age. The WHO probe (see Figure 1.3.1) was used.

Overall, it was found that 55% of the adults examined had no pocketing, 37% had a pocket or pockets of between 4 mm and 5.5 mm and 8% had a pocket or pockets of 6 mm or deeper. The methodology used makes it impossible to compare these results with those obtained in the NHANES 2009/2010 survey. There were wide variations in the percentage of adults assessed as having a healthy periodontium with a range from 9% in the West Midlands to 36% in the East of England. Two examiners recorded over 70% of those they examined as periodontally healthy. It is entirely possible that these apparent variations were due to examiner inconsistency and did not reflect the true picture.

> ### KEY POINT 13
> As the report of the survey points out, this could reflect inter-examiner variation (an under recording of disease) rather than a difference in the pattern of disease (NHS Information Centre 2009).

> ### KEY POINT 14
> In other countries, it is rare to find periodic national oral health surveys, let alone periodontal surveys. Furthermore, when they have been performed, they used a variety of techniques, both to recruit the population sample and in the clinical assessment.

TABLE 1.3.3	Modified from WHO periodontal examination criteria 2013
Score	Criteria
0	Healthy periodontium
1	Gingival bleeding but no pocket depth greater than 3.5 mm
2	Pocket of between 3.5 mm and 5.5 mm
3	Pocket greater than 5.5 mm in depth

These problems were highlighted in a systematic review of published studies which concluded that as far as Europe was concerned, more comparable and representative data on periodontal disease and tooth loss from all major countries are needed to get a clear picture on periodontal health in Europe (König et al. 2010).

Positive Developments

The fifth edition of *Oral Health Surveys: Basic Methods* (WHO 2013) recommends that a full mouth assessment should be performed using the WHO probe and the recording criteria and scores in Table 1.3.3.

In addition, at a minimum, loss of attachment should be assessed at all upper and lower first and second molars and the upper right and lower left central incisors (WHO 2013).

KEY POINT 15
WHO has suggested the need for full mouth examination of the periodontium when epidemiological studies are performed and also indicated the irrelevance of assessing calculus in these studies, as it is not a disease.

A group of North American and European periodontal epidemiologists (Holfreter et al. 2015) have published standards for reporting chronic periodontitis prevalence and severity in epidemiological studies – proposed standards from the Joint EU/USA Periodontal Epidemiology Working Group. Among other things, this publication recommends that, when conducting periodontal epidemiological surveys, the key indicators to record are the prevalence and extent of clinical attachment loss, probing depth and bleeding on probing at site and tooth level using the Centre for Disease Control/American Academy of Periodontology case definition.

KEY POINT 16
In order to achieve comparable data, there is a need for all future periodontal epidemiological studies to use the same standardised methods.

Possible Future Developments

As has been demonstrated in this chapter, periodontal epidemiology has developed and evolved over the last 70 years and will doubtless continue to do so. In the next 10 years changes may occur as a result of two developments; the first is the newest classification scheme for periodontal and peri-implant diseases and conditions (Caton et al. 2018). This may lead to changes in the case definitions used and the data recorded in periodontal epidemiology. However, because the new scheme requires the availability of radiographs for all subjects/patients, there may be no immediate changes in periodontal epidemiological methods. The second is that Papapanou and Susin (2017) have suggested that additional dimensions should be included in periodontal epidemiology, such as the assessment of impaired function, aesthetics and the effect on general health and quality of life. The authors believe that such a multidimensional approach would lead to improved understanding of the epidemiology and effects of periodontitis and its consequences.

Multiple choice questions on the contents of this chapter are available online at Elsevier eBooks+.

References

Ainamo J, Barmes D, Beaggrie G, Cutress T, Martin J, Sardo-Infirri J. Development of the World Health Organisation (WHO) Community Periodontal Index of Treatment Need (CPITN). *Int Dent J.* 1982;32:281–291.

Carlos JP, Wolfe MD, Kingman A. The extent and severity Index: a simple method for use in epidemiologic studies on periodontal disease. *J Clin Periodontol.* 1986;13:500–505.

Caton JG, Armitage G, Berglundh T, Chapple ILC, Jepson S, Kornman KS, Mealey BL, Papapanou PN, Sanz M, Tonetti MS. A new classification scheme for periodontal and peri-implant diseases and conditions - introduction and key changes from the 1999 classification. *J Periodontol.* 2018;89(suppl 1):S1–S8.

Eke PJ, Dye BA, Wei L, Thornton-Evans GD, Genco RJ, et al. Prevalence of periodontitis in adults in the United States: 2009 and 2010. *J Dent Res.* 2012;91:914–920.

Holtfreter B, Albandar JM, Dietrich T, Dye BA, Eaton KA, Eke PI, Papapanou PN, Kocher T. Joint EU/USA Periodontal Epidemiology Working Group. Standards for reporting chronic periodontitis prevalence and severity in epidemiologic studies: proposed standards from the Joint EU/USA Periodontal Epidemiology Working Group. *J Clin Periodontol.* 2015;42(5):407–412.

König J, Holtfreter B, Kocher T. Periodontal health in Europe: future trends based on treatment needs and the provision of periodontal services – position paper 1. *Eur J Dent Educ.* 2010;14(suppl 1):1–20.

Leroy R, Eaton KA, Savage A. Methodological issues in epidemiological studies of periodontitis – how can it be improved? *BMC Oral Health.* 2010;10:8.

MacMahon B, Pugh TF, Ipsen J. *Epidemiologic Methods.* Boston: Little and Brown; 1960.

NHS Information Centre for Health and Social Care. *Adult Dental Health Survey 2009. London, Health and Social Care Information Centre*; 2011. Available from https://digital.nhs.uk/data-and-information/publications/statistical/adult-dental-health-survey-2009-summary-report-and-thematic-series. (accessed 31.05.21).

Page RC, Eke PI. Case definitions for use in population-based surveillance of periodontitis. *J Periodontol.* 2007;78:1387–1399.

Papapanou PN. The prevalence of periodontitis in the US: forget what you were told. *J Dent Res.* 2012;91:907–908.

Papapanou PN, Susin C. Periodontitis epidemiology: is periodontitis under-recognised, over-diagnosed, or both? *Periodontology 2000.* 2017;75:45–51.

Porta M, Last JT. *Dictionary of Epidemiology.* 5th ed. USA: Oxford University Press, Oxford United Kingdom; 2008.

Ramfjord SP. Indices for the prevalence and incidence of periodontal disease. *J Periodontol.* 1959;30:51–59.

Russell AL. A system of classification and scoring for prevalence surveys of periodontal disease. *J Dent Res.* 1956;35:350–359.

Savage A, Eaton KA, Moles DR, Needleman I. A systematic review of definitions of periodontitis and methods that have been used to identify the disease. *J Clin Periodontol.* 2009;36:458–467.

Tonetti MS, Claffey N. Advances in the progression of periodontitis and proposal of definitions of a periodontitis case and disease progression for use in risk factor research. Group C consensus report of the 5th European Workshop in Periodontology. *J Clin Periodontol.* 2005;32(suppl 6):210–213.

World Health Organization. *Oral Health Surveys: Basic Methods.* 3rd ed. Geneva: WHO; 1989.

World Health Organization. *Oral Health Surveys: Basic Methods.* 4th ed. Geneva: WHO; 1997.

World Health Organization. *Oral Health Surveys: Basic Methods.* 5th ed. Geneva: WHO; 2013.

1.4

HOST RESPONSE AND SUSCEPTIBILITY

PAUL COOPER AND MARTIN LING

CHAPTER OUTLINE

Introduction

Definitions

Host Susceptibility

Host Response to the Bacterial Biofilm

Normal Host Response

The Pathogenesis of Periodontal Lesions

Cell Signalling

Innate Immunity

Acquired Immunity

The Contribution of Genes to Host Responses

Acknowledgements

OVERVIEW OF THE CHAPTER

This chapter explains the factors that contribute to a susceptible host response and the host's innate immune response to the plaque biofilm. It then goes on to describe the immunopathology of the host response in periodontitis and to explain the contribution of genes to host susceptibility.

By the end of the chapter the reader should be able to:

- Describe the factors which contribute to a susceptible host response
- Explain the host's innate immune response to the plaque biofilm
- Describe the immunopathology of the host response in periodontitis
- Explain the contribution of genes to host susceptibility.

The chapter covers the following topics:

- Introduction
- Definitions
- Host susceptibility
- Host response to the bacterial biofilm
- Normal host response
- The pathogenesis of periodontal lesions
- Cell signalling
- Innate immunity
- Acquired immunity
- The contribution of genes to host responses

Introduction

Periodontal diseases, as a group, are one of the most prevalent of human chronic inflammatory conditions, and they are a major cause of tooth loss, particularly in developed countries. They are also one of the most complex of human diseases, involving a range of aetiological factors, including microbial, genetic and environmental factors.

Without bacteria there would be no periodontitis, but bacteria are also important to oral health with over 1200 species (including uncultivable species) described in the mouth. However, certain key bacteria, which are referred to as "periopathogenic" organisms, such as *Porphyromonas gingivalis* and *Aggregatibacter actinomycetemcomitans,* are strongly associated with periodontitis progression.

> ### KEY POINT 1
>
> Periodontitis is an inflammatory disease initiated by bacteria, but it is the host response that causes the majority of the damage to the periodontium.

Whereas bacteria in the biofilm trigger the disease process and are part of the causal pathway of periodontal destruction, the response of the host to the bacteria is key to the development of periodontitis and to disease progression (Figure 1.4.1). In the past, it was thought that the presence of bacteria, and their toxins, were principally responsible for the tissue damage seen in periodontitis and that the host response had only a relatively small part to play in this destructive process. That understanding is now reversed, and it is now thought that the host response is the principal determinant of disease progression. It has been estimated that 20% of the tissue destruction in periodontitis is explained directly by bacterial action (Grossi et al. 1994) and that about 80% of the damage occurring in periodontal diseases is attributable to the host response.

The host response includes both inflammatory and immune components, comprising innate and acquired immunity.

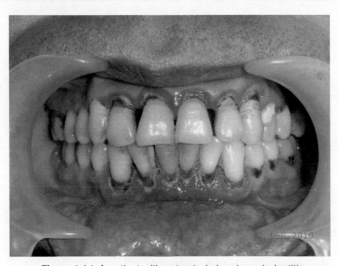

• **Figure 1.4.1** A patient with untreated chronic periodontitis.

Periodontitis results from an imbalance between the oral bacterial flora and the host response (Figure 1.4.2). There is a delicate balance between host and bacterial factors in health, and there is the potential for dysregulation of this balance which can result in disease. Genetic and environmental factors are key to upsetting this balance.

Overall, the host response to the oral microbial biofilm is designed to be protective, but underactivity, or indeed overactivity, of specific aspects of the response can lead to tissue destruction. The host response is largely determined by genetics, and some individuals display an inappropriate or dysregulated host response. In addition, and rarely, certain inherited conditions may affect the periodontal tissues and act as a systemic risk factor for periodontitis.

Evidence now suggests that most of the damage seen in periodontitis is the direct result of the inflammatory and immune response of the individual to the bacterial biofilm and that over 50% of susceptibility to periodontitis can be explained by genetic factors (Michalowicz et al. 2000). Thus it has been stated that "periodontitis is an inflammatory disease initiated by the oral microbial biofilm. However, it is the host response to the biofilm that destroys the periodontium" (Van Dyke 2008).

It is probably inaccurate therefore to describe periodontitis as an "infection" in the traditional sense, mainly because the causative organisms are mostly commensal and rarely invade the tissues; instead it is ". . . more accurately categorised as a non-resolving inflammation that is ineffective in eliminating the initiating pathogens" (Chapple 2009). It should be thought of as a disease that is initiated by the accumulation of pathogenic bacteria, but one that is propagated by a dysregulated immune response and includes aspects of autoimmunity.

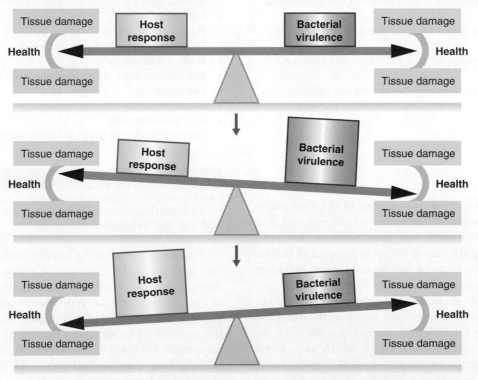

• **Figure 1.4.2** The interaction between bacteria and the host response.

Definitions

Pathogen: An organism that causes disease.

Commensal: Non-disease-causing microorganism that is part of the resident flora.

Opportunistic pathogen: Microorganism not normally pathogenic (can be commensal) but can become pathogenic if the local environment changes.

Virulence factors: Molecules expressed and/or secreted by pathogens to enable colonisation, evasion of the host's immune response, cellular entry/exit or derive nutrition from the host.

Host Susceptibility

A susceptible host is an individual who is at risk of developing disease if he or she is exposed to a causative agent; in the case of periodontitis this is the bacterial biofilm. Host susceptibility results from a number of risk factors that are involved in the host response (Figure 1.4.3).

KEY POINT 3

A susceptible host is someone who is at greater risk of developing a disease when exposed to a causative agent.

Such factors include genetic factors, including those that contribute to impaired neutrophil function, or environmental factors, such as smoking, poorly controlled diabetes or a poor diet. In health, a balance is achieved between the oral bacteria and the host response, but such equilibrium may easily be disrupted in a susceptible host, leading to inflammation and tissue damage.

Bacterial virulence can increase as a result of an increase in bacterial load and/or change in composition. The bacteria present may express virulence factors and toxins. These molecules may be expressed by the pathogens to:

- enable colonisation and multiplication
- evade the host's immune response
- enable intracellular entry/exit
- derive nutrition from the host.

The host inflammatory and immunological response to oral bacteria will ultimately determine how the individual responds to these bacterial factors and whether this response is inappropriate in such a way as to cause collateral tissue damage.

In addition to these host-related factors, there may also be local site-based factors within the mouth, usually in the form of plaque retention factors, such as the presence of calculus or overhanging restorations. Although such local risk factors may contribute to the accumulation of bacterial biofilm, remember that this alone is insufficient to progress gingivitis to a form of periodontitis; it is necessary for the host to be susceptible for this to happen.

There are thus many factors related to both the host and bacteria in the mouth that can contribute to periodontal tissue destruction. Most commonly, it is factors on both sides of the equation that lead to periodontitis.

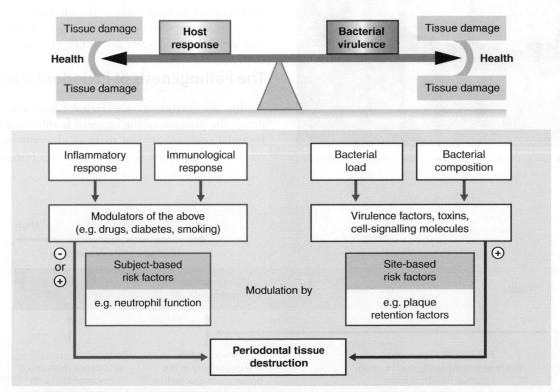

• **Figure 1.4.3** Bacterial/host factors that can affect the delicate balance between the host and the oral microflora.

Host Response to the Bacterial Biofilm

A normal host response to the accumulation of bacterial biofilm invariably results in gingivitis, which is ubiquitous in all populations. This is a reversible inflammatory condition and can be resolved with clinical intervention and does not lead to any periodontal tissue loss. Sometimes, the host response to the bacterial biofilm may be inappropriate (hypo-responsive or, more likely, hyper-responsive), and host-mediated damage occurs in the periodontal tissues (Figure 1.4.4).

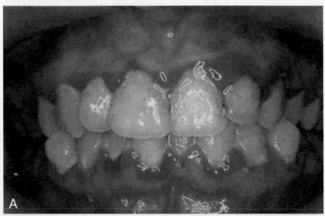

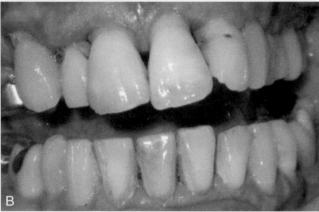

• **Figure 1.4.4** Gingivitis (A) does not necessarily lead to periodontitis (B).

Normal Host Response

There are two main components of the normal host response to plaque bacteria:

Innate or natural immunity: This is the first line of defence. It is rapid but may cause collateral tissue damage if not regulated or controlled correctly.

Acquired or specific immunity: This occurs at the same time as the innate immune response but takes longer to develop and is more specific and more efficient.

Both types of immunity are involved in the host's response to the biofilm and occur at the same time. The innate system is constantly in function and more rapidly mobilised in response to a bacterial threat, whereas the acquired system involves specific cell–cell interactions, which take more time.

> ### KEY POINT 4
> The normal host response involves both innate and acquired immunity.

Early gingival inflammation largely involves the innate system, whereas the acquired system becomes involved in moderate-to-advanced gingivitis and periodontitis (i.e. longer-term, chronic disease).

In a less periodontally susceptible host, the response to the microbial biofilm may be minimal and results only in gingivitis, which is a reversible condition. However, in the presence of systemic and local risk factors, gingivitis may progress to periodontitis, in which irreversible tissue damage occurs (Figure 1.4.5). The more susceptible the host the more damage that will occur and the more advanced the resulting periodontitis. In most cases, periodontitis is chronic but, in the most susceptible individuals, aggressive periodontitis may develop (see Chapter 2.1 and Figure 1.4.5).

The Pathogenesis of Periodontal Lesions

Within the gingival crevice (Figure 1.4.6), the host tissues detect the presence of the bacterial biofilm and respond to bacterial components and toxin production by the bacteria within the biofilm (Figure 1.4.7). This initiates both the

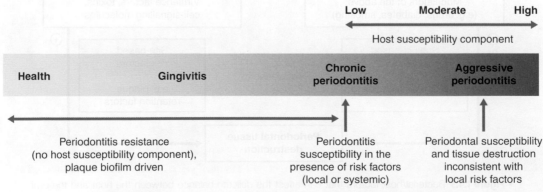

• **Figure 1.4.5** Factors affecting the progression of gingivitis to periodontitis.

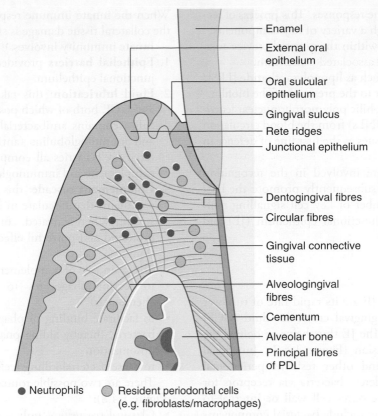

● Neutrophils   ● Resident periodontal cells
                      (e.g. fibroblasts/macrophages)

• **Figure 1.4.6** The microanatomy of the dentogingival area.

Labels (top figure):
- Enamel
- External oral epithelium
- Oral sulcular epithelium
- Gingival sulcus
- Rete ridges
- Junctional epithelium
- Dentogingival fibres
- Circular fibres
- Gingival connective tissue
- Alveologingival fibres
- Cementum
- Alveolar bone
- Principal fibres of PDL

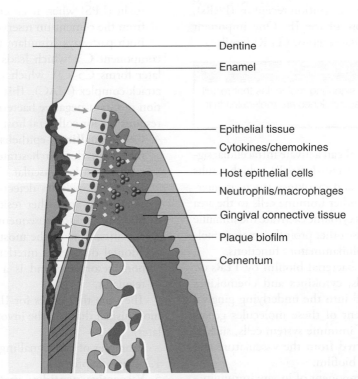

• **Figure 1.4.7** Bacterial interaction with host epithelial cells.

Labels (bottom figure):
- Dentine
- Enamel
- Epithelial tissue
- Cytokines/chemokines
- Host epithelial cells
- Neutrophils/macrophages
- Gingival connective tissue
- Plaque biofilm
- Cementum

innate and acquired immune responses. This process of recognition is achieved through a variety of key components:

- Bacteria form a biofilm within the gingival crevice adjacent to root dentine and associated cementum.
- Bacterial components (such as lipopolysaccharide [LPS]/ endotoxin) alert the host to the presence of the biofilm.
- The host releases neutrophilic polymorphonuclear leucocytes (neutrophils or PMNLs) from the blood circulation and adjacent gingival tissues as the first line of defence in the host response.
- Various resident cells are involved in the recognition of biofilm bacteria and subsequently promote the host response through a number of key cell signalling molecules initially via the junctional epithelium (JE) and sulcular epithelium (SE).

Cell Signalling

The unique features of the JE are its rapid rate of turnover and permeability to both gingival crevicular fluid (GCF) and PMNLs (diapedesis). The JE thus helps to defend the host against bacterial invasion (Figure 1.4.7). Junctional and sulcular epithelium and other resident periodontal cells, such as fibroblasts, detect bacteria via receptors for molecules derived from the outer cell wall or internal to the bacteria. These molecules include bacterial components such as LPS, lipoteichoic acids and bacterial DNA and are known collectively as pathogen-associated molecular patterns (PAMPs). PAMPs can be detected by bacterial-sensing receptors, known as pathogen recognition receptors (PRRs), on human cells, such as those of the JE. One important example of PRRs is the Toll-like receptor (TLR) family.

KEY POINT 5

In general, chemokines are cell signalling molecules that recruit other inflammatory cells whereas cytokines are molecules that activate inflammatory cells.

Binding of a PAMP to a TLR can activate intracellular signalling pathways (e.g. nuclear factor-kappaB), which results in the release of chemokines and cytokines (such as interleukins). Chemokines recruit other immune cells to the area where they are needed whereas cytokines activate the immune cells, stimulating them to release other proinflammatory molecules, which perform key proinflammatory functions.

After the detection of the bacterial biofilm by TLRs on the host's oral epithelial cells, cytokines and chemokines are produced and are released into the underlying gingival connective tissue. The gradient of these molecules generated results in recruitment of immune system cells, such as neutrophils, which are attracted from the vasculature and migrate towards the bacterial biofilm.

This is an example of a component of innate immunity.

Innate Immunity

Innate immunity, although rapid, remains crudely indiscriminate relative to the specificity of the acquired system.

When the innate immune response becomes dysregulated, the collateral tissue damage is significant.

Innate immunity involves:

1. **Epithelial barriers** provided by the oral, sulcular and junctional epithelium.
2. **Fluid lubrication**: this takes the form of both saliva and GCF, both of which possess antibacterial properties. Saliva contains antibacterial enzymes such as lysozyme and immunoglobulins (antibody) which bind to bacteria. GCF carries all components of serum, including complement and immunoglobulins.
3. **Complement cascade**: this is a series of 20 serum glycoproteins that circulate in inactive forms in the bloodstream. When activated, complement components have profound and powerful effects in stimulating inflammation.

The main role of complement activation is:

- to recruit phagocytes to the area (diapedesis and chemotaxis)
- to facilitate binding of phagocytes (e.g. neutrophils) to bacteria, thereby aiding phagocytosis – a process called opsonization
- to cause bacterial killing (cell lysis).

There are two possible routes for complement activation (Figure 1.4.8):

- Classical pathway – only activated by the formation of antigen–antibody complexes (i.e. after initiation of the acquired immune response)
- Alternate pathway – activated directly by bacterial endotoxin (LPS) when it enters the periodontal tissues and from the cementum reservoir.

Both pathways stimulate the activation of complement component C3, which leads to the activation of C5 and later forms C5–C9, which is also termed the membrane attack complex (MAC). This is responsible for the destruction of Gram-negative bacteria, but it is also thought to be responsible for collateral host cell damage.

4. **Cell signalling**: epithelial cells release cell-signalling molecules that orchestrate the inflammatory response resulting in key vascular changes in early inflammation. Signalling includes detection of bacteria (e.g. by TLRs on JE cells and other resident periodontal cells such as fibroblasts) and subsequent release of cytokines and chemokines. One of the most important cytokines in periodontal diseases is interleukin-1 (IL-1) as it stimulates bone resorption and is a powerfully proinflammatory regulator.

The gene that codes for IL-1 has different forms (polymorphisms) that may be involved in host susceptibility (see later).

Examples of cell signalling molecules are listed in Table 1.2.1. in Chapter 1.2.

5. **Vasoactive peptides**: vasoactive peptides such as histamine play an important role in the development of inflammation.

Histamine is released from mast cells on stimulation (by either complement C3a and C5a or prostaglandin E2 [PGE2]) and causes vasodilation to recruit more blood cells

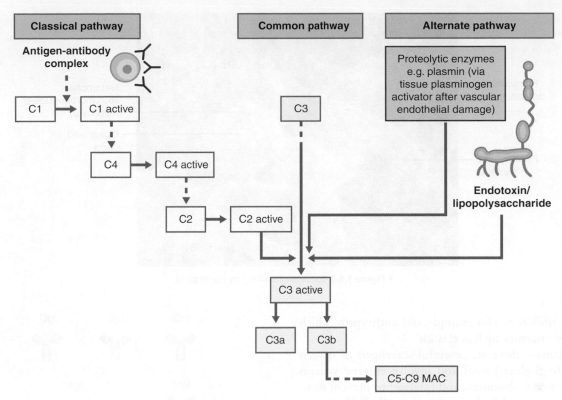

• **Figure 1.4.8** Complement activation pathways.

and plasma proteins (e.g. complement and antibody) to the area of infection.

Histamine also increases vascular permeability and, because vasodilation slows down blood flow within the vessels, this allows defence cells to migrate out of midstream circulation, contact the endothelial cells lining the blood vessels and then leave the circulation and enter adjacent tissues (diapedesis and subsequently chemotaxis).

6. **Adhesion molecule expression** facilitates inflammatory cell contact with vascular endothelial cells and migration to infected areas. This is a tightly controlled process directed by signalling molecules in very specific sequences and pathways.

Examples of important adhesion molecules are intercellular adhesion molecules I and II (ICAM-I and II), endothelial adhesion molecule 1 (ELAM-I) and leucocyte function antigen-1 (LFA-1).

7. **Neutrophils (PMNLs):** the neutrophil is an immune defence cell that destroys invading bacteria, ideally by internalizing them (phagocytosis) prior to destroying them.

It is the most abundant and important defence cell in the periodontal tissues.

Once the neutrophils arrive at the site of infection, they kill bacteria by either intra- or extracellular methods. Intracellular killing involves the same methods as extracellular killing, except the neutrophils release their enzymes and oxygen radicals (a process called degranulation) safely within themselves and inside special membrane-bound structures called phagosomes.

> ### KEY POINT 6
> The neutrophil (PMNL) is the most abundant and important cell in the innate host defence system.

The sequence of neutrophil activity is as follows:
- Rolling – slowing down of neutrophils (PMNLs) within the bloodstream occurs due to vasodilation after the release of vasoactive peptides. Selectins on the neutrophils then make initial "make and break" contacts with complementary ligands on the endothelial cells lining the vessel wall.
- Margination – as the neutrophil slows down, the receptor binding increases and eventually the neutrophils become immobilized on the vascular endothelium by adhesion of integrins on the neutrophil to integrin receptors on the endothelium.
- Diapedesis – other cell-to-cell adhesions allow the neutrophil to pass through the "leaky" blood vessel wall and enter the tissues.
- Chemotaxis – the neutrophil then moves along a chemical gradient through the tissue towards the area of infection.

Neutrophil intracellular killing: after intracellular killing of bacteria, the neutrophils go through a process of programmed cell death (apoptosis) whereby they essentially self-digest to prevent harmful contents entering the host tissues.

The enzymes and oxygen radicals, if released by neutrophils, may damage host tissue and bacteria, and the PMNL therefore contains:

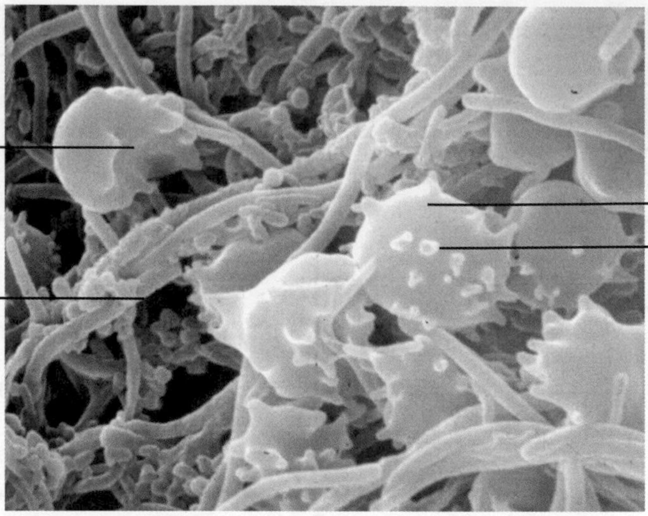

• Figure 1.4.9 Extracellular killing by neutrophils.

• Enzyme inhibitors – for example, α-1 antitrypsin, which neutralize enzymes such as elastase
• Antioxidants – these are powerful scavengers of oxygen radicals (e.g. glutathione) and involve enzyme systems (e.g. superoxide dismutase and catalase) to prevent damage to the neutrophils during oxygen radical release.

Neutrophil extracellular killing (Figure 1.4.9): when the bacterial mass is too large for the neutrophil to phagocytose, it degranulates extracellularly and releases its enzymes, oxygen radicals and neutrophil extracellular traps (NETs) over the bacterial mass in an effort to kill and contain it. If this occurs in the gingival crevice, it may cause damage to the crevicular epithelium. Where a massive neutrophil response is present in the tissues, inadvertent release of these chemicals is believed to be the major cause of periodontal tissue damage and subsequently contributes to bone loss. Notably, NETs are relatively newly described and are formed from the release of the neutrophil's DNA, which is decorated with antimicrobial proteins and enzymes derived from the granules. Whereas these DNA webs entrap and lead to the killing of the bacteria, they can also cause further damage to the host periodontal tissues (Cooper et al. 2013).

8. **Macrophages**: macrophages not only scavenge dead cells (bacteria and neutrophils) but also play an important role in bridging the gap between innate and acquired immunity. As phagocytes, they function in a similar manner to neutrophils, but they also act as antigen presenting cells (APCs), thereby stimulating acquired, or specific, immunity.

Acquired Immunity

Acquired immunity occurs at the same time as the innate immune response but is more specific and efficient.

Cell mediators include:
• T lymphocytes – require direct contact with bacteria for killing

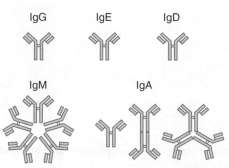

• Figure 1.4.10 Immunoglobulins.

• B lymphocytes – form humoral immune response as they produce immunoglobulins (Ig) which, with complement and phagocytes, kill bacteria (Figure 1.4.10)
• Immunoglobulins – include five main classes: IgG, IgA, IgM, IgD and IgE.

In periodontitis, IgG (in gingival crevicular fluid) and IgA (in saliva) are considered the most important.

The Contribution of Genes to Host Responses

The host response to the bacterial biofilm depends not only on the nature and virulence of the bacterial pathogens but also on genetic factors. Because the pathogenesis of periodontitis largely involves host responses to periodontal microorganisms, it follows that genetic variations modulate host responses which can influence disease progression.

Genetic variation influencing the host response to environmental or systemic risk factors for periodontitis could also influence the effects of such factors on disease.

The host's response to the biofilm is complex, and the host's innate and acquired immune response can lead to the development of periodontitis. Local factors can be managed to reduce risk, but there is usually a significant genetic factor involved in the host's susceptibility to periodontitis.

TABLE 1.4.1   Inherited conditions with additional risk for the development of periodontitis

Condition	Associated gene	Underlying defect of periodontal relevance
Down's syndrome	Chromosome 21	Defects of neutrophil chemotaxis, killing and phagocytosis. Depressed T-cell antigen-induced killing
Chronic granulomatous disease	Gp91 protein p91-PHOX on chromosome b558	Failure of the "respiratory burst" in phagocytosis. Oxygen radicals are not produced, and bacteria survive
Insulin-dependent juvenile diabetes	IDDM1 gene located on chromosome 6	Hyperglycaemia reduces neutrophil function. Monocytes are hyper-reactive and excess IL-1, PGE2, TNF-α and oxygen radicals are produced. Collagen solubility and vascularity changes negatively affect the healing ability
Papillon–Lefèvre syndrome	Cathepsin C gene on chromosome 11	Defects of neutrophil chemotaxis and phagocytosis
Ehlers–Danlos syndrome	Gene mutation encoding for fibrous proteins (e.g. COL1A1) or enzymes	Altered collagen structure and function. Type VIII is associated with severe periodontal destruction
Chediak–Higashi syndrome	Lysosomal trafficking regulator gene on chromosome 1	Defects of phagocyte chemotaxis, degranulation and membrane fusion results in loss of the adult dentition
Job syndrome	STAT3 gene on chromosome 17	Excessive IgE and histamine release by mast cells and IgE immune complex formation. Results in abnormal neutrophil chemotaxis as a result of an altered cytokine profile

KEY POINT 7

There is understood to be a significant genetic contribution to the host's susceptibility to periodontitis.

Twin, sibling pair and family studies demonstrate that periodontitis has a significant genetic component (Michalowicz et al. 2000).

Genetic single nucleotide polymorphisms (SNPs) have been linked to risk of periodontal tissue breakdown. There is extensive research aimed at identifying the association between gene polymorphisms and periodontitis susceptibility. IL-1 gene polymorphisms are examples of SNPs that have been shown to be associated with periodontitis in some people. IL-1 is a key cytokine in periodontal disease pathogenesis, and "overproduction" of this cytokine has been identified in chronic periodontitis patients. In the future, it may be possible to develop "periodontitis susceptibility tests" based on screening SNPs that may identify patients at risk of developing periodontitis. Such a test already exists for IL-1 but is not widely employed because of a lack of generalizability of results from IL-1 SNP studies.

In addition to SNPs, certain inherited conditions may affect the periodontal tissues and act as risk factors for periodontitis. These are shown in Table 1.4.1.

Ultimately, periodontitis is the result of a complex interaction between the bacterial biofilm, the environment, the host's lifestyle and genetic factors. The environmental factors can be effectively controlled by oral hygiene, and, to some extent, lifestyle factors can also be controlled or managed. A host's genetic susceptibility cannot easily be controlled. However, genetics could help identify those patients who are more susceptible and therefore help with prevention, early diagnosis, and management of the disease. Ultimately, susceptible individuals could be targeted with preventative treatments to minimise disease risk.

KEY POINT 8

Periodontitis is the result of a complex interaction between the bacterial biofilm, the host's lifestyle and genetic factors.

Acknowledgements

This chapter is based on a session within e-Den which Professor Cooper and Dr. Ling produced in 2011. Acknowledgement is given to the Faculty of Dental Surgery of the Royal College of Surgeons of England for giving permission for material from the e-Den session to be used in this chapter.

Multiple choice questions on the contents of this chapter are available online at Elsevier eBooks+.

References

Chapple ILC. Periodontal diagnosis and treatment – where does the future lie? *Periodontol.* 2009;51:9–24.

Cooper PR, Palmer LJ, Chapple IL. Neutrophil extracellular traps as a new paradigm in innate immunity: friend or foe? *Periodontol 2000.* 2013;63(1):97–165.

Grossi SG, Zambon JJ, Ho AW, Koch G, Dunford RG, Machtei EE, et al. Assessment of risk for periodontal disease. 1. Risk indicators for attachment loss. *J Periodontol.* 1994;65:260–267.

Michalowicz BS, Diehl SR, Gunsolley JC, Sparks BS, Brooks CN, Koertge TE, et al. Evidence of a substantial genetic basis for risk of adult periodontitis. *J Periodontol.* 2000;71:1699–1707.

Van Dyke TE. The management of inflammation in periodontal disease. *J Periodontol.* 2008;79:1601–1608.

Further reading

Chapple ILC, Gilbert AD. *Understanding Periodontal Diseases: Assessment and Diagnostic Procedures in Practice.* Quintessence London; 2002.

Henderson B, Curtis M, Seymour R, Donos N. *Periodontal Medicine and Systems Biology.* Wiley-Blackwell Chichester; 2009.

1.5

THE ROLE OF BIOFILMS IN HEALTH AND DISEASE

PHILIP D MARSH

CHAPTER OUTLINE

OVERVIEW OF THE CHAPTER

This chapter describes the role of dental biofilms (previously referred to as dental plaque) in periodontal health and disease. The chapter discusses the significance of a biofilm lifestyle on the properties of oral microorganisms and explains why clinicians need to be aware of this when they plan their treatment.

By the end of the chapter the reader should:

- Understand the significance of the term "biofilm" and appreciate the benefits to the host of the microorganisms found naturally in the mouth (the oral microbiome)
- Be aware of the main groups of microorganisms found in the healthy mouth
- Describe the shifts in composition of the subgingival microbiome that occur in periodontal diseases
- Understand the mechanisms by which these subgingival biofilms cause disease and are more difficult to treat.

The chapter covers the following topics:

- Introduction
- What are biofilms?
- Biofilms in the mouth
- Methods to determine the microbial composition and function of dental biofilms
- Microbial composition of dental biofilms in health
- Stages in the formation of dental biofilms
- Reduced sensitivity of biofilms to antimicrobial agents
- Benefits of the resident oral microbiome
- Microbial composition of dental biofilms in periodontal diseases
- Contemporary perspectives on the aetiology of periodontal diseases
- Concluding remarks

Introduction

The mouth, like all other surfaces in the body, is colonised by a characteristic and natural community of microorganisms, termed the oral microbiome or the oral microbiota (Kilian et al. 2016), which is composed predominantly of bacteria but can also include viruses, fungi, mycoplasmas, *Archaea* and even protozoa. The oral microbiome is normal and confers important benefits to the host (see later) and exists on surfaces as structurally organised, multispecies biofilms (Marsh et al. 2016).

> ### KEY POINT 1
> The mouth harbours characteristic communities of microorganisms, the presence of which are normal and beneficial to the host. These microbial communities grow on oral surfaces as biofilms.

The resident oral microbiome plays a direct and active role in the normal development of the physiology, nutrition and defence systems of the host (Kilian et al. 2016, Marsh et al. 2016). A dynamic balance exists between the resident microbiome and the host in health (symbiosis), whereas disease results from a breakdown (dysbiosis) of this delicate relationship (Curtis et al. 2020, Hajishengalis et al. 2020). Therefore it is important that the factors that regulate and influence this intimate relationship between the host and their microorganisms are understood, and those that are driving dysbiosis in individual patients are identified and rectified. Thus oral care should involve effective plaque control techniques that maintain dental biofilms at levels compatible with oral health to retain the beneficial properties of the resident microbiome, while reducing the risk of dental disease from excessive plaque accumulation (Marsh 2012). These levels may vary between individual patients.

> ### KEY POINT 2
> The resident oral microbiome and the host exist in a natural and mutually beneficial relationship (symbiosis). Disease results from a breakdown of this relationship after a deleterious shift in the composition of the microbiome (dysbiosis).

What are Biofilms?

In nature, microorganisms preferentially attach to surfaces (inanimate and living) usually as multispecies communities. This is a fundamental survival stratagem for microbes (Nobbs et al. 2011). Once attached, microbes grow and form three-dimensional structures, termed *biofilms,* embedded in an extracellular matrix of sticky polymers (Zijnge et al. 2010, 2012, Mark Welch et al. 2016, 2019, Bowen et al. 2018). Biofilms are ubiquitous and are found in water distribution pipes and machinery, on contact lenses, implants and catheters, as well as on oral surfaces, especially teeth (dental plaque), dentures and implants (Figure 1.5.1). The significance of dental plaque as an example of a biofilm is that discoveries made on biofilms in general may also be applicable to dental plaque.

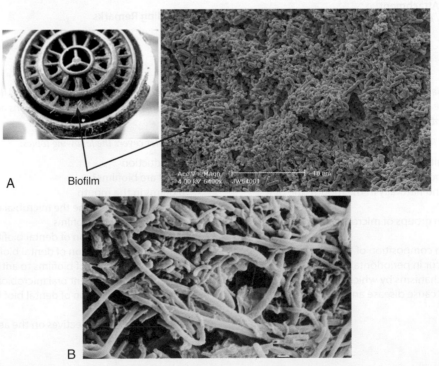

• **Figure 1.5.1** Examples of biofilms. (A) A biofilm forming on a hospital tap outlet and (B) a dental biofilm on a tooth surface. (Courtesy Dr. Jimmy Walker, PHE.)

Dental plaque is a classic example of both a biofilm and a microbial community. Plaque is composed of numerous interacting microbial species; on average, there are 20 to 50 species present in even a small sample of dental biofilm (Aas et al. 2005). There are numerous advantages for microorganisms to exist as a biofilm and as a microbial community. These include:

- Biofilms are more tolerant of environmental stresses, the host defences and antimicrobial agents
- Microbial communities have a greater tolerance of antimicrobial agents and the host defences because of cross-protection, i.e. one species can protect a neighbouring species, for example, by producing a neutralizing enzyme
- Microbial communities display an enhanced pathogenic potential; groups of different bacteria can combine to pool their weak virulence determinants in order to cause disease ("pathogenic synergism")
- Microorganisms that exist within a community exhibit a broader habitat range (e.g. obligate anaerobes can survive in an overtly aerobic environment) and increased metabolic diversity and efficiency (e.g. they can catabolize substrates collectively which individual organisms are unable to utilize)
- Therefore the properties of a microbial community such as dental plaque are greater than the sum of the activities of the component species.

Biofilms in the Mouth

Biofilms are found on all surfaces in the mouth, but the largest and most diverse biofilms are found on teeth (dental plaque). The composition and structure of the biofilms are directly influenced by the anatomy and biological properties of the surface to which they attach. Therefore each surface will have a biofilm with a characteristic microbial composition that reflects, and is a product of, the local environment (Aas et al. 2005, Marsh et al. 2016, Papaioannou et al. 2009).

Biofilms that form on mucosal surfaces are restricted by desquamation, whereas non-shedding surfaces, such as teeth (or dentures, implants and restorations, etc.), permit extensive biofilm development. Dental plaque preferentially forms at retention and stagnant sites because these provide protection from removal forces in the mouth, e.g. saliva flow, mastication, and such sites are also the most susceptible to disease.

Methods to Determine the Microbial Composition of Dental Biofilms

The method of sampling dental biofilms depends on the anatomy of the site. When plaque is processed, care must be taken to disperse the biofilm, which, by definition, is a diverse collection of interacting microorganisms that are tightly bound to one another, without adversely killing fastidious bacteria, such as obligate anaerobes, that may be present in the sample. Fissures can be sampled with a fine probe or toothpick. Dental floss, abrasive strips or dental probes can be used for approximal surfaces whereas the gingival crevice can be sampled with a paper point, curette or scaler.

There are three main approaches to determine the microbial composition of plaque biofilms; these are: microscopy, conventional culture techniques and molecular biology–based (culture-independent) methods. Microscopy can give a rapid and cheap assessment of the microbial diversity within the biofilm, e.g. the enumeration of motile bacteria such as spirochaetes, but generally cannot identify the microbes unless specific stains are available, e.g. antibody- or nucleotide-based probes labelled with a signalling molecule such as a fluorescent dye (for example, fluorescent in situ hybridization [FISH]) (Mark Welch et al. 2016, 2019). Confocal laser scanning microscopy enables biofilms to be viewed in their natural hydrated state and has shown that all biofilms, including dental plaque, have a more open architecture than thought from previous electron microscopy images and a functionally organised structure (Mark Welch et al. 2016, 2019).

As stated previously, bacteria are the most abundant group of microorganisms in the oral microbiome, but significant numbers of fungi can be present too (Dewhirst et al. 2010, Hong et al. 2015, Marsh et al. 2016). Initially, bacteria and fungi were characterised using traditional approaches which involved prolonged culture on selective and nonselective agar plates, under different atmospheric conditions; the microbial colonies that grew then had to be further cultured in pure culture and undergo additional biochemical tests to obtain an identification. These steps are laborious, time consuming and expensive, and over time it became apparent that there was a large discrepancy between the number of microorganisms in a sample that could be grown by these conventional methods and those that were observed directly by microscopy. Only about 50% of the resident oral microbiome can currently be grown in pure culture in the laboratory (Wade & Prosdocimi 2020). The "missing" microbes have been referred to as "unculturable"', but our inability to culture them is due mainly to our ignorance of the growth requirements of some species and our naivety in attempting to isolate microbes in pure culture as these have evolved over millennia to grow with other species as part of a community (Wade et al. 2016).

Contemporary approaches are using molecular (i.e. culture-independent) methods to detect and identify microorganisms (Diaz et al. 2017, Wade & Prosdocimi 2020). These rely on detecting the nucleic acid signatures that are specific to each species and range from targeted approaches such as PCR, DNA–DNA checkerboard systems or microarrays that identify preselected microbial groups to the more current and preferable open-ended approaches in which all of the microbial DNA in a sample is digested, amplified, sequenced, reassembled and finally mapped against a reference database of relevant genomes (metagenomics), so that the whole diversity of the microbiome is revealed (Wade & Prosdocimi 2020) (Figure 1.5.2). These culture-independent approaches are not without their own bias, however, as it can be more difficult to lyse and extract DNA from some organisms, and because the primers used for amplification are not optimised for all species (Wade et al. 2016, Wade & Prosdocimi 2020). Nevertheless, the introduction of these culture-independent approaches has changed our understanding of the richness and diversity of the oral microbiome in health and disease (Marsh et al. 2016, Wade et al. 2016) and could lead eventually to chairside kits and services to help diagnose oral diseases and monitor the outcome of treatment (Meuric et al. 2017, Belibasakis et al. 2019, Chen et al. 2021).

Rather than just cataloguing the types of microorganism that are present at a site, complementary molecular approaches are also being used to monitor gene expression so as to determine the metabolic and functional activity in a sample (e.g. by using metatranscriptomics, proteomics and metabolomics). In the future, more emphasis may be placed on what microorganisms are "doing" (i.e. their function and activity) rather than providing a list of merely "who" is present (Takahashi 2015, Espinoza et al. 2018). It is likely that different combinations of species within a microbial community will perform similar tasks, and this might explain why there is not always a clear consensus when comparing the composition of dental biofilms in health and disease from different studies.

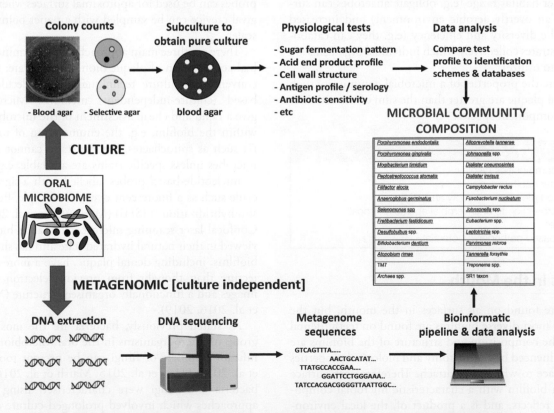

• **Figure 1.5.2** Schematic to show the stages in determining the microbial composition of dental biofilms using traditional culture or contemporary molecular-based (metagenomic) approaches. Theoretically, a metagenomic approach can be quicker than conventional culture as many species grow slowly; also approximately half of the oral microbiome cannot be cultured at present.

The accumulated data from numerous studies of different oral surfaces and sites from around the world have resulted to date in the identification of around 770 different types of microorganism (sometimes referred to as different taxa or phylotypes) from the mouth; of these, 57% are officially named, 13% unnamed but cultivable and 30% are known only as currently "unculturable" phylotypes. A single individual may harbour between 50 to 300 species. It is beyond the scope of this chapter to describe the properties of members of the resident oral microbiome, and the reader is recommended to refer to specialist texts for more detail (for example, Marsh et al. 2016), or to the two curated oral 16S rRNA databases: the Human Oral Microbiome Database (HOMD; http://www.homd.org) and the Core Oral Microbiome Database (CORE; http://microbiome.osu.edu).

Molecular (culture-independent) approaches are being adopted because:

- there is less bias compared with culture
- "unculturable" and novel species can be detected; these can account for >50% of the microorganisms that are present, especially at subgingival sites
- the techniques can be comparatively quick and are not as labour intensive as traditional culture
- microbial signatures of health and disease can be identified (Meuric et al. 2017, Chen et al. 2021).
  A limitation of molecular approaches is that:
- they are semiquantitative at best
- viable bacteria are not isolated, from which to determine their properties, including antibiotic sensitivities
- some approaches will detect dead as well as viable cells.

Microbial Composition of Dental Biofilms in Health

The microbial composition of biofilms on distinct surfaces on teeth varies markedly because of differences in local environmental conditions (nutrition, pH, O_2, host defences, etc.) (Aas et al. 2005, Papaioannou et al. 2009, Marsh et al. 2016).

Fissures

The microbiota of fissures is composed mainly of Gram-positive and facultatively anaerobic bacteria that have a saccharolytic metabolism (i.e. gain energy from the catabolism of carbohydrates including dietary sugars); the majority of the bacteria are streptococci, especially extracellular polysaccharide-producing species. Obligately anaerobic Gram-negative bacteria are either absent or detected only rarely and in low numbers; *Veillonella* species are the most commonly isolated Gram-negative organism from this site. Saliva has a large influence on the properties of the microbiota of fissures.

Approximal Surfaces

These surfaces have high numbers of Gram-positive and facultatively anaerobic bacteria, particularly *Actinomyces* spp.

and streptococci. Obligately anaerobic bacteria are common (e.g. *Veillonella*, *Prevotella* and *Fusobacterium* spp.) and present in relatively high proportions, although spirochaetes are usually absent.

Gingival Crevice

This site contains biofilms with the highest species diversity in the healthy mouth and with the greatest numbers of obligately anaerobic bacteria, many of which are Gram negative or are *Eubacterium*-like. Many of the currently "unculturable" bacteria are found subgingivally. Common bacteria associated with the healthy gingival crevice are members of the mitis and anginosus groups of streptococci and Gram-positive rods such as species of *Actinomyces*, *Rothia* and *Corynebacterium*. Gram-negative genera that are commonly detected include *Neisseria*, *Lautropia*, *Haemophilus*, *Capnocytophaga*, *Fusobacterium*, *Prevotella* and *Veillonella* (Abusleme et al. 2013, Hong et al. 2015, Diaz et al. 2016). The ecology of the crevice is influenced by the flow and properties of gingival crevicular fluid (GCF). GCF introduces not only components of the host defences (neutrophils, complement, antibodies), but also host molecules that can be degraded and used as important substrates. Many of the microbial residents are proteolytic and derive their energy from the hydrolysis of these host proteins and peptides and from the catabolism of amino acids; others also require heme as an essential cofactor for growth, which can be obtained from haemoglobin and other host molecules in GCF.

Stages in the Formation of Dental Biofilms

The formation of dental plaque can be subdivided into a series of arbitrary stages although, as biofilm formation is a dynamic process, some of these stages will occur simultaneously (Figure 1.5.3).

KEY POINT 6

Stages in the formation of dental plaque:
1. conditioning film formation: adsorption of host molecules on to dental surfaces (the acquired pellicle)
2. transport of microbes to surface: passive or active
3. reversible phase: long-range, weak, physicochemical forces
4. irreversible phase: strong, short-range adhesin-receptor interactions
5. secondary colonisation: co-aggregation/co-adhesion
6. biofilm maturation: growth and extracellular matrix formation
7. detachment: facilitates colonisation at other sites.

Stage 1. Conditioning Film Formation

Microorganisms rarely come into contact with clean enamel. Within seconds of being cleaned, molecules are adsorbed onto the tooth surface, forming a surface-conditioning film

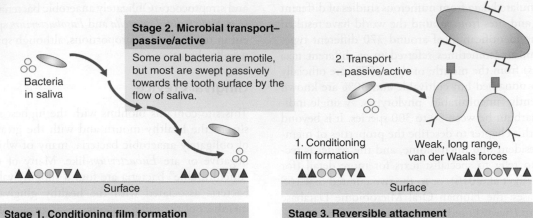

Stage 2. Microbial transport–passive/active

Some oral bacteria are motile, but most are swept passively towards the tooth surface by the flow of saliva.

Bacteria in saliva

Surface

2. Transport – passive/active

1. Conditioning film formation

Weak, long range, van der Waals forces

Surface

Stage 1. Conditioning film formation

The conditioning film (also referred to as the acquired pellicle) starts to form within seconds immediately after a surface is cleaned. It is composed of salivary proteins, glycoproteins and bacterial glucans and enzymes.

A

Stage 3. Reversible attachment

Once bacteria are close to the tooth surface, weak long-range (>10–20 μm) forces between the molecules on the microbial cell surface and those in the conditioning film can hold the cell reversibly near to the tooth.

B

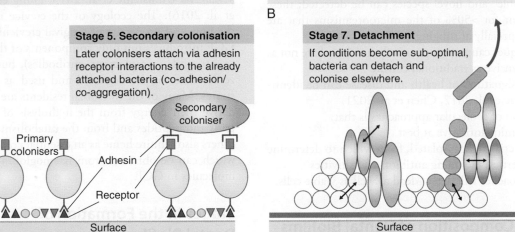

Stage 5. Secondary colonisation

Later colonisers attach via adhesin receptor interactions to the already attached bacteria (co-adhesion/co-aggregation).

Secondary coloniser

Primary colonisers

Adhesin

Receptor

Surface

Stage 4. Irreversible attachment

Attachment can become irreversible if specific molecules on the bacterial cell surface (termed "adhesins") are able to bind to complementary molecules in the acquired pellicle (termed "receptors").

C

Stage 7. Detachment

If conditions become sub-optimal, bacteria can detach and colonise elsewhere.

Surface

Stage 6. Biofilm maturation

The attached bacteria grow, form micro-colonies, and interact both synergistically (e.g. food webs, cell–cell signalling, etc.) and antagonistically (e.g. inhibitor production, etc.). The metabolism of the early colonisers modifies the environment in the biofilm, thereby making conditions suitable for the attachment and growth of later colonisers (e.g. obligate anaerobes). An extracellular matrix is synthesised.

D

• **Figure 1.5.3** Stages in the development of dental biofilms. (A) Stage 1: A conditioning film (the acquired pellicle) forms immediately on a cleaned tooth surface. Stage 2: Microorganisms are generally transported passively to the tooth surface. (B) Stage 3: Microorganisms may be held reversibly close to the tooth surface by weak, long-range physicochemical forces of attraction. (C) Stage 4: Attachment becomes more permanent if specific and stronger stereochemical molecular interactions occur between adhesins on the bacterium and receptors in the acquired pellicle. Stage 5: Secondary colonisers attach to primary colonisers, also by adhesin-receptor interactions (co-adhesion), thereby increasing the diversity of the developing biofilm. (D) Stage 6: Growth of attached cells results in biofilm maturation, facilitating interbacterial interactions (synergistic and antagonistic) and biofilm matrix formation. Stage 7: If conditions become sub-optimal, cells can detach and colonise elsewhere.

(termed the acquired enamel pellicle). This film contains salivary glycoproteins, phosphoproteins and lipids, including statherin, amylase, proline-rich peptides (PRPs), host defence components and bacterial components such as glucosyltransferases and glucan (Figure 1.5.3A) (Hannig et al. 2005); it is to these molecules that the early microbial colonisers (predominantly bacteria) attach. Depending on the site, pellicle can also contain components from GCF.

Stage 2. Transport of Microorganisms

Microorganisms are generally transported passively to the tooth surface by the flow of saliva (see Figure 1.5.3A); a few oral bacterial species are motile (e.g. possess flagella), and these are mainly located subgingivally.

Stage 3. Reversible Attachment

Long-range, relatively weak physicochemical forces of attraction are generated as the cell approaches the pellicle-coated surface. These are generated by the interactions between the electrical charge on the molecules on the surface of the colonising bacteria and the charge on the conditioning film and can hold the cell reversibly close to the tooth (see Figure 1.5.3B) (Busscher et al. 2008).

Stage 4. Irreversible Attachment

The adherence of the reversibly attached cells can become stronger, and more likely to be permanent, if molecules (adhesins) on early bacterial colonisers (mainly streptococci, e.g. *Streptococcus mitis, Streptococcus oralis*) can bind to complementary receptors in the acquired pellicle (Busscher et al. 2008, Nobbs et al. 2011) (see Figure 1.5.3). *Actinomyces, Haemophilus* and *Neisseria* spp. are also commonly isolated early on, but obligately anaerobic species are detected only rarely at this stage and are usually in low numbers. Individual species express multiple adhesins; in Gram-positive bacteria, several families of surface proteins can act as adhesins, including serine-rich repeat, antigen I/II and pilus families. Adhesins in Gram-negative bacteria include autotransporters, extracellular matrix–binding proteins and pili (Nobbs et al. 2011). Once attached, these early colonisers divide and form microcolonies, and their metabolism starts to modify the local environment in the biofilm.

Stage 5. Secondary Colonisation

Over time, the composition of the biofilm becomes more diverse; there is a shift away from dominance by streptococci to increasing proportions of *Actinomyces*, other Gram-positive bacilli and obligate anaerobes. Some organisms that were unable to colonise the pellicle-coated tooth surfaces are able to attach to already adherent pioneer species by further adhesin-receptor interactions (termed co-aggregation or co-adhesion) (see Figure 1.5.3C) (Kolenbrander et al. 2006, 2010). *Fusobacterium nucleatum* is a key organism in dental biofilm development, as this species can coadhere to most oral bacteria and acts, therefore, as an important bridging organism between early and late colonising species. Co-adhesion may help ensure that bacteria are co-located with other organisms with complementary metabolic functions. Thus the composition of the biofilm changes over time due to a series of complex interactions; these changes are termed microbial succession.

Stage 6. Biofilm Maturation

The microbial diversity of the biofilm increases still further over time because of consecutive waves of microbial succession and subsequent growth, eventually leading to a stable "climax microbial community" and a "mature" biofilm (see Figure 1.5.3D). The metabolism of the early colonising bacteria can modify the biofilm environment (e.g. consumption of oxygen and production of reduced fermentation products), which can increase the probability of colonisation by more fastidious species (e.g. obligate anaerobes). Some of the attached bacteria can synthesize extracellular polymers (the plaque matrix) that can consolidate attachment of the biofilm (Bowen et al. 2018). The matrix is more than a mere scaffold for the biofilm; the matrix can bind and retain molecules, including enzymes, and retard the penetration of charged molecules (including antimicrobial agents) into the biofilm (Bowen et al. 2018). The matrix can contain extracellular DNA (eDNA) (Jakubovics & Burgess 2015), soluble and insoluble polysaccharides (glucans, fructans, etc.) (Koo et al. 2013) and lipoteichoic acid, the differing proportions of which will influence the biological properties of the biofilm (Koo et al. 2013, Bowen et al. 2018).

Biofilms are spatially and functionally organised, and the heterogeneous conditions within the biofilm induce novel patterns of bacterial gene expression, whereas the close proximity of different species provides the opportunity for multiple types of synergistic and antagonistic interaction (Jakubovics 2015, Marsh & Zaura 2017, Bowen et al. 2018). Examples of these interactions include:

(a) The development of food chains (in which the terminal product of metabolism of one organism is used as a primary nutrient by secondary feeders) and metabolic cooperation among species to catabolize structurally complex host macromolecules. These interactions increase the metabolic efficiency of the microbial community and contribute to the stability and resilience of oral biofilms (Marsh & Zaura 2017, Rosier et al. 2018).

(b) Cell–cell signalling. Plaque bacteria can communicate with one another in a cell density–dependent manner via small diffusible molecules. Gram-positive bacteria secrete small peptides to coordinate gene expression among cells of a similar species, whereas autoinducer-2 (AI-2) is produced by several genera of oral Gram-positive and Gram-negative bacteria, implying that AI-2 may signal across a broader species range (Jakubovics 2010, Leung et al. 2015, Nobbs & Jenkinson 2015). Several putative periodontal pathogens (*Fusobacterium nucleatum, Prevotella intermedia, Porphyromonas gingivalis, Aggregatibacter actinomycetemcomitans*) secrete a signal related to AI-2.

(c) Physically close cell-cell associations, such as "corn-cob" (in which coccal-shaped cells attach along the tip of filamentous organisms), and "test-tube brush" structures (rod-shaped bacteria sticking out perpendicularly from bacterial filaments), develop (Zijnge et al. 2010). Lactobacilli formed the central axis of some of the "test-tube brushes", with organisms such as *Tannerella, F. nucleatum* and *Synergistes* spp. radiating from this central cell. Corncobs can form between streptococci and *Corynebacterium matruchotii* and between *Veillonella* spp. and *Eubacterium* spp. (Zijnge et al. 2010).

(d) Horizontal gene transfer, including the sharing of antibiotic resistance genes (Marsh & Zaura 2017).

(e) Antagonism between competing species, for example, by the production of inhibitory molecules (bacteriocins, hydrogen peroxide, organic acids, etc.). The production of such inhibitory molecules will also contribute to "colonisation resistance" in which the resident oral microbiome is able to prevent the growth of potentially invading organisms (Marsh & Zaura 2017).

As the biofilm matures, bacterial metabolism results in the development of gradients within dental biofilms in parameters that are critical to microbial growth (nutrients, pH, oxygen, etc.). Such environmental heterogeneity will allow fastidious bacteria to survive in plaque and enable microorganisms to coexist that would be incompatible with one another in a more homogeneous environment.

Stage 7. Detachment From Surfaces

Bacteria can "sense" adverse changes in environmental conditions, and these may act as "cues" to induce genes involved in active detachment from the biofilm, for example, by the upregulation of proteases to cleave their adhesins from the cell surface (see Figure 1.5.3D).

Reduced Sensitivity of Biofilms to Antimicrobial Agents

All biofilms display a reduced sensitivity to antimicrobial agents compared with the same cells growing in conventional liquid culture (Mah 2012, Koo et al. 2017, Uruen et al. 2020). For example, concentrations of chlorhexidine need to be 10- to 50-fold greater than the minimum inhibitory concentration (MIC) in order to eliminate a biofilm of an oral bacterium such as *Streptococcus sanguinis*. Older biofilms are even more tolerant of antimicrobial agents than younger biofilms. Generally, this is a phenotypic response, as these cells display their original sensitivity when resuspended from the biofilm into liquid broth (mechanisms for this are listed later), and so the reduced sensitivity should be

referred to as "tolerance". Microorganisms can become truly "resistant" to antimicrobial agents because of the increased probability of gene transfer occurring in biofilms. Recipients of an antibiotic resistance gene are truly resistant to the agent irrespective of whether they are in a biofilm or not (Uruen et al. 2020).

KEY POINT 7
- Oral biofilms are difficult to treat
- Biofilms are many times more tolerant of antimicrobial agents than the same cells in planktonic liquid culture.

The mechanisms that underpin this enhanced tolerance of biofilms to antimicrobial agents include:

- limited penetration of charged molecules, e.g. due to the binding of antimicrobials to the biofilm matrix
- inactivation by production of neutralizing enzymes (e.g. cross-protection by neighbouring cells that secrete catalase or β-lactamase that degrade hydrogen peroxide or penicillin, respectively)
- quenching of the agent, e.g. by binding to cells at the biofilm surface
- unfavourable environments for the antimicrobial to function in the depths of the biofilm
- expression of a novel phenotype, e.g. the drug target is no longer expressed during growth in the biofilm
- the slow growth rates of bacteria in biofilms (slow-growing organisms are generally less susceptible than faster-growing cells)
- horizontal gene transfer (e.g. drug resistance plasmids; this is an example of increased "resistance" to an antimicrobial agent). In a biofilm, cells are close to one another, which facilitates effective gene transfer (Uruen et al. 2020).

Benefits of the Resident Oral Microbiome

The resident oral microbiome confers important benefits to the host and plays an essential role in the normal development of the physiology, nutrition and defences of the host (Sanz et al. 2017).

KEY POINT 8
The oral microbiome provides significant benefits to the host by:
- Resisting colonisation (in which the resident microbiome prevents colonisation by exogenous species)
- Downregulating proinflammatory host responses to beneficial species (Devine et al. 2015)
- Regulating gastrointestinal and cardiovascular systems.
Thus it is essential to control oral biofilms, and not eliminate them, to maintain the beneficial properties of the oral microbiota.

- One of the principal functions of a resident microbiome is the ability to prevent colonisation by exogenous (and often pathogenic) microorganisms. This property, termed "colonisation resistance", is due to the resident microbes being more effective at:

- attaching to host receptors
- competing for endogenous nutrients
- creating unfavourable growth conditions to discourage attachment and multiplication of invading organisms, and
- producing antagonistic substances (hydrogen peroxide, bacteriocins, etc.).

- Attempts to boost colonisation resistance using replacement therapy (in which resident organisms are deliberately reimplanted), for example, after periodontal therapy or by using probiotics or prebiotics (molecules that boost the growth of beneficial resident microbes), are being explored (Devine & Marsh 2009).
- The biological mechanisms are being identified that permit a constructive coexistence between the host and the resident microbiome. The host is actively engaged in cross-talk with its resident microbiome in order to maintain a symbiotic relationship. The host has evolved systems to enable it to tolerate resident microorganisms without initiating a damaging inflammatory response, while also being able to mount an efficient defence against pathogens (Devine et al. 2015).
- The resident oral bacteria play an important role in maintaining many important aspects of the gastrointestinal and cardiovascular systems via the metabolism of dietary nitrate. Approximately 25% of ingested nitrate is secreted in saliva where facultatively anaerobic oral resident bacteria reduce nitrate to nitrite. Nitrite affects a number of key physiological processes including the regulation of blood flow, blood pressure, gastric integrity and tissue protection against ischaemic injury. Nitrite can be further converted to nitric oxide in the acidified stomach, and this has antimicrobial properties and contributes to defence against enteropathogens; nitric oxide also regulates gastric mucosal blood flow and promotes mucus formation (Koch et al. 2017, Rosier et al. 2020).

Microbial Composition of Dental Biofilms in Periodontal Diseases

Numerous studies with different designs and a variety of populations and sites have consistently shown that the microbiota from periodontal pockets is markedly different from that found at healthy sites, even in the same mouth (Diaz et al. 2016). The conclusion from these studies is that, unlike some medical infections, there is a not a single pathogen responsible for periodontal disease but that inflammation is a consequence of an increased biomass with higher numbers and proportions of obligate anaerobes, many of which are Gram-negative bacteria expressing a proinflammatory phenotype and with a proteolytic metabolism.

Some of the microbiological features of distinct forms of periodontal diseases are described in the following sections.

Gingivitis

Dental biofilm-induced gingivitis is a nonspecific, reversible inflammatory response to an increased accumulation of biofilm around the gingival margin due to poor oral hygiene. Gingivitis is usually eradicated if effective oral hygiene is restored, and the tissues become clinically normal again. The consensus is that there are no specific pathogens associated with gingivitis (Marsh et al. 2016). The increase in biomass provides a more suitable environment for the growth of fastidious species including obligate anaerobes, many of which have inflammatory molecules on their cell surface resulting in the biofilm having a raised inflammatory potential. Not all sites with gingivitis progress to more advanced forms of periodontal diseases, but it is accepted that gingivitis does precede periodontitis. Gingival diseases can also be modified by systemic factors.

Periodontitis

Numerous cross-sectional microbiological culture studies on periodontal pockets from different patient groups from various geographical regions have recovered highly diverse microbial communities, with increased proportions of proteolytic and obligately anaerobic bacteria, many of which are Gram negative. These bacteria are difficult to recover, grow and identify in the laboratory, and there is often conflicting evidence as to which organisms might be playing an active role in disease (Diaz et al. 2016, Marsh et al. 2016). Some of the bacteria that have been implicated are listed in Table 1.5.1.

Despite the enormous diversity of bacterial species isolated from these studies, certain trends and microbial associations began to be discerned. Socransky and colleagues (Socransky et al.1998, Socransky & Haffajee 2002, 2005) analysed and compared the microbiota from over 13,000 samples from patients with and without periodontitis, using an early culture-independent approach (checkerboard DNA–DNA hybridization technique with probes against 40 preselected subgingival species). They found that certain combinations or "complexes" of bacteria were associated with different states of periodontal health or disease. The strongest association with advanced periodontitis was with three bacterial species (*Porphyromonas gingivalis*, *Treponema denticola* and *Tannerella forsythia*), and these were designated the "red complex". Their presence was often preceded by other consortia which included various *Prevotella* species, *Fusobacterium nucleatum*, *Campylobacter* species and *Eubacterium nodatum* (designated the "orange complex"). Other bacterial groupings were associated with periodontal health ("purple", "yellow" and "green" complexes) (Socransky et al. 1998). These studies helped to shift the focus away from trying to identify a single pathogen and supported concepts in which complex consortia of microorganisms were responsible for disease (Lamont et al. 2018, Curtis et al. 2020, Hajishengallis & Lamont 2021).

TABLE 1.5.1	Identified species that have been implicated with periodontitis
Species implicated with periodontitis	
Bacteroidales species	Prevotella spp.
Porphyromonas endodontalis	Alloprevotella tannerae
Porphyromonas gingivalis	Johnsonella spp.
Mogibacterium timidium	Dialister pneumosintes
Peptostreptococcus stomatis	Dialister invisus
Filifactor alocis	Campylobacter rectus
Anaeroglobus germinatus	Fusobacterium nucleatum
Selenomonas spp.	Johnsonella spp.
Fretibacterium fastidiosum	Eubacterium spp.
Desulfobulbus spp.	Leptotrichia spp.
Bifidobacterium dentium	Parvimonas micros
Atopobium rimae	Tannerella forsythia
TM7	Treponema spp.
Archaea spp.	SR1 taxon

The presence or detection of these microorganisms does not necessarily mean that they are playing a direct or active role in the aetiology of disease.
(Perez-Chaparro et al. 2014, Diaz et al. 2016)

In recognition of the diversity of the subgingival microbiota and the fact that perhaps less than 50% can be cultured, most contemporary studies are using open-ended, culture-independent metagenomic approaches, which do not have the limitation of detecting only a predetermined set of species, as occurred with checkerboard DNA–DNA hybridization techniques. Such studies have further emphasised the complexity of the microbiota associated with disease and have discovered the presence of a large number of novel bacteria (Table 1.5.1), some of which have no or few cultivable examples, and several are currently unnamed. Most studies attempting to correlate the bacterial composition of subgingival biofilms with periodontal health or disease are, of necessity, cross-sectional in design. A major challenge in such studies is to determine which bacteria are playing an active role in disease, which are present as a result of disease and which are merely bystander organisms. The lack of consistency in microbial composition of subgingival biofilms isolated from diseased sites when the data from different studies are compared might be a result of the technical methods used to sample, process and analyze the samples, but it could also indicate that consortia with a different composition can produce the same clinical signs (Perez-Chaparro et al. 2014). To date, the field has been obsessed

with accurately naming the members of these communities, whereas it could be more instructive in the future if the "function" or "role" of each organism within the consortium was determined (Takahashi 2015, Espinoza et al. 2018), as it is probable that bacteria with different "names" could be performing identical "functions" within a community. Hence, we might see a greater consensus across studies looking at diseased sites if we reported by microbial function rather than by bacterial name. Most tissue destruction in periodontitis is a result of the exaggerated inflammatory response to the developing subgingival biofilm (see later).

Some younger patients can present with a more aggressive form of periodontitis despite only low amounts of biofilm present at affected sites; these patients may have functional abnormalities associated with their neutrophils. Affected sites can have high numbers of *Aggregatibacter* (formerly *Actinobacillus*) *actinomycetemcomitans*. This bacterium produces a powerful leukotoxin, enzymes capable of degrading collagen and cell-surface-associated material that can cause bone resorption (Belibasakis et al. 2019, Norskov-Lauritsen et al. 2019). A virulent clone (JP2) of *A. actinomycetemcomitans* has been identified that overproduces the leukotoxin and is found endemically in Northwest Africa; the presence of this clone significantly increases the risk of adolescents suffering from aggressive periodontitis (Belibasakis et al. 2019, Norskov-Lauritsen et al. 2019).

Necrotizing Periodontal Diseases

Necrotizing ulcerative gingivitis (NUG)

NUG, also described as Vincent's disease, trench mouth or acute necrotizing gingivitis, is a severe form of necrotizing inflammation of the interdental papillae, accompanied by spontaneous gingival bleeding and intense pain. In smears of the affected tissues, microorganisms (resembling spirochaetes and fusiform bacteria – the characteristic fuso-spirochaetal complex) can be seen invading the host gingival tissues. Culture-independent approaches have confirmed the predominance of a diverse range of *Treponema* species (spirochaetes) in lesions, many of which cannot be cultivated, but showed that the "fusiform" bacteria could belong to a broader range of genera including *Leptotrichia*, *Capnocytophaga* and *Tannerella* in addition to *Fusobacterium* spp. (Dewhirst et al. 2000, Paster et al. 2002, Gmur et al. 2004). Culture-based studies also recovered *Prevotella intermedia*. Metronidazole is effective in eliminating the fuso-spirochaetal complex from infected sites, and this is associated with rapid clinical improvement.

Necrotizing ulcerative periodontitis

Necrotizing ulcerative periodontitis is a painful condition that affects a small proportion of HIV-positive subjects. Molecular approaches detected a wide range of bacteria including *Bulleida extructa*, *Dialister*, *Fusobacterium*, *Selenomonas*, *Veillonella* spp., members of the TM7 phylum and anaerobic streptococci (Paster et al. 2002).

Contemporary Perspectives on the Aetiology of Periodontal Diseases

It is now accepted that disease is a consequence of a wholescale shift in the balance and composition of the entire subgingival microbial community, with the emergence and increased abundance of many species that are apparently absent in health or present as only minor constituents of the normal subgingival microbiome (Diaz et al. 2016, Lamont et al. 2018). An intriguing question, therefore, is the origin of these potential pathogens. Previous theories have suggested that disease-associated microbial species could be (a) acquired exogenously, (b) translocated from reservoir sites such as the buccal mucosa or tongue, or (c) present at healthy sites but in numbers too low to be detected. The application of sensitive molecular techniques has detected several of the putative pathogens (e.g. *P. gingivalis, A. actinomycetemcomitans*) at noninflamed, healthy sites but, whichever theory applies to the origins of these putative periodontopathogens, a dramatic change to the environment of the habitat would be necessary for the balance of the microbiota to be shifted to the extent seen in disease in which these species are able to out-compete the resident beneficial bacteria. In other ecosystems, such dramatic shifts in microbiota are associated with a major alteration to the habitat, such as to the nutrient status (e.g. the overgrowth of algae in rivers after the wash-off of nitrogenous fertilizers from neighbouring farm land), pH (e.g., the disruption of aquatic life in lakes by "acid rain") or immune status (e.g. reactivation of dormant *Mycobacterium tuberculosis* in the lungs of HIV-infected patients).

Support for the concept that a change in environment can drive the enrichment of generally minor but potentially pathogenic components of the microbiota has come from a biofilm model system that attempted to replicate some of the environmental changes associated with inflammation, particularly those that affect the availability of nutrients suitable for proteolytic bacteria. Biofilm samples were taken from healthy oral sites in adult human volunteers (tongue, supragingival plaque) and grown in human saliva; this medium was then supplemented with serum as a surrogate for the increased flow of GCF that occurs during the inflammatory response, and after just 3 weeks metagenomic analyses could detect most of the pathogens, including unculturable species, that are now implicated with periodontitis (Naginyte et al. 2019), including many of those listed in Table 1.5.1. Several of the species that were enriched were present in such low numbers that they were below the level of detection in the original biofilm samples. At these low levels, these bacteria would have no or minimal clinical impact.

In disease, the host mounts an inflammatory response when plaque biofilm accumulates beyond levels that are compatible with health, and this leads to substantial changes in the subgingival environment. There is an increase in the flow of GCF which introduces components of the host defences into the crevice. However, GCF also contains an array of complex host molecules, including transferrin, haemoglobin, etc., that can be exploited as primary nutrient sources by the proteolytic Gram-negative anaerobes which also have the potential to act as periodontal pathogens (see previous discussion) (Naginyte et al. 2019). Also, organisms such as *Prevotella intermedia* and *Porphyromonas gingivalis* have an absolute requirement for haemin for growth and derive this cofactor from the catabolism of host glycoproteins, such as haemoglobin, using proteases such as interpain and gingipains, respectively. An increase in haemin availability can dramatically alter the phenotype of bacteria; *P. gingivalis* displays increased protease activity, changes in the structure of its lipopolysaccharide and is more virulent when grown in a surplus of haemin. A further consequence of this proteolytic metabolism is an increase in local pH and a fall in the redox potential, which also promotes the upregulation of some of the virulence factors associated with these putative pathogens and favours their growth at the expense of the species associated with gingival health (i.e. these environmental changes increase the competitiveness of the potential pathogens).

Combinations of bacteria in these dysbiotic microbial communities display "pathogenic synergism" in that weakly pathogenic species combine forces to overcome the host defences and drive inflammation and tissue damage. Microbial proteolytic activity in the pocket can also target and degrade host defence molecules which can result in a deregulated and ultimately exaggerated inflammatory response, causing bystander damage to the subgingival tissues (Curtis et al. 2020, Hajishengallis et al. 2020). This uncontrolled response provides an even broader range of host molecules for the increasingly metabolically versatile microbial community. Most of the tissue damage is due to this excessive and subverted host response. If sustained, the combined selective pressures of changed nutrient supply, elevated pH and lower redox potential together with an impaired inflammatory response will lead to a substantial rearrangement of community structure and subsequent damage to the periodontal tissues.

Thus a cyclical situation develops in which, if the host fails to control the initial microbial insult, the nature of its response to the subgingival biofilm inadvertently provides conditions that will further select for the pathogens that will subsequently continue to drive the inflammatory response. This concept was encapsulated initially in the "ecological plaque hypothesis" (Marsh 2003) (Figure 1.5.4),

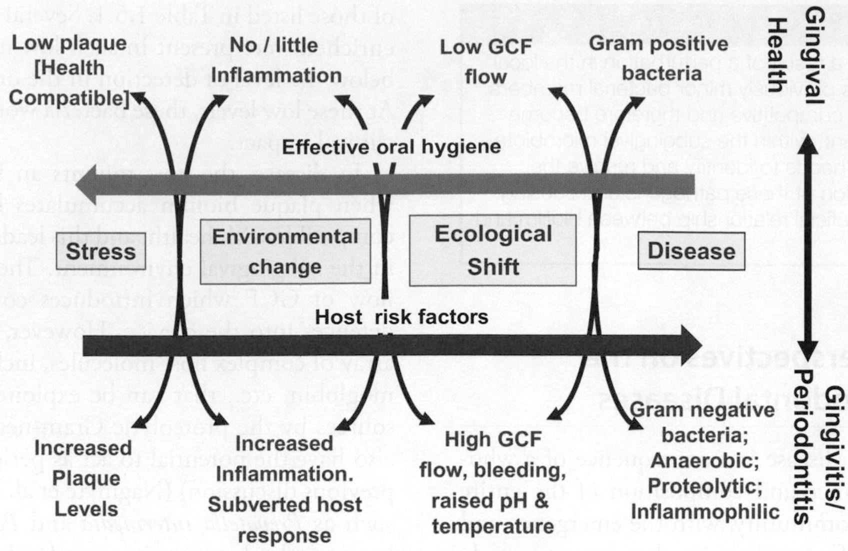

Gingival Health

Gingivitis/ Periodontitis

Low plaque [Health Compatible]

No / little Inflammation

Low GCF flow

Gram positive bacteria

Effective oral hygiene

Stress

Environmental change

Ecological Shift

Disease

Host risk factors

Increased Plaque Levels

Increased Inflammation. Subverted host response

High GCF flow, bleeding, raised pH & temperature

Gram negative bacteria; Anaerobic; Proteolytic; Inflammophilic

• **Figure 1.5.4** The "ecological plaque hypothesis" and periodontal diseases. Biofilm accumulation induces an inflammatory host response which causes a change in local environmental conditions that favours the growth of proteolytic and anaerobic Gram-negative bacteria. Diseases could be prevented by not only targeting the putative pathogens, but also by interfering with the factors driving their selection. Effective oral hygiene will favour healthy interactions between the host and the biofilm (symbiosis), while host risk factors (e.g. smoking, neutrophil defects) may increase the likelihood of disease (dysbiosis).

in which there is recognition of a direct link between local environmental conditions in the host and the activity and composition of the biofilm community. Any change to the host environment will induce a response in the microbiota and vice versa. Implicit in this hypothesis is that although disease can be treated by targeting the putative pathogens directly (e.g. with antimicrobial agents), long-term prevention will only be achieved by interfering with the underlying changes in host environment that drive the deleterious shifts in the microbiota (Marsh 2003). With increasing knowledge, this theory has been further refined with greater emphasis on the damage caused by the deregulated inflammatory response (the polymicrobial synergy and dysbiosis model) while reinforcing the concept that the change in the subgingival environment will drive dysbiosis (Lamont & Hajishengallis 2015). Also, it is recognised that some organisms such as *P. gingivalis* may play a role in disease that is disproportionately more significant than their numbers within the subgingival microbial community, and for this reason they have been termed "keystone pathogens" (Hajishengallis et al. 2012). The presence of the keystone pathogen may be dependent on the activity of neighbouring species, for example, in terms of provision of nutrients or inactivation of the host defences, and these are described as "accessory pathogens". The keystone pathogens, supported by accessory pathogens, combine to subvert host immunity and cause the emergence of a detrimental and dysbiotic microbiota which drives the exaggerated and deregulated inflammatory response resulting in further tissue destruction (Curtis et al. 2020, Hajishengallis et al. 2020, Hajishengallis & Lamont 2021). A bidirectional and cyclical (positive feedback loop) process develops in which the inflammatory response further enriches for inflammophilic

and inflammatory microorganisms which accentuates dysbiosis and perpetuates the inflammatory response (Rosier et al. 2018, Curtis et al. 2020, Hajishengallis et al. 2020, Hajishengallis & Lamont 2021) (Figure 1.5.5). Approaches to break this cycle can be via traditional treatments, such as mechanical periodontal therapy (e.g. root surface debridement) augmented by improved oral hygiene practices, and lifestyle changes (e.g. elimination of risk factors such as smoking), but newer adjunctive strategies are being developed that could modulate an excessive and exaggerated host response to reduce these detrimental aspects of inflammation and promote resolution and tissue healing (Curtis et al. 2020, Hajishengallis et al. 2020, Van Dyke et al. 2020).

> ### KEY POINT 10
> Periodontal diseases are a result of a perturbation in the local environment that enables previously minor components of the biofilm to become more competitive, and therefore more numerically dominant, within the subgingival microbiota. These microorganisms are able to subvert and disrupt the inflammatory response, leading to tissue damage and further inflammation; this process is termed dysbiosis. Effective disease control needs to identify and resolve the factors driving the selection of these pathogens and causing the disruption of the normally beneficial relationship between biofilm and the host.

Concluding Remarks

The mouth supports the growth of diverse communities of microorganisms that grow as structurally and functionally organised biofilms. These communities, and those present at other habitats in the body, play an active and critical role in the normal development of the host and in the maintenance of health. Clinicians need to be aware of the beneficial

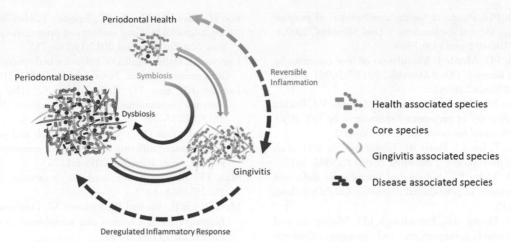

• Figure 1.5.5 The bidirectional relationship between the subgingival microbiome and the inflammatory and immune response (Curtis et al. 2020). The subgingival symbiotic microbiota in health is dominated by health-associated species (green) but species linked with gingivitis (orange) and periodontitis (red) are present in low abundance. Core species are found in both health and disease. Gingivitis is characterised by an increased biomass (green and orange arrows) comprising both green and particularly orange species and an associated increase in inflammation. In periodontitis, biomass increases further (green, orange and red arrows), and the red species become increasingly dominant in the dysbiotic microbiota. Furthermore, the gene expression profiles (transcriptome) of the green and orange species are modified with increased expression of virulence determinants. This is accompanied by the development of a deregulated inflammatory response and tissue destruction. Interventions which are able to resolve the inflammatory response may also be important in the reversal of the dysbiotic microbiota. Reprinted from *Periodontology 2000*, 83(1):12, Curtis. et al. (2020), with permission from John Wiley & Sons.

functions of the resident oral microbiota, so that treatment strategies are focused on the control rather than the elimination of these natural biofilms. Oral care should attempt to maintain plaque biofilm at levels compatible with health in order to retain the beneficial properties of the resident oral microbiota while preventing microbial overload that increases the risk of dental disease.

The microbiota at sites with periodontal breakdown is radically different from that at healthy sites, with a more diverse community of microorganisms, many of which are Gram negative, inflammophilic and highly proteolytic, and some are novel, often unnamed and even unculturable at present. The microbiota shifts from being in "symbiosis" with the host to undergoing "dysbiotic" changes and driving a damaging inflammatory response, thereby predisposing sites to tissue damage. Disease is a consequence of the activity of consortia of interacting species that act in consort to overcome the host defences. Combinations of different bacteria could produce the same clinical signs if the component species have the same "function" within the community. Most tissue damage is caused by an excessive and inappropriate response by the host to the microbial challenge. The ecological plaque hypothesis and the polymicrobial and dysbiosis model argue that changes in local environmental conditions drive the selection of previously minor components of the subgingival microbiota (some of which are termed keystone pathogens), resulting in a more inflammatory and inflammophilic microbial community. The resultant exaggerated and subverted inflammatory response is responsible for the damage to the host tissues. Effective treatment would need to identify and rectify the

factors that are driving the "dysbiosis", otherwise the deleterious changes to the microbiota will reoccur, risking further episodes of disease.

Multiple choice questions on the contents of this chapter are available online at Elsevier eBooks+.

References

Aas JA, Paster BJ, Stokes LN, Olsen I, Dewhirst FE. Defining the normal bacterial flora of the oral cavity. *J Clin Microbiol.* 2005;43:5721–5732.

Abusleme L, Dupuy AK, Dutzan N, Silva N, Burleson JA, Strausbaugh LD, et al. The subgingival microbiome in health and periodontitis and its relationship with community biomass and inflammation. *ISME Journal.* 2013;7:1016–1025.

Belibasakis GN, Bostanci N, Marsh PD, Zaura E. Applications of the oral microbiome in personalized dentistry. *Archs Oral Biol.* 2019;104:7–12.

Belibasakis GN, Maula T, Bao K, Lindholm M, Bostanci N, Oscarsson J, et al. Virulence and pathogenicity properties of *Aggregatibacter actinomycetemcomitans. Pathogens.* 2019;8. https://doi.org/10.3390/pathogens8040222.

Bowen WH, Burne RA, Wu H, Koo H. Oral biofilms: Pathogens, matrix, and polymicrobial interactions in microenvironments. *Trends Microbiol.* 2018;26:229–242.

Busscher HJ, Norde W, van der Mei HC. Specific molecular recognition and nonspecific contributions to bacterial interaction forces. *Appl Environ Microbiol.* 2008;74:2559–2564.

Chen T, Marsh PD, al-Hebshi NN. SMDI: An index for measuring subgingival microbial dysbiosis. *J Dent Res.* 2022;101:331–338. accepted for publication.

Curtis MA, Diaz PI, van Dyke TE. The role of the microbiota in periodontal disease. *Periodontol 2000.* 2020;83:14–25.

Devine DA, Marsh PD. Prospects for the development of probiotics and prebiotics for oral applications. *J Oral Microbiol.* 2009;1. https://doi.org/10.3402/jom.v1i0.1949.

Devine DA, Marsh PD, Meade J. Modulation of host responses by oral commensal bacteria. *J Oral Microbiol.* 2015;7:26941. https://doi.org/10.3402/jom.v7.26941.

Dewhirst FE, Tamer MA, Ericson RE, Lau CN, Levanos VA, Boches SK, et al. The diversity of periodontal spirochetes by 16S rRNA analysis. *Oral Microbiol Immunol.* 2000;15:196–202.

Dewhirst FE, Chen T, Izard J, Paster BJ, Tanner AC, Yu WH, et al. The human oral microbiome. *J Bacteriol.* 2010;192:5002–5017.

Diaz PI, Hoares A, Hong BY. Subgingival microbiome shifts and community dynamics in periodontal diseases. *J Calif Dent Assoc.* 2016;44:421–435.

Diaz PI, Hong BY, Dupuy AK, Strausbaugh LD. Mining the oral mycobiome: Methods, components, and meaning. *Virulence.* 2017;8:313–323.

Espinoza JL, Harkins DM, Torralba M, Gomez A, Highlander SK, Jones MB, et al. Supragingival plaque microbiome ecology and functional potential in the context of health and disease. *mBio.* 2018;9. https://doi.org/10.1128/mBio.01631-18.

Gmur R, Wyss C, Xue Y, Thurnheer T, Guggenheim B. Gingival crevice microbiota from Chinese patients with gingivitis or necrotizing ulcerative gingivitis. *Eur J Oral Sci.* 2004;112:33–41.

Hajishengallis G, Darveau RP, Curtis MA. The keystone-pathogen hypothesis. *Nat Rev Microbiol.* 2012;10:717–725.

Hajishengallis G, Chavakis T, Lambris JD. Current understanding of periodontal disease pathogenesis and targets for host-modulation therapy. *Periodontol 2000.* 2020;84:14–34.

Hajishengallis G, Lamont RJ. Polymicrobial communities in periodontal disease: their quasi-organismal nature and dialogue with the host. *Periodontol 2000.* 2021;86:210–230.

Hannig C, Hannig M, Attin T. Enzymes in the acquired enamel pellicle. *Europ J Oral Sci.* 2005;113:2–13.

Hong BY, Furtado Araujo MV, Strausbaugh LD, Terzi E, Ioannidou E, Diaz PI. Microbiome profiles in periodontitis in relation to host and disease characteristics. *PLoS ONE.* 2015;10:e0127077.

Jakubovics NS. Talk of the town: interspecies communication in oral biofilms. *Mol Oral Microbiol.* 2010;25:4–14.

Jakubovics NS. Intermicrobial interactions as a driver for community composition and stratification of oral biofilms. *J Mol Biol.* 2015;427:3662–3675.

Jakubovics NS, Burgess JG. Extracellular DNA in oral microbial biofilms. *Microbes Infect.* 2015;17:531–537.

Kilian M, Chapple IL, Hannig M, Marsh PD, Meuric V, Pedersen AM, et al. The oral microbiome - an update for oral healthcare professionals. *Br Dent J.* 2016;221:657–666.

Koch CD, Gladwin MT, Freeman BA, Lundberg JO, Weitzberg E, Morris A. Enterosalivary nitrate metabolism and the microbiome: Intersection of microbial metabolism, nitric oxide and diet in cardiac and pulmonary vascular health. *Free Radic Biol Med.* 2017;105:48–67.

Kolenbrander PE, Palmer RJ, Rickard AH, Jakubovics NS, Chalmers NI, Diaz PI. Bacterial interactions and successions during plaque development. *Periodontol 2000.* 2006;42:47–79.

Kolenbrander PE, Palmer Jr RJ, Periasamy S, Jakubovics NS. Oral multispecies biofilm development and the key role of cell-cell distance. *Nat Rev Microbiol.* 2010;8:471–480.

Koo H, Falsetta ML, Klein MI. The exopolysaccharide matrix: a virulence determinant of cariogenic biofilm. *J Dent Res.* 2013;92:1065–1073.

Koo H, Allan RN, Howlin RP, Stoodley P, Hall-Stoodley L. Targeting microbial biofilms: current and prospective therapeutic strategies. *Nat Rev Microbiol.* 2017;15:740–755.

Lamont RJ, Hajishengallis G. Polymicrobial synergy and dysbiosis in inflammatory disease. *Trends Mol Med.* 2015;21:172–183.

Lamont RJ, Koo H, Hajishengallis G. The oral microbiota: dynamic communities and host interactions. *Nat Rev Microbiol.* 2018;16:745–759.

Leung V, Dufour D, Levesque CM. Death and survival in *Streptococcus mutans:* differing outcomes of a quorum-sensing signaling peptide. *Front Microbiol.* 2015;6:1176.

Mah TF. Biofilm-specific antibiotic resistance. *Future Microbiol.* 2012;7:1061–1072.

Mark Welch JL, Rossetti BJ, Rieken CW, Dewhirst FE, Borisy GG. Biogeography of a human oral microbiome at the micron scale. *PNAS.* 2016;113:791–800.

Mark Welch JL, Dewhirst FE, Borisy GG. Biogeography of the oral microbiome: the site-specialist hypothesis. *Annu Rev Microbiol.* 2019;73:335–358.

Marsh PD. Are dental diseases examples of ecological catastrophes? *Microbiol.* 2003;149:279–294.

Marsh PD. Contemporary perspective on plaque control. *Br Dent J.* 2012;212:601–606.

Marsh PD, Lewis MAO, Rogers H, Williams DW, Wilson M. *Marsh and Martin's Oral Microbiology.* 6th ed. Edinburgh, Elsevier Editora Ltda, 2018.

Marsh PD, Zaura E. Dental biofilm: ecological interactions in health and disease. *J Clin Periodontol.* 2017;44(Suppl 18):S12-S22.

Meuric V, Le Gall David S, Boyer E, Acuna-Amador L, Martin B, Fong SB, et al. Signature of microbial dysbiosis in periodontitis. *Appl Environ Microbiol.* 2017;83. https://doi.org/10.1128/AEM.00462-17.

Naginyte M, Do T, Meade J, Devine DA, Marsh PD. Enrichment of periodontal pathogens from the biofilms of healthy adults. *Sci Rep.* 2019;9(1):5491. https://doi.org/10.1038/s41598-019-41882-y.

Nobbs AH, Jenkinson HF. Interkingdom networking within the oral microbiome. *Microbes Infect.* 2015;17:484–492.

Nobbs AH, Jenkinson HF, Jakubovics NS. Stick to your gums: mechanisms of oral microbial adherence. *J Dent Res.* 2011;90:1271–1278.

Norskov-Lauritsen N, Claesson R, Birkeholm Jensen A, Aberg CH, Haubek D. *Aggregatibacter actinomycetemcomitans:* clinical significance of a pathobiont subjected to ample changes in classification and nomenclature. *Pathogens.* 2019;8(4). https://doi.org/10.3390/pathogens8040243.

Papaioannou W, Gizani S, Haffajee AD, Quirynen M, Mamai-Homata E, Papagiannoulis L. The microbiota on different oral surfaces in healthy children. *Oral Microbiol Immunol.* 2009;24:183–189.

Paster BJ, Russell MK, Alpagot T, Lee AM, Boches SK, Galvin JL, et al. Bacterial diversity in necrotizing ulcerative periodontitis in HIV-positive subjects. *Ann Periodontol.* 2002;7:8–16.

Perez-Chaparro PJ, Goncalves C, Figueiredo LC, Faveri M, Lobao E, Tamashiro N, et al. Newly identified pathogens associated with periodontitis: a systematic review. *J Dent Res.* 2014;93:846–858.

Rosier BT, Marsh PD, Mira A. Resilience of the oral microbiome in health: mechanisms that prevent dysbiosis. *J Dent Res.* 2018;97:371–380.

Rosier BT, Buetas E, Moya-Gonzalvez EM, Artacho A, Mira A. Nitrate as a potential prebiotic for the oral microbiome. *Sci Rep.* 2020;10(1):12895.

Sanz M, Beighton D, Curtis MA, Cury JA, Dige I, Dommisch H, et al. Role of microbial biofilms in the maintenance of oral health and in the development of dental caries and periodontal diseases. Consensus report of group 1 of the Joint EFP/ORCA workshop on the boundaries between caries and periodontal disease. *J Clin Periodontol.* 2017;44(Suppl 18):S5-S11.

Socransky SS, Haffajee AD. Dental biofilms: difficult therapeutic targets. *Periodontol 2000.* 2002;28:12–55.

Socransky SS, Haffajee AD. Periodontal microbial ecology. *Periodontol 2000.* 2005;38:135–187.

Socransky SS, Haffajee AD, Cugini MA, Smith C, Kent Jr RL. Microbial complexes in subgingival plaque. *J Clin Periodontol.* 1998;25:134–144.

Takahashi N. Oral microbiome metabolism: from "who are they?" to "what are they doing?". *J Dent Res.* 2015;94:1628–1637.

Uruen C, Chopo-Escuin G, Tommassen J, Mainar-Jaime RC, Arenas J. Biofilms as promoters of bacterial antibiotic resistance and tolerance. *Antibiotics (Basel).* 2020;10(1). https://doi.org/10.3390/antibiotics10010003.

Van Dyke TE, Bartold PM, Reynolds EC. The nexus between periodontal inflammation and dysbiosis. *Front Immunol.* 2020;11:511.

Wade W, Thompson H, Rybalka A, Vartoukian S. Uncultured members of the oral microbiome. *J Calif Dent Assoc.* 2016;44:447–456.

Wade WG, Prosdocimi EM. Profiling of oral bacterial communities. *J Dent Res.* 2020;99:621–629.

Zijnge V, van Leeuwen MB, Degener JE, Abbas F, Thurnheer T, Gmur R, et al. Oral biofilm architecture on natural teeth. *PLoS ONE.* 2010;5:e9321.

Zijnge V, Ammann T, Thurnheer T, Gmur R. Subgingival biofilm structure. *Front Oral Biol.* 2012;15:1–16.

1.6

PERIODONTAL RISK – MODIFYING AND PREDISPOSING FACTORS

IAIN CHAPPLE AND MIKE MILWARD

CHAPTER OUTLINE

OVERVIEW OF THE CHAPTER

This chapter conceptualises periodontitis as a complex non-communicable disease (NCD) and explains how such diseases exhibit not just a single cause but multiple component causes or risk factors. It describes and defines risk factors, risk predictors and risk indicators for periodontitis. It reviews both modifying (formerly "systemic") and predisposing (formally "local") factors for periodontitis in line with the 2017 World Workshop Classification (WWC) system and their mechanisms of action. It then details digital risk assessment programmes and online risk assessment tools.

By the end of the chapter the reader should be able to:

- Understand causality in the context of complex diseases and how that relates to risk factors
- Describe and define risk factors, risk predictors and risk indicators
- List the critical stages in the development of periodontal tissue destruction and how these relate to risk factors that patients possess or have been exposed to
- Identify the key risk factors for periodontitis and the evidence base for each
- Define basic terminology and discuss the different types of risk factors for periodontitis, including their mechanisms of action
- Enable the clinician to assess risk at the patient level as a vital part of Step 1 of periodontal therapy in the S3-level periodontal treatment guideline (2020–2021)
- Introduce digital risk assessment programmes and online risk assessment tools to their practice.

This chapter covers the following topics:

- Introduction
- Risk factors, markers and predictors
- Complex diseases and causal theory
- Risk assessment and the "at risk" patient
- Classification of risk factors
- Risk factors in periodontitis progression
- Modifying (systemic risk) factors
- Predisposing (local risk) factors
- Mechanisms of common risk factors
- Periodontal risk assessment
- The role of risk assessment and risk factor control in behaviour change as part of Steps 1–4 of the international S3-level treatment guideline.

Introduction

Inflammatory periodontal diseases are complex NCDs. They are one of the most prevalent chronic diseases of humans, affecting 7.4–11.2% of adults globally (Kassebaum 2014, 2017). The incidence of severe periodontitis globally was 6 million in 2015, resulting in 3.5 million disability-associated life years (DALYs) compared with 1.89 million DALYs for untreated caries in deciduous and adult teeth (Kassebaum 2014). Patients vary greatly in their risk for developing disease because of the interaction between microbial, genetic, environmental and lifestyle factors. Risk assessment, as a means of attempting to identify the level of risk faced by individual patients for the development of periodontitis over their lifespan, has become a fundamental part of modern preventive practice.

By assessing patients' level of risk, the practitioner can implement individual patient-centred (rather than generic) plans for managing an individual patient's periodontitis and can also help determine an appropriate supportive care recall frequency, based upon risk status. This will therefore allow limited healthcare resources to be targeted at patients with greater risk of developing disease. Rosling and colleagues demonstrated in a 12-year supportive care (SPT) study that planning SPT interval frequency and length according to individual patient risk virtually eliminated tooth loss due to periodontitis in "normal susceptibility" patients and led to an average loss of two teeth to periodontitis during the 12-year SPT period for "high susceptibility" patients (Rosling et al. 2001).

Risk Factors, Markers and Predictors

Risk factors for a disease have been defined as certain characteristics of a person or their environment which, when present, directly result in an increased likelihood of that person getting the disease, and when absent directly result in a decreased likelihood (Beck et al. 1995). They are causally associated with a disease. Examples for periodontitis are genetics, smoking, stress and sub-optimally controlled diabetes.

> **KEY POINT 1**
>
> Risk factors are characteristics of a person or their environment which, when present, directly result in an increased likelihood of that person getting the disease, and when absent directly result in a decreased likelihood.

Risk markers or predictors are not causally related to a disease, but their presence is more a consequence of the disease being present. Examples in periodontitis are bleeding on probing, suppuration, tooth mobility, interproximal recession and evidence of past disease. Risk markers imply the presence of disease and are often used to detect early stages of disease, before overt clinical signs become apparent.

> **KEY POINT 2**
>
> Risk markers or predictors are not causally related to a disease, but their presence is more a consequence of the disease being present.

Complex Diseases and Causal Theory

The majority of NCDs are complex diseases, meaning they do not have a single cause but multiple component causes or true "risk factors", which aggregate towards a critical threshold, above which the disease is triggered. In periodontitis, plaque accumulation is not *the* cause of periodontitis, otherwise 100% of the population would exhibit the disease, yet the Sri-Lankan Tea Worker study by Löe and colleagues (1986) demonstrated natural resistance to the disease in a small proportion of individuals (11%), and a high susceptibility (8%) in a similarly small number, with the remainder exhibiting a spectrum of medium risk of disease progression (81%).

> **KEY POINT 3**
>
> The majority of NCDs are complex diseases, meaning they do not have a single cause but multiple component causes or true "risk factors", which aggregate towards a critical threshold, above which the disease is triggered.

Rothman (2002) described what is today still regarded as the most plausible theory for causality of complex diseases, the "causal pie" hypothesis (Figure 1.6.1). For a disease to manifest in an individual there must be a "sufficient cause", made up of multiple "component causes" or risk factors. In the figure each pie represents a patient with disease; the disease only arises when the pie is full of slices. Slice "A" is common to each patient and is a necessary component cause, but insufficient on its own to cause the disease: for periodontitis this would be the plaque biofilm. Slice D may be tobacco smoking, slice G may be glycaemia or hyperglycaemia in a diabetes patient and slice I may represent stress without coping strategies. Key to this concept is that component causes differ between individuals, providing heterogeneity of disease expression, and importantly, that eliminating one risk factor may stabilise the disease as the pie is no longer full.

> **KEY POINT 4**
>
> For a complex disease to manifest in an individual there must be a "sufficient cause", made up of multiple "component causes" or risk factors.

Risk Assessment and the "At Risk" Patient

An "at risk" patient is someone who has a higher-than-average probability of developing a specific disease over a specific period of time; they either possess or have been exposed to risk factors for that disease. Thus

Sufficient versus necessary cause theory for complex diseases

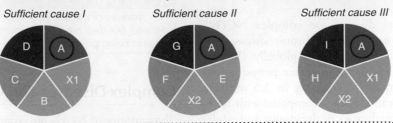

Causal pies. Each combination is sufficient for the disease to develop. "A" is a necessary cause because it is present in every pie. The rest (X1, X2, C, etc.) are component causes that could belong to different sufficient causes or appear as a joint element (e.g. sufficient cause III).

• **Figure 1.6.1** Rothman's "causal pie" model for complex diseases. "A" is a necessary cause but insufficient on its own to cause the disease. A sufficient cause is needed for disease to manifest and consists of aggregated component causes or risk factors, forming a full pie.

a 20-cigarette-per-day smoker with poor oral hygiene is potentially at high risk for periodontitis and/or necrotising gingivitis (NG).

One of the strongest predictors of future disease activity is the amount of disease the patient presents with at the first consultation, taking their age into account. For example, a 25-year-old with 40% generalised horizontal bone loss is at far greater risk of tooth loss due to periodontitis than a 70-year-old with the same amount of bone loss. This concept underpins the "grading" of periodontitis within the 2017 WWC (Papapanou et al. 2018).

To help understand the role of systemic risk factors in the pathogenesis of periodontitis, the "critical pathway model of pathogenesis" was described by Salvi et al. (1997). This pathway (updated in Figure 1.6.2) identifies nine critical stages that must be present for disease to develop and progress. As discussed in Chapters 1.2 and 1.4, it has been estimated that merely 20% of the tissue destruction in periodontitis is explained directly by bacterial action (Grossi et al. 1994); the remainder being attributable to a dysregulated host immune-inflammatory response.

> ### KEY POINT 5
> Approximately 20% of the tissue damage seen in periodontitis is due to direct bacterial action; the remainder is due to a dysregulated host immune-inflammatory response.

Classification of Risk Factors

Risk factors can be described in a variety of ways:
- True or putative
- Modifying or predisposing
- Modifiable or non-modifiable.

True or Putative

True risk factors for a disease have a causal association, that is, when present, they increase the likelihood of the disease developing, but when they are removed the disease

improves. One example might be plaque biofilm levels around the teeth. Note that true risk factors do not imply absolute cause and effect (Rothman 2002), simply that they increase the likelihood of disease if present. In the case of the oral plaque biofilm, high biofilm levels do not cause periodontitis in all patients, only those who have some periodontal susceptibility.

Putative risk factors for a disease are those factors that are associated with the occurrence of a disease, as observed in cross-sectional studies. Such factors do not satisfy the criteria for true risk factors because there is a lack of evidence from longitudinal studies (which may not have been performed) that removal of the risk factor will improve the disease state. Examples might be stress or nutritional factors.

Modifying or Predisposing Factors

Modifying factors (systemic risk factors) for periodontitis are those characteristics present in an individual which negatively influence the immune-inflammatory response to a given dental plaque biofilm burden, resulting in exaggerated or "hyper" inflammation (Chapple et al. 2018). Examples include those affecting the host response either directly or indirectly. They may be environmental factors (e.g. stress), lifestyle factors (e.g. nutrition or smoking) or those relating to general health (e.g. diabetes status, immunodeficiency or other conditions such as leucocyte adhesion defects).

Predisposing factors (formerly local risk factors) for periodontitis are those that encourage plaque accumulation at a specific site by either inhibiting its removal during daily oral hygiene practices and/or creating a biological niche that encourages increased plaque accumulation and consequent inflammation (Chapple et al. 2018). They include biofilm retention factors, which may be anatomical in nature (e.g. root grooves, enamel pearls) or relate to poor restoration margins, imbricated teeth or dental appliances that are close to the gingival margin and oral dryness due to some medications or autoimmune disease.

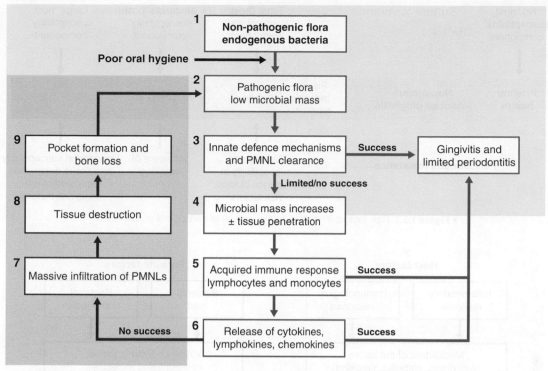

• **Figure 1.6.2** The "critical pathway model" (Salvi et al. 1997) updated to recognise the interplay between gingival inflammation, dysbiosis and periodontal tissue damage.

Modifiable or Non-Modifiable

Modifiable risk factors for a disease are those that can be influenced by the patient or the clinician. These may be systemic or environmental in nature and include smoking cessation, improving diabetes control, improved diet and reducing biofilm levels through improved oral hygiene, or correction of local risk factors such as restorations with subgingival ledges.

Non-modifiable risk factors for a disease are those that cannot be influenced by the patient and essentially relate to genetic traits or characteristics. In the future, gene therapy may change this.

Risk Factors in Periodontitis Progression

Periodontitis risk can be described as part of a spectrum with resistance at the left and the highest risk states at the right (Figure 1.6.3). In the 2017 WWC, periodontitis is graded to embrace risk, the grade representing the patient's lifetime experience of periodontitis in relation to their age. Baseline grading is determined by dividing percentage bone loss at the worst affected site by the patient's age. Grade C represents rapid progression, grade B, a moderate rate of progression and grade A, a slow rate. If a patient is a current smoker or has poorly controlled diabetes, this increased the grade from the baseline grade allocated (Tonetti et al. 2018). The British Society of Periodontology and Implant Dentistry (BSP) created a simpler implementation (BSPi) of the staging and grading system (Dietrich et al. 2019), which has been shown to predict tooth loss due to periodontitis as well, and indeed slightly better than the 2017

WWC (Dukka et al. 2021). The BSPi grades in the same manner as the 2017 WWC but employs a different threshold for defining grade B disease and does not modify the grade by risk factors but lists those risk factors present without assigning a weight to them, as part of a "diagnostic statement".

Modifying and predisposing factors have an important part to play in the progression of periodontal breakdown, and control can only be achieved if a proper assessment is made of the factors involved. Figure 1.6.4 shows how systemic (subject-based) and local (site-based) risk factors underpin the disease process.

Systemic Risk (Modifying) Factors

If applying the strict definition of the term "true risk factors", there is only one true risk factor that has been unequivocally demonstrated for periodontitis, which is dental plaque. Plaque biofilm accumulation has been shown to cause gingivitis, but strictly speaking this cannot be extrapolated to include periodontitis, other than by inference. However, although there is abundant evidence that biofilm reduction improves periodontal outcomes, the amount of reduction required varies from patient to patient. Table 1.6.1 shows the principal risk factors for periodontitis and our current understanding of the evidence for their risk status.

Genetics

Studies of monozygous twins indicate that genetics may explain about 50% of periodontitis prevalence

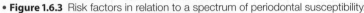

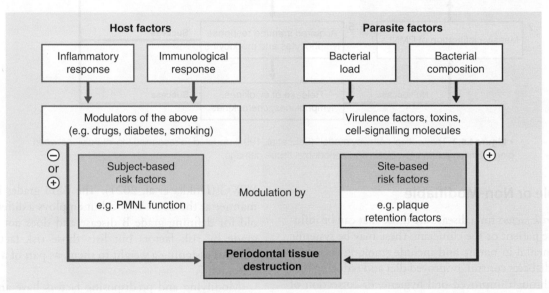

• **Figure 1.6.3** Risk factors in relation to a spectrum of periodontal susceptibility.

• **Figure 1.6.4** How systemic (subject-based) modifying and local (site-based) predisposing risk factors underpin the periodontitis process.

TABLE 1.6.1

Levels of evidence for the common risk factors in periodontitis

	Good evidence, putative risk factor	Some evidence, putative risk factor	Some evidence, true risk factor	Good evidence, true risk factor
Genetics	✓			
Age		✓		
Nutrition	✓			
Smoking	✓			
Diabetes			✓	
Stress		✓		
Poor oral hygiene				✓

(Michalowicz et al. 2000). Evidence is stronger for grade C forms of periodontitis, where the attachment loss is inconsistent with local risk factors (formerly called aggressive periodontitis). However, genetics cannot be described as a "true" risk factor because intervention studies

employing gene therapies have not been performed to assess their efficacy in improving periodontal outcomes.

Periodontitis is a complex disease and, just as it is regarded as being polymicrobial and poly immune-inflammatory in nature, it can also be regarded as being polygenetic and epigenetic.

Polymorphisms (different forms) of specific genes of the immune-inflammatory responses have also been associated with periodontitis and include those affecting single nucleotides. These are referred to as single nucleotide polymorphisms (SNPs) and occur when one base pair may be different. This can result in a difference in the gene product (e.g. a cytokine or cell surface receptor). An example is the SNP for the neutrophil receptor that binds antibody, the FcγR11a receptor. This may confer high or low avidity to the receptor's ability to bind antibody. A compound genotype of interleukin 1β (IL-1β) is also reported which codes for excess IL-1β cytokine production.

In addition, epigenetic influences are becoming important in the study of periodontitis. These are the effects of agents such as enzymes produced by bacteria, micronutrients or oxygen radicals which are able to modify genes by processes such as methylation, reducing their expression and preventing the gene from being expressed correctly.

Age

Age was not previously regarded as a risk factor for periodontitis, more that as we get older our lifetime exposure to risk factors increases and therefore more periodontitis is seen in older patients – approximately 60% of over 60-year-olds in the UK have some periodontitis, and older patients have more severe disease (14% versus 8% respectively) (White et al. 2012).

Age is a difficult risk factor to evaluate because it is not possible to make patients younger; therefore interventions that aim to test the true nature of age as a risk factor are not possible. However, as people age their immune system starts to weaken – a phenomenon called "immune senescence", reducing our ability to kill pathogens and increasing the collateral tissue damage caused. For this reason, evidence is accumulating to suggest that age may indeed emerge as a true modifying factor for periodontitis.

It is also important to recognise that the population of the developed world is ageing and patients expect to keep their teeth longer. The World Health Organization has set a target to define successful dentistry as the retention of 20 teeth at 80 years of age. Periodontitis will therefore become more prevalent in older patients.

Nutrition

There is considerable interest in nutrients as both agonists and antagonists of inflammatory processes (Chapple 2009). Evidence demonstrates that refined carbohydrate intake drives systemic or "meal-induced" inflammation (Monnier et al. 2006).

Several association studies demonstrate that blood levels of certain antioxidant micronutrients are inversely related to periodontitis prevalence; for instance, low vitamin C is estimated to account for 4% of attachment loss seen in certain populations (Chapple & Matthews 2007). Blood total antioxidants show similar results. Evidence from intervention studies is emerging that demonstrates marginal improvements in periodontal outcomes demonstrated following adjunctive use of micronutrients, either as phytonutrients in capsules of dried fruit and vegetable concentrates (Chapple et al. 2012), or through non-adjunctive twice daily consumption of vitamin C and associated micronutrients within kiwi fruit in the absence of periodontal instrumentation (Graziani et al. 2018). The role of poor nutrition as a risk factor for periodontitis remains under-researched at present but could represent a "component cause" in certain patients.

Smoking

Smoking is as close as any risk indicator can get to being a true risk factor. It has been estimated that 42% of periodontitis may be attributable to smoking (Tomar & Asma 2000).

Smoking has both topical and systemic effects which place patients at greater risk of periodontitis progression.
- Local effects:
  - Reduced tissue vascularity
  - Impaired polymorphonuclear leukocyte (PMNL) chemotaxis and function (phagocytosis)
- Systemic effects:
  - Decreased salivary IgA
  - Decreased serum IgG
  - Decreased helper T cells

Smokers have been shown to have more pockets, deeper pockets (especially palatally), more recession, more bone loss and increased tooth loss in comparison to non-smokers (Fig. 1.6.5). Smokers may also experience more bone loss in upper anterior regions than non-smokers (Baharin et al. 2006). Smokers have also been shown to have less marginal bleeding that can have the effect of masking early critical signs (bleeding gums) of periodontitis. The evidence associating smoking with periodontitis is thus robust. However, there remains limited evidence from substantial and sufficiently powered intervention studies that demonstrate improved periodontal outcomes after smoking cessation.

Odds ratios (ORs) for periodontitis in smokers vary between a three- and seven-fold increased relative risk for disease. A dose response exists between smoking and periodontal risk – 10 cigarettes/day increasing risk by 5% and 20 per day increasing risk by 10%. Moreover, serum levels of the stable nicotine metabolite cotinine correlate with attachment loss, probing pocket depth and alveolar crest height.

The healing response to non-surgical and surgical periodontal therapy is poorer in smokers, and maintenance patients who smoke are twice as likely to lose teeth as non-smokers.

Based upon the moderate success of smoking cessation counselling demonstrated by Ramseier et al. (2020), the S3-level treatment guideline 1.6 strongly recommends smoking cessation counselling in the management of periodontitis (Sanz et al. 2020, West et al. 2021).

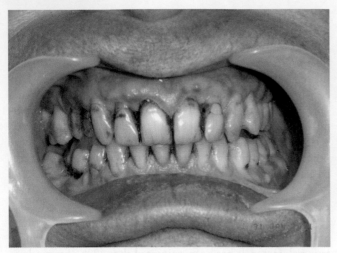

• **Figure 1.6.5** Generalised periodontitis in a heavy smoker.

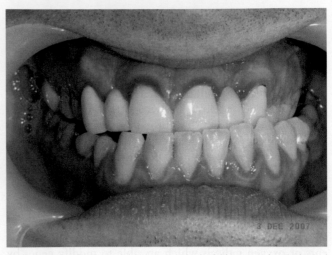

• **Figure 1.6.6** Poor oral hygiene and gingivitis around subgingival crown margins.

Diabetes and Obesity

There is reportedly a "bi-directional relationship" between diabetes mellitus and periodontitis (Taylor 2001), whereby the presence of one condition adversely affects the other. Severe periodontitis adversely affects glycaemic control in diabetes and glycaemia in non-diabetes patients, and there is a direct and dose-dependent relationship between periodontitis severity and diabetes complications. Emerging evidence supports an increased risk for diabetes onset in patients with severe periodontitis and mechanisms appear to involve elevated systemic inflammation (acute-phase and oxidative stress biomarkers) resulting from the entry of periodontal organisms and their virulence factors into the circulation (Chapple & Genco 2013). Whereas the 2020 to 2021 S3-level guidelines returned an open recommendation (recommendation 1.10) for interventions aimed at weight loss through lifestyle modification, indicating insufficient evidence currently, there was a strong recommendation (recommendation 4.19) for the promotion of diabetes control interventions in periodontitis patients during maintenance therapy (Sanz et al. 2020, West et al. 2021). In support of this a consensus report and guidelines produced jointly by the EFP and International Diabetes Federation in 2018 strongly advise joint care pathways for physicians and dental professionals in managing diabetes for periodontal benefit (Sanz et al. 2018), and in the UK an NHS commissioning standard was published in 2020 requiring the same joined-up approach (NHSE 2019).

> ### KEY POINT 6
> Control of periodontitis can only be achieved if systemic and local risk factors are properly assessed and managed.

Stress

The evidence for stress per se as a risk factor for periodontitis is weak; however, there is evidence that poor coping strategies may negatively affect periodontitis (Wimmer et al. 2002).

It has also been demonstrated that patients under financial stress and strain had greater levels of periodontitis, but those who had good coping strategies had no more disease than unstressed controls.

Stress triggers neuroendocrine responses via the hypothalamic–pituitary–adrenal (HPA) axis. This in turn triggers the activation of complement and the release of proinflammatory cytokines.

There is also evidence that certain periodontal pathogens are able to utilise stress hormones like noradrenaline and adrenaline to acquire iron for growth and virulence (Roberts et al. 2005). Additionally, they appear to produce an autoinducer of their own growth in response to the same stress hormones (Roberts et al. 2002), indicating that certain periodontal bacteria can take advantage of a stressed host.

Poor Oral Hygiene

The evidence for the oral biofilm as a true risk factor for gingivitis is strong (see Figure 1.6.6), based upon the original experimental gingivitis study of Löe et al. (1965). In this study, volunteers were prevented from tooth brushing for 21 days to allow plaque accumulation. Gingivitis developed, and when the biofilm was removed the gingivitis resolved.

A study in 2009, however, challenged the simplicity of this paradigm (Baumgartner et al. 2009). Ten volunteers placed on a diet free from simple refined sugars were prevented from brushing for 4 weeks, and while oral biofilm accumulated significantly, bleeding scores significantly reduced. Thus the bacterial biofilm is a "component cause" of gingivitis, but there appear to be other factors, equally as powerful, such as simple refined sugar intake, which contribute towards disease by driving inflammation.

Biofilm accumulation is essential for periodontitis to develop but, as it does not cause periodontitis in all patients, it is regarded as the trigger for disease initiation but not the sole cause. The amount of biofilm necessary to induce periodontitis, or cause periodontitis progression, varies between patients and, in any individual, the biofilm needs to reach a "threshold" level for disease to occur. Some patients will never develop periodontitis (Löe et al. 1986) even if they never brush their teeth, because they are inherently resistant to disease development.

Using the experimental gingivitis model, Bamashmous et al. (2021) demonstrated three unique clinical inflammatory phenotypes, which they termed "high", "low" and "slow", in relation to the development of gingival inflammation. They mapped various host mediators and microbial species in the three groups and demonstrated that key inflammatory mediators were not associated with clinical gingival inflammation in the slow group, where higher levels of Gram-positive commensal organisms were evident. The low clinical response group exhibited low host mediators compared with the high responder group, despite a similar microbial profile in plaque. Interestingly, neutrophil and bone activation modulators were down-regulated in all response groups, indicating protective tissue and bone responses during the development of experimental gingivitis. Similar work by Scott and colleagues enabled the mapping of the clinical and biological phenotypes of experimental gingivitis patients (Scott et al. 2012).

Periodontal Risk Assessment

Periodontal risk is multifactorial and risk assessment for patients dictates that different analytical levels of risk should be employed at different stages of treatment. Thus multilevel risk assessment is necessary (Figure 1.6.7) and can be mapped to the steps of care under the S3-level treatment guidelines (West et al. 2021).

At the start of treatment, analysis is at the patient level but, as treatment progresses, increasing levels of detail can be employed.

Risk Assessment – The Third Dimension

Risk assessment should help clinicians to formulate an effective management plan for a periodontitis patient and to establish the frequency of recall intervals for supportive care.

Traditionally, periodontitis management and treatment planning have been based on a detailed patient history and examination, but including risk assessment as a third dimension will tailor a more appropriate treatment plan for an individual patient (Figure 1.6.8).

Risk Assessment Technologies

Risk assessment should form a fundamental part of any preventative practice.

Risk assessment tools are already a component of comprehensive dental and periodontal evaluations as well as part of all periodic dental and periodontal examinations in many practices (Busby et al. 2013).

There are different ways of assessing risk, including online tools that offer consistent and accurate scoring and visual biofeedback to patients. This reduces the need for complex therapy, in turn leading to an improvement in oral health with reduced healthcare costs for the patient. One

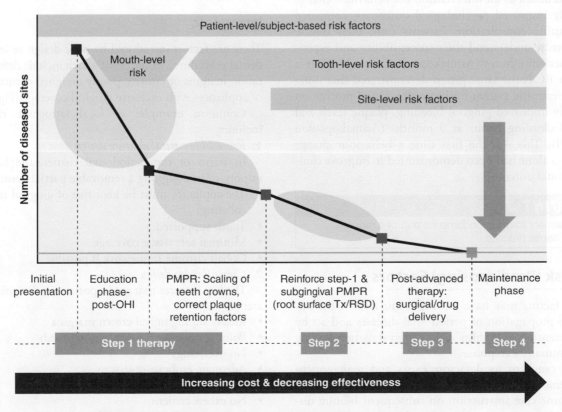

• **Figure 1.6.7** Multilevel risk assessment, taking the treatment stage into account.

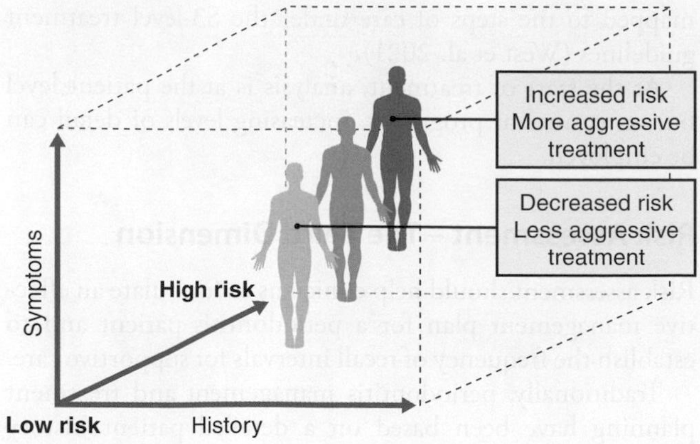

• **Figure 1.6.8** Risk assessment as a third dimension in patient management.

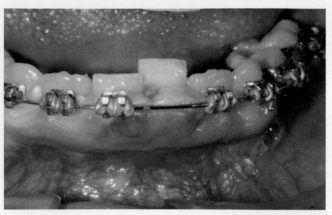

• **Figure 1.6.9** Biofilm retention around an orthodontic appliance is acting as a local risk factor.

study investigating the use of a periodontal risk calculator (PRC) concluded that risk scores determined using a PRC predict future periodontal status with a high degree of accuracy and validity (Page et al. 2003). The 11th European Workshop in Periodontology assessed risk assessment tools via systematic reviews and in their consensus stated that the PRC and another system called the PRA (periodontal risk assessment) could improve clinicians' ability to identify, communicate and manage periodontitis patients (Lang et al. 2015). Perhaps more importantly, Asimakopoulou and colleagues (2015) demonstrated in a randomised controlled trial (RCT) in primary care dental practice that using a risk assessment tool (PRC/PreViser) to provide personalised biofeedback as an intervention for behaviour change significantly improved psychological outcomes, compared with a routine consultation. Patients took their disease more seriously, understood their susceptibility and experienced higher self-efficacy (Asimakopoulou et al. 2015). In a subsequent RCT, the same group demonstrated that using the same electronic system for biofeedback and motivation significantly improved gingival bleeding, plaque levels and interdental cleaning habits at 3 months (Asimakopoulou et al. 2019). This was the first time a behaviour change intervention alone had been demonstrated to improve clinical periodontal outcomes.

> ### KEY POINT 7
> Risk assessment forms a fundamental part of a modern preventive dental practice.

Local Risk (Predisposing) Factors

Local risk factors may have an important role in the initiation and propagation of periodontal diseases and act by allowing retention of biofilm at the gingival margin leading to an inflammatory response.

A wide range of local factors exists and management involves removal or modification of the factor along with detailed home care instruction on subsequent biofilm disruption by the patient.

> ### KEY POINT 8
> Local risk factors act by allowing plaque retention in localised areas.

Local risk factors include:
- Iatrogenic (restorations, appliances, crown and bridge)
- Anatomical (e.g. root groove)
- Root caries
- Tooth malalignment
- False/true pockets
- High frenal attachment
- Calculus
- Oral dryness.

Iatrogenic

These are factors introduced by poor design or execution of dental procedures, examples of which include defective restoration margins or crowns, poorly designed dentures, bridges or appliances with excessive gingival coverage (Figure 1.6.9).

Common examples of local iatrogenic risk factors include:

1. *Removable partial denture design*
   In terms of the periodontal tissues, the key features important in designing a removable partial denture are:
   - The appliance must be kept free of gingival margins (no colleting)
   - Tooth supported
   - Minimal soft tissue coverage
   - Cobalt chrome framework if possible
2. *Crown/bridge design*
   The key features that are important in designing a crown are:
   - Ideally supragingival crown margins
   - Point contact with neighbouring teeth
   - No overhangs
   - Adequate embrasure space
   - No occlusal trauma
   - No excess cement
   - Instructions to patient in cleaning

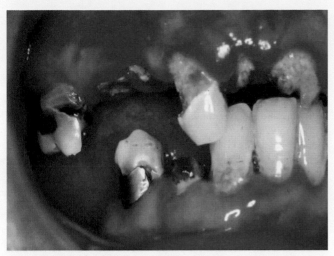

• **Figure 1.6.10** Root caries, subgingival restoration margins and calculus acting as local risk factors for periodontitis.

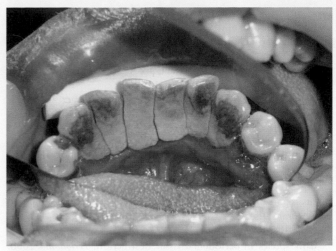

• **Figure 1.6.11** Significant supragingival calculus formation impeding adequate biofilm control.

3. *Bridge pontic design*

The key features that are important in designing a bridge pontic are:
- Ideally supragingival margins
- No overhangs
- Adequate embrasure space
- Adequate support of abutment teeth
- Hygienic pontic design.

Anatomical

Anatomical factors may result in biofilm retention due to anatomical anomalies of the dental hard tissues; examples include furcation involvement, root grooves and enamel projections.

Root Caries

The presence of caries on the root surface can result in local biofilm accumulation adjacent to the gingival tissues (Figure 1.6.10).

Tooth Position

When crowding of the dentition is present, this can result in difficulty in biofilm removal.

False/True Pockets

Pocketing results in difficulty in biofilm removal, resulting in plaque accumulation.

High Frenal Attachment

The presence of a high frenal attachment can result in compromised oral hygiene in the area and biofilm retention.

Calculus

The presence of calculus deposits may result in biofilm accumulation (Figure 1.6.11).

Oral Dryness

The 2017 WWC identified oral dryness as a key predisposing factor for periodontal disease. A lack of salivary flow, availability or alterations in saliva rheology can cause reduced cleansing of tooth surfaces and enhanced biofilm accumulation. Mouth breathing or an incompetent lip seal have similar effects (Mizutani et al. 2015).

Acknowledgement

This chapter is based on a session within e-Den which Professor Chapple and Professor Milward produced in 2011. Acknowledgement is given to the Faculty of Dental Surgery of the Royal College of Surgeons of England for giving permission for material from the e-Den session to be used in this chapter.

Multiple choice questions on the contents of this chapter are available online at Elsevier eBooks+.

References

Asimakopoulou K, Daly B, Kutzer Y, Ide M. The effects of providing periodontal disease risk information on psychological outcomes – a randomized controlled trial. *J Clin Periodontol.* 2015;42:350–355.

Asimakopoulou K, Nolan M, McCarthy C, Newton T. The effect of risk communication on periodontal treatment outcomes: a randomized controlled trial. *J Periodontol.* 2019;90:94895.

Baharin B, Palmer RM, Coward P, Wilson RF. Investigation of periodontal destruction patterns in smokers and non-smokers. *J Clin Periodontol.* 2006;33:485–490.

Bamashmous S, Kotsakis GA, Kernsa KA, et al. Human variation in gingival inflammation. *PNAS.* 2021;118(27):e2012578118.

Baumgartner S, Imfeld T, Schicht O, Rath C, Persson RE, Persson GR. The impact of the stone age diet on gingival conditions in the absence of oral hygiene. *J Periodontol.* 2009;80:759–768.

Beck JD, Koch GG, Offenbacher S. Incidence of attachment loss over 3 years in older adults – new and progressing lesions. *Community Dent Oral Epidemiol.* 1995;23:291–296.

Busby M, Chapple EC, Matthews R, Chapple ILC. Practitioner evaluation of a novel online integrated oral health and risk assessment tool: a practice pilot. *Br. Dent. J.* 2013;215:115–120.

Chapple ILC. Potential mechanisms underpinning the nutritional modulation of periodontal inflammation. *JADA.* 2009;140:178–184.

Chapple ILC, Genco RJ. Diabetes and periodontal diseases: consensus report of the Joint EFP/AAP Workshop on Periodontitis and Systemic Diseases. *J Clin Periodontol.* 2013;40(s14):106–112.

Chapple ILC, Matthews JB. The role of reactive oxygen and antioxidant species in periodontal tissue destruction. *Periodontol 2000.* 2007;43:160–232.

Chapple ILC, Milward MR, Ling-Mountford N, Weston P, Carter K, Askey K, et al. Adjunctive daily supplementation with encapsulated fruit, vegetable and berry juice powder concentrates and clinical periodontal outcomes: a double-blind RCT. *J Clin Periodontol.* 2012;39:62–72.

Chapple ILC, Genco RJ, Glogauer M, Goldstein M, Griffin TJ, Holmstrup P, et al. Periodontal health and gingival diseases and conditions on an intact and a reduced periodontium: consensus report of workgroup 1 of the 2017 World Workshop on the Classification of Periodontal and Peri-Implant Diseases and Conditions. *J Clin Periodontol.* 2018;45(suppl 20):S68S77.

Dietrich T, Ower P, Tank M, et al. British Society of Periodontology. Periodontal diagnosis in the context of the 2017 classification system of periodontal diseases and conditions - implementation in clinical practice. *Br Dent J.* 2019;11(226):1622.

Dukka H, Dietrich T, Saleh MHA, et al. The Prognostic Performance of the 2017 World Workshop Classification on Staging and Grading of Periodontitis compared to the British Society of Periodontology's implementation. *J Periodontol.* 2021 Jul 27. 2021. https://doi.org/10.1002/JPER.21-0296. Online ahead of print. PMID: 34314515.

Graziani F, Discepoli N, Gennai S, et al. The effect of twice daily kiwifruit consumption on periodontal and systemic conditions before and after treatment: a randomized clinical trial. *J Periodontol.* 2018;89:285–293.

Grossi SG, Zambon JJ, Ho AW, et al. Assessment of risk for periodontal disease. 1. Risk indicators for attachment loss. *J Periodontol.* 1994;65:260–267.

Kassebaum NJ, Bernabé E, Dahiya M, Bhandari B, Murray CJL, Marcenes W. Global burden of severe periodontitis in 1990-2010: a systematic review and meta-regression. *J Dent Res.* 2014;93:104553.

Kassebaum NJ, Smith AGC, Bernabé E, Fleming TD, Reynolds AE, Vos T, et al. Global, regional, and national prevalence, incidence, and disability-adjusted life years for oral conditions for 195 countries, 1990-2015: a systematic analysis for the global burden of diseases, injuries, and risk factors. *J Dent Res.* 2017;96:3807.

Lang NP, Suvan JE, Tonetti MS. Risk factor assessment tools for the prevention of periodontitis progression. A systematic review. *J Clin Periodontol.* 2015;42(suppl 16):S5970.

Löe H, Theilade E, Jensen SB. Experimental gingivitis in man. *J Periodontol.* 1965;36:177–187.

Löe H, Boysen AH, Morrison E. Natural history of periodontal disease in man Rapid, moderate and no loss of attachment in Sri Lankan laborers 14 to 46 years of age. *J Clin Periodontol.* 1986;13:431440.

Michalowicz BS, Diehl SR, Gunsolley JC, et al. Evidence of a substantial genetic basis for risk of adult periodontitis. *J Periodontol.* 2000;71:1699–1707.

Mizutani S, Ekuni D, Tomofuji T, et al. Relationship between xerostomia and gingival condition in young adults. *J Periodontal Res.* 2015;50:74–79.

Monnier L, Colette C, Boniface H. Contribution of postprandial glucose to chronic hyperglycaemia: from the glucose "triad" to the trilogy of "sevens". *Diabetes Metab.* 2006;32(Spec2):11–16.

NHSE. *Commissioning Standard: Dental care for people with diabetes*; 2019. https://www.england.nhs.uk/wp-content/uploads/2019/08/commissioning-standard-dental-care-for-people.pdf.

Page RC, Martin J, Krall EA, Mancl L, Garcia R. Longitudinal validation of a risk calculator for periodontal disease. *J Clin Periodontol.* 2003;30:819–827.

Papapanou PN, Sanz M, Buduneli N, Dietrich T, Feres M, Fine DH, et al. Periodontitis: consensus report of workgroup 2 of the 2017 world workshop on the classification of periodontal and peri-implant diseases and conditions. *J Clin Periodontol.* 2018;45(suppl 20):S162S170.

Ramseier CA, Woelber JP, Kitzmann J, Detzen L, Carra MC, Bouchard P. Impact of risk factor control interventions for smoking cessation and promotion of healthy lifestyles in patients with periodontitis: a systematic review. *J Clin Periodontol.* 2020;47(suppl 22):90–106.

Roberts A, Matthews JB, Socransky SS, Freestone PP, Williams PH, Chapple IL. Stress and periodontal diseases: effects of catecholamines on the growth of periodontal bacteria in vitro. *Oral Microbiol Immunol.* 2002;17:296–303.

Roberts A, Mathews JB, Socransky SS, Freestone PP, Williams PH, Chapple IL. Stress and periodontal diseases: growth responses of periodontal bacteria to Escherichia coli stress-associated autoinducer and exogenous Fe. *Oral Microbiol Immunol.* 2005;20:47–53.

Rosling B, Serino G, Hellstrom MK, Socransky SS, Lindhe J. Longitudinal periodontal tissue alterations during supportive therapy. Findings from subjects with normal and high susceptibility to periodontal disease. *J Clin Periodontol.* 2001;28:241249.

Rothman KJ. Measuring interactions. In: Rothman KJ, ed. *Epidemiology: An Introduction.* New York: Oxford University Press; 2002:168–180.

Salvi GE, Lawrence HP, Offenbacher S, Beck JD. Influence of risk factors on the pathogenesis of periodontitis. *Periodontol 2000.* 1997;14:173–201.

Sanz M, Ceriello A, Buysschaert M, Chapple I, Demmer RT, Graziani F. Scientific evidence on the links between periodontal diseases and diabetes: consensus report and guidelines of the joint workshop on periodontal diseases and diabetes by the International Diabetes Federation and the European Federation of Periodontology. *Diabetes Res Clin Pract.* 2018;137:231241. https://doi.org/10.1016/j.diabres.2017.12.001. and J Clin Periodontol. 45, 138149.

Sanz M, Hererra D, Kebschull M, et al. Treatment of stage I–III periodontitis—The EFP S3 level clinical practice guideline. *J Clin Periodontol.* 2020;47:4–60.

Scott A, Milward MR, Brock GR, et al. Mapping biological to clinical phenotypes during the development (21 days) and resolution (21 days) of experimental gingivitis. *J Clin Periodontol.* 2012;39:123–131.

Taylor GW. Bidirectional interrelationships between diabetes and periodontal diseases: an epidemiological perspective. *Ann Periodontol.* 2001;6:99–112.

Tomar SL, Asma S. Smoking-attributable periodontitis in the United States: findings from NHANES III. National Health and Nutrition Examination Survey. *J Periodontol.* 2000;71:743–751.

Tonetti MS, Greenwell H, Kornman KS. Staging and grading of periodontitis: framework and proposal of a new classification and case definition. *J Periodontol.* 2018;89(suppl 1):S159–S172.

White DA, Tsakos G, Pitts NB, et al. Adult Dental Health Survey 2009: common oral health conditions and their impact on the population. *Br Dent J.* 2012;213:567–572.

West N, Chapple I, Claydon N, et al. BSP implementation of European S3 - level evidence-based treatment guidelines for stage I-III periodontitis in UK clinical practice. *J Dentistry.* 2021;106:105362.

Wimmer G, Janda M, Wieselmann-Penkner K, Jaske N, Polansky R, Pertl C. Coping with stress: its influence on periodontal disease. *J Periodontol.* 2002;73:1343–1351.

Periodontal Diagnosis and Prognosis

SECTION 2

Periodontal Diagnosis and Prognosis

2.1

Classification and Diagnosis of Periodontal Diseases

PHILIP OWER

CHAPTER OUTLINE

OVERVIEW OF THE CHAPTER

This chapter will describe the various systems that have been devised to classify periodontal diseases, the objective of disease classification being to help clinicians develop the most appropriate therapeutic approaches for patients with these conditions, although the important distinction between classification and diagnosis will be discussed. Numerous classification systems have been devised in the past, and inevitably the increase in knowledge about the pathogenesis of periodontal diseases over the years has necessitated the revision of classification systems. The only systems that will be described in any detail in this chapter are those that are in current usage, namely those that arose from World Workshop proceedings in 1999 (Armitage 1999) and 2017 (Tonetti et al. 2018). The British Society of Periodontology and Implant Dentistry (BSP) modification of the 2017 World Workshop classification system will be explained in detail, as this is the most appropriate system to be used in a general practice setting.

This chapter covers the following topics:

- Background
- Classification is not the same as diagnosis
- Previous classification systems
- The 1999 classification system
- The 2017 classification system

- Staging and grading in the 2017 classification system
- Implementation of the 2017 classification system in clinical practice
- The BSP implementation of the 2017 classification system in general practice
- Establishing the periodontal diagnosis
- Summary

Introduction

Classification of any disease is important in terms of helping to determine the most accurate diagnosis and thus the most appropriate care for a patient, as well as forming the basis for research into disease pathology, aetiology and epidemiology. Diseases may be classified in terms of cause, pathogenesis or symptoms. In the case of periodontal diseases, which present as a wide range of conditions affecting the tooth-supporting tissues, classification is, and has been, most commonly defined in terms of pathological loss of tooth support and presenting symptoms. Many classification systems for periodontal diseases have existed in the past, but as ongoing research has contributed to the knowledge of these diseases, so classification systems have had to adapt to this new knowledge.

Classification Is Not the Same as Diagnosis

A common misconception of classification is that the name given to a disease forms the diagnosis and that, in turn, a specific treatment approach is then indicated. However, the name given to a disease is just that, a label, and this is not the same as a comprehensive diagnosis, which should take into account a variety of other factors. Classification is thus historical and tells the clinician little or nothing about the patient's current disease status. For example describing a patient as having *chronic periodontitis* (using the older classification system) doesn't tell the clinician anything about whether the disease is stable or progressive, mild, moderate or advanced, how the disease is distributed or what led the patient to develop the condition in the first place. Thus treating a patient on this basis alone would not necessarily manage their condition appropriately. A proper diagnosis on the other hand includes the classification term but should also include information about the patient's current disease status and the risk profile of the patient. It is only by arriving at this detailed diagnosis that the most appropriate treatment plan can be formulated for the patient. In this example the patient may be classified as having *chronic periodontitis*, but a full diagnosis may be *generalised moderate chronic periodontitis, widespread pocketing and bleeding on probing with smoking and uncontrolled diabetes as risk factors*. It is only the full diagnosis that can help the clinician to formulate the most appropriate treatment plan for that individual patient. In recent years the failure to diagnose periodontal diseases has become one of the most common reasons for dental litigation in the UK (Briggs 2014).

> ### KEY POINT 1
> Classification is not the same as diagnosis; diagnosis includes the classification term but should also include information about the patient's current disease status and the risk profile of the patient.

Previous Classification Systems

The first attempt to classify diseases of the periodontium was made by Pierre Fauchard in 1728. Since then many classification systems have been devised to reflect developing understanding of the causes and effects of these common conditions. The term *pyorrhoea* (from the Greek, meaning "discharge of matter") was first used in the early 20th century, and this is still a term that clinicians may hear used by some older patients today. In 1977 the American Academy of Periodontology (AAP) Classification system (Ranney 1977) identified a more aggressive form of periodontitis seen in younger patients with low levels of plaque, often affecting first molars and incisors. The term *juvenile periodontitis* was used to describe this particular group of patients, distinguishing this condition from the more common form, *adult periodontitis*. This distinction was further developed in subsequent classification systems in 1989 (American Academy of Periodontology 1989), 1993 and

1999. The 1999 World Workshop in Periodontics Classification System (Armitage 1999) was in widespread use up until 2017 when a new World Workshop on the Classification of Periodontal and Peri-implant Diseases and Conditions was held, co-sponsored by the AAP and the European Federation of Periodontology (EFP), with the proceedings of this workshop being published in 2018. The 1999 and 2017 classification systems are the main systems in current use globally, although it is anticipated that the latest system will gradually become the predominant system used to classify periodontal and peri-implant diseases. The 1999 system will be described briefly, and the 2017 system will be described in more detail in this chapter.

> ### KEY POINT 2
> The most common classification systems in current use for periodontal diseases are the 1999 and 2018 systems, but the latter will become predominant.

The 1999 Classification System

The 1999 World Workshop in Periodontics proposed a classification system (Armitage 1999) which was in use for 19 years. The main difference between this system and numerous predecessors was that it dispensed with age as a criterion. Previous classification systems had related more aggressive forms of periodontitis to age, but the 1999 system sought to identify this type of disease, which was often seen in younger patients, based on clinical, radiographic and historical findings alone. In addition, refractory periodontitis (that is, periodontitis not responding to therapy) was no longer recognised. This emphasised evidence at the time that indicated that it should be possible to identify why a patient did not respond to treatment as expected. Periodontitis was classified as chronic (generalised and localised), aggressive (generalised and localised), necrotising and as a manifestation of systemic disease. The full 1999 classification system was as follows:

I. Gingival diseases
- Dental plaque-induced gingival diseases
- Non-plaque-induced gingival lesions

II. Chronic periodontitis
- Localised
- Generalised

III. Aggressive periodontitis
- Localised
- Generalised

IV. Periodontitis as a manifestation of systemic diseases
- Associated with haematological disorders
- Associated with genetic disorders
- Not otherwise specified

V. Necrotising periodontal diseases
- Necrotising ulcerative gingivitis
- Necrotising ulcerative periodontitis

VI. Abscesses of the periodontium
- Gingival abscess
- Periodontal abscess
- Pericoronal abscess

- Periodontitis associated with endodontic lesions
- Combined periodontic-endodontic lesions

VII. Developmental or acquired deformities and conditions
- Localised tooth-related factors that modify or predispose to plaque-induced gingival diseases/periodontitis
- Mucogingival deformities and conditions around teeth
- Mucogingival deformities and conditions on edentulous ridges
- Occlusal trauma

KEY POINT 3

1999 Classification system – major groups:
I. Gingival diseases
II. Chronic periodontitis
III. Aggressive periodontitis
IV. Periodontitis as a manifestation of systemic disease
V. Necrotising periodontal diseases
VI. Periodontal abscesses
VII. Developmental or acquired deformities or conditions

The principal clinical and radiographic signs and symptoms of the categories in the 1999 classification system were as follows.

I. Gingival Diseases

- Mostly plaque-induced, chronic gingivitis being the most common.
- Characterised by gingival inflammation (redness, oedema, bleeding) but with no loss of attachment (LOA) or radiographic bone loss.

II. Chronic Periodontitis

- Inflammation of the gingivae as above but with evidence of LOA and radiographic bone loss.
- Mild (LOA 1–2 mm), moderate (LOA 3–4 mm) or severe (LOA over 5 mm).
- Radiographic evidence of bone loss, typically horizontal.
- Generalised (more than 30% of sites affected) or localised (less than 30% of sites affected).

III. Aggressive Periodontitis

- Rapid LOA (more than 2 mm per year) and bone loss.
- Bone loss usually vertical.
- Often familial aggregation.
- Localised if no more than two teeth apart from first molars and incisors affected (that is all eight incisors and all four first molars as well as two other teeth), otherwise generalised (Highfield 2009).
- Tissue destruction greater than would be expected given plaque and calculus levels.

IV. Periodontitis as a Manifestation of Systemic Diseases

Periodontitis that may be associated with systemic disorders; see Chapter 2.4.

V. Necrotising Periodontal Diseases

- Necrotising ulcerative gingivitis presenting as interdental ulcers (giving a "punched-out" appearance) but with no bone loss, often in younger patients with smoking, stress and poor diet as common factors.
- Necrotising ulcerative periodontitis as above but with the addition of bone loss.

VI. Abscesses Arising from the Periodontium

Abscess formation affecting the gingiva only, or both the gingival and periodontal tissues, and requiring specific treatment strategies.

VII. Developmental or Acquired Deformities and Conditions

- Tooth-related factors that modify the risk of plaque-related gingival and/or periodontal disease such as enamel pearls and diverticulated roots.
- Mucogingival deformities and conditions around teeth that modify the risk of plaque-related gingival and/or periodontal disease, such as recession defects.
- Mucogingival deformities and conditions on edentulous ridges.
- Occlusal trauma modifies the response of the gingival and periodontal tissues to plaque.

The 2017 Classification System

With advances in knowledge from both clinical and laboratory research over the last two decades the time was right for the introduction of a new classification system, both for periodontal diseases and also for those affecting the peri-implant tissues. The international workshop that took place in 2017 comprised four main working groups, which considered:
- Periodontal health, gingival diseases and conditions
- Periodontitis
- Other conditions affecting the periodontium
- Peri-implant diseases and conditions.

Table 2.1.1 shows the four working groups and their subject areas. The full consensus reports of the four working groups are freely available online at https://onlinelibrary.wiley.com/toc/1600051x/2018/45/S20, and a summary of the differences between the 1999 and 2017 classification systems was published by the AAP in 2018 (Caton et al. 2018). The recommendations of Working Group 4 (peri-implant diseases and conditions) will be considered in Chapter 7.3.

The main differences between the 2017 classification system and the 1999 system are as follows:
- For the first time in any classification system, periodontal health was clearly defined.
- Chronic and aggressive periodontitis were replaced with a model based on stages and grades.
- A *personalised medicine* approach was adopted.
- Peri-implant diseases and conditions were included.

World Workshop on the Classification of Periodontal and Per-implant Diseases and Conditions 2017 – Working Groups

Classification of periodontal and peri-implant diseases and conditions 2017

Periodontal diseases and conditions

Periodontal health, gingival diseases and conditions	Periodontitis	Other conditions affecting the periodontium
Chapple, Mealey, et al. 2018 consensus Rept link	Papapanou, Sanz et al. 2018 consensus Rept link	Jepsen, Caton et al. 2018 consensus Rept link
Trombelli et al. 2018 case definitions link	Jepsen, Caton et al. 2018 consensus Rept link	Papapanou, Sanz et al. 2018 consensus Rept link
	Tonetti, Greenwell, Kornman. 2018 case definitions link	

Periodontal health and gingival health	Gingivitis: Dental biofilm-induced	Gingival diseases: Non-dental biofilm-induced	Necrotizing periodontal diseases	Periodontitis	Periodontitis as a manifestation of systemic disease	Systemic disease or conditions affecting the periodontal supporting tissues	Periodontal Abscesses and Endodontic-Periodontal lesions	Mucogingival deformities and conditions	Traumatic occlusal forces	Tooth and prosthesis related factors

Peri-implant diseases and conditions
Berglundh, Armitage et al. 2018 consensus Rept link

Peri-implant health	Peri-implant mucositis	Peri-implantitis	Peri-implant soft and hard tissue deficiencies

Reprinted from *Journal of Clinical Periodontology* 45(S20):8, Maurizio S Tonetti et al. (2018), with permission from John Wiley & Sons.

KEY POINT 4

Main changes in the 2018 classification system:
- Periodontal health clearly defined.
- Aggressive periodontitis not recognised as a separate condition.
- Periodontitis classified in terms of stages and grades.
- Peri-implant diseases and conditions included.

Perhaps the most radical of these principal differences was the replacement of the long-recognised distinction between chronic and aggressive periodontitis with a universal system that sought to capture the severity, extent and rate of progression of a patient's disease, based on the lack of scientific evidence that these were distinct conditions. In other words, although chronic and aggressive periodontitis were in the past regarded as separate conditions, they are now recognised as variations on the same spectrum of disease. However, it was also considered that there was a specific clinical phenotype of extreme periodontal destruction affecting the molars and incisors of young patients, previously referred to as localised juvenile periodontitis, that was now being described as a molar/incisor pattern (MIP) of disease.

Staging and Grading in the 2017 Classification System

The 2017 classification system uses a staging and grading system (similar to that used in cancer diagnoses) in which staging describes the severity of disease in an individual patient (based on the worst-affected site in the mouth) and grading describes the level of that individual's susceptibility to disease. An important underlying principle of staging is that it is carried out at initial assessment and that patients cannot subsequently reduce their stage, a consequence of

periodontal destruction (attachment and bone loss) being an irreversible process.

KEY POINT 5

Staging describes the severity of disease in a patient.
Grading describes the level of that individual's susceptibility to disease.

Staging involves assessment of the following:
- site of greatest attachment loss
- bone loss (single worst site)
- tooth loss (due to periodontitis)
- other factors (maximum pocket depth, pattern of bone loss, furcation involvement, ridge defects, occlusal trauma, restorative needs).

Grading involves assessment of the following:
- bone and attachment loss over a 5-year period
- the ratio of percentage bone loss to age
- the relationship between biofilm volume and level of periodontal destruction
- levels of smoking
- blood glucose status.

This detailed system of periodontal classification has been summarised in a downloadable practice resource from the AAP that can be found at https://www.perio.org/2017wwdc. The original staging and grading guidance from Tonetti et al. (2018) is reproduced in Appendix 1. However, it should be appreciated that the staging and grading of a periodontal patient only reflects that patient's historical disease experience and that staging and grading alone does not inform the clinician about the patient's current disease status, which is indicated principally by probing pocket depths (PPD) and bleeding on probing (BoP). Not taking these commonly measured clinical features into account as part of the diagnosis risks misdiagnosing the periodontal patient; for example, the treatment needs of an untreated periodontal patient with pocketing and bleeding will be very different from those of a treated periodontal patient with little pocketing or bleeding, even though their staging and grading may be identical. In addition it should be remembered that a periodontal patient is a periodontal patient for life, and even apparently stable patients can experience recurrent episodes of periodontal destruction if their personal and professional periodontal maintenance slips or if their risk factor profile changes. Staging and grading of periodontitis therefore has its limitations and should not be used as a diagnostic tool in isolation.

Implementation of the 2017 Classification System in Clinical Practice

There is no doubt that the 2017 classification system is a more detailed and scientifically robust diagnostic tool than previous systems. Such a system should result in more appropriate therapeutic strategies and more personalised treatment plans for periodontal patients. However, whereas the 2017 system lends itself to research and specialist practice, after publication of the World Workshop proceedings in 2018 some doubts were raised about the practicalities of adopting such a complex system in general dental practice. Guidance on the implementation of the new system in clinical practice and education was published in 2019 (Tonetti & Sanz 2019), but concerns remained that the system, as recommended by the World Workshop, was still too complex to be used in a general practice setting. In 2018 the British Society of Periodontology and Implant Dentistry (BSP) formed a working group to consider these difficulties, and in 2019 the BSP published an adaptation of the 2017 classification that would allow dentists and hygienists to adopt a more practical approach to implement the new system in such settings (Dietrich et al. 2019). Following publication, this modified implementation scheme has received widespread acceptance in the profession, not only in the UK but also globally.

KEY POINT 6

The British Society of Periodontology and Implant Dentistry has modified the 2017 World Workshop classification system for use in general dental practice.

The BSP Implementation of the 2017 Classification System in General Practice

One of the objectives of the BSP implementation of the 2017 World Workshop classification system was to describe how the BSP's Basic Periodontal Examination (BPE) Guidelines (British Society of Periodontology 2016), which have been widely used by UK clinicians as a means of screening all patients for periodontal status for many years, could be integrated into the new system. The BPE guidelines are described in more detail in Chapter 2.2, but as part of the BSP's implementation recommendations for the new

classification system, an infographic was produced to show how the workflow between BPE screening and a full periodontal diagnosis could be achieved. This infographic can be downloaded from the BSP website at www.bsperio.org.uk and is reprinted in Appendix 2. A summary of the algorithm used to prepare the infographic is shown in Figure 2.1.1. The BPE system is designed to distinguish between gingival and periodontal health, and gingivitis and periodontitis, and to indicate when further investigation of periodontal conditions needs to be carried out. Periodontal patients (BPE code 3 and 4) will require a detailed medical and dental history, more detailed oral examination and further investigations such as special tests and radiographs that will allow differentiation between different types of disease (gingivitis, periodontitis, periodontitis associated with systemic disease, necrotising periodontal disease and so on) and, when appropriate, a full periodontal diagnosis will then need to be performed, as shown in Fig 2.1.1.

The BSP implementation of the 2017 classification system accepts the four stages of severity (I – mild, II – moderate, III – severe, IV – very severe) and the three grades of progression (A – slow, B – moderate, C – rapid), but the attribution of stage/grade to an individual patient has been simplified to enable clinicians to do so quickly and consistently. Recognising that clinicians in general practice already routinely assess periodontal disease severity by means of pocket depths (not attachment levels, which are rarely used in a practice setting) and bone levels, and that the bone level is the most useful and objective determinant for severity, the BSP implementation plan proposed bone level (at the worst affected site) as the sole determinant for severity, depending on whether the bone loss was less than 15% or was within the coronal, middle, apical third of the root (see Table 2.1.2). This method of stage assessment requires radiographs, but these are highly likely to be in existence in any event as a result of routine patient examinations (which periodically require the taking of bitewing radiographs) and the BPE because the BSP's BPE Guidelines (British Society of Periodontology 2016) require the existence of suitable radiographs for all BPE code 3 and 4 sextants (see Chapter 2.2). It was also recognised, in the BSP modification proposals, that the radiograph was a crucial component of grading in the World Workshop system, specifically the extent of bone loss in relation to the age of the patient, a ratio that most clinicians would be assessing instinctively; for example 20% bone loss in an 80- or 90-year-old patient would not cause the clinician any great alarm, unlike the same amount of loss in a 20- or 30-year-old. The comparison of successive radiographs (as proposed in the World Workshop) is often impractical in the general practice setting and such information adds little useful information to that obtained from the percentage bone loss/age ratio alone. Similarly, the inclusion of specific risk factors (biofilm volume, smoking and diabetes) in grade determination, as proposed in the World Workshop, also provides little additional information because the percentage bone loss/age ratio shows a patient's lifelong exposure to such risk factors, although

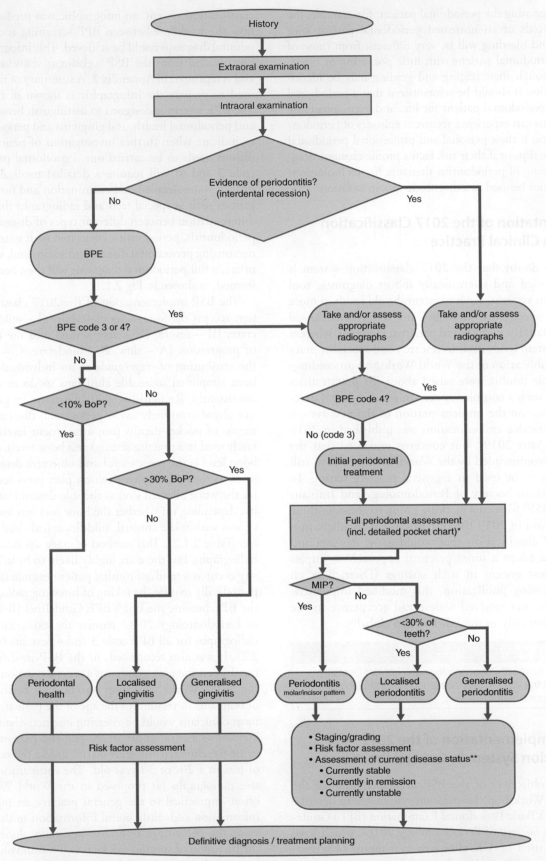

• **Figure 2.1.1** Algorithm for screening and assessment of periodontal status. *BPE*, Basic periodontal examination; *BoP*, bleeding on probing; *MIP*, molar incisor pattern. *A diagnosis of periodontitis requires radiographic bone loss at two non-adjacent teeth that cannot be attributed to causes other than periodontitis. **See Table 2.1.4. (*Reprinted by permission from Springer Nature: Br. Dent. J. Periodontal diagnosis in the context of the 2017 classification system of periodontal diseases and conditions - implementation in clinical practice, Dietrich, T., Ower, P., et al., copyright 2019.*)

TABLE 2.1.2   Staging of periodontitis (BSP modification 2019)

	Stage I (early/mild)	Stage II (moderate)	Stage III (severe)	Stage IV (very severe)
Maximum % interproximal bone loss	<15% or <2 mm**	Coronal third	Mid third	Apical third
Extent	Describe as: • Localized (up to 30% of teeth) • Generalised (more than 30% of teeth) • Molar/incisor pattern			

** Measurement in mm from cemento-enamel junction if only bitewing radiograph available (bone loss) or if no radiographs clinically justified (clinical attachment level)
(Reprinted by permission from Springer Nature: Br. Dent. J. Periodontal diagnosis in the context of the 2017 classification system of periodontal diseases and conditions - implementation in clinical practice, Dietrich, T., Ower, P., et al., copyright 2019.)

TABLE 2.1.3   Grading of periodontitis (BSP modification 2019)

	Grade A (slow)	Grade B (moderate)	Grade C (rapid)
Maximum % bone loss/age	<0.5	0.5–1.0	>1.0

(Reprinted by permission from Springer Nature: Br. Dent. J. Periodontal diagnosis in the context of the 2017 classification system of periodontal diseases and conditions - implementation in clinical practice, Dietrich, T., Ower, P., et al., copyright 2019.)

assessment of these risk factors will inevitably form part of the diagnosis, if not the classification of disease. The BSP therefore recommended that the ratio of percentage bone loss to age was the main determinant for grade, or rate of progression of periodontal destruction (see Table 2.1.3). However the ranges of the percentage bone loss/age ratios for grade assessment suggested by the World Workshop, which were estimates, did not seem to be of practical use in a general practice setting, and the BSP modification of the grading ratios is slightly different. The reasoning behind this departure from the World Workshop recommendation is complex and is fully explained by Dietrich et al. (2019), to which readers are referred. In practical terms, using the BSP modification of the classification system means that grade can be quickly determined as follows:

• Grade A If the maximum percentage bone loss is less than half the patient's age in years (e.g. <30% in a 60-year-old)
• Grade B All other situations
• Grade C If the maximum percentage bone loss is greater than the patient's age in years (e.g. >30% in a 29-year-old)

Establishing the Periodontal Diagnosis

Staging and grading therefore establishes the severity of disease and the level of patient susceptibility, but in order for a full diagnosis to be made, and for an appropriate and personalised treatment approach to be selected, the current status and the risk factor profile of the patient needs to be assessed.

Current status was described by the World Workshop in terms of a stable patient, an unstable patient or a patient with residual inflammation. The BSP modification describes stable, unstable and "in remission" periodontal patients, further adapting cancer diagnosis principles. Furthermore, unlike the World Workshop assessment of current status, which depends on measurement of attachment levels, the BSP recommended determination of current status by PPD and BoP measurements, parameters that have always been routinely used in the general practice setting. The criteria for determining current status are shown in Table 2.1.4, although it should be noted that the BSP also recognised that periodontal patients in long-term supportive care may have pockets of 5 or 6 mm with no BoP, and such patients may well be considered stable, emphasizing the importance of clinical discretion when estimating current status.

Risk factor profile is a crucial part of establishing a working periodontal diagnosis because such factors will need to be addressed in the earliest stages of treatment planning if successful outcomes are to be achieved. Both systemic and local risk factors (such as tooth position, poor restorations, calculus deposits) need to be considered. Chief among systemic risk factors are diabetic status and smoking habits, probably the most important factors that need to be assessed, and for which the strongest evidence base in the pathogenesis of periodontitis exists but other, less strongly evidence-based factors are also likely be involved and should be commented upon. Such putative systemic risk factors include diet, genetics, obesity and stress (see Chapter 1.6).

Full and proper periodontal diagnosis, which includes a stage/grade classification, informs and indeed dictates the appropriate management of the periodontitis patient; a full periodontal diagnosis should therefore contain the following elements:

TABLE 2.1.4	Determining the current status of a periodontitis patient (BSP modification 2019)		
	Stable	In Remission	Unstable
BoP	<10%	>10%	>10%
PPD	<4mm	<4mm	>5mm
4mm sites with	no BoP	no BoP	BoP

BoP: bleeding on probing; PPD: probing pocket depths.

- Distribution generalised, localised or molar/incisor pattern
- Classification stage/grade
- Current status stable, in remission or unstable
- Risk factor profile

KEY POINT 7

Diagnosis should include:
- Distribution
- Classification
- Current status
- Risk factor profile

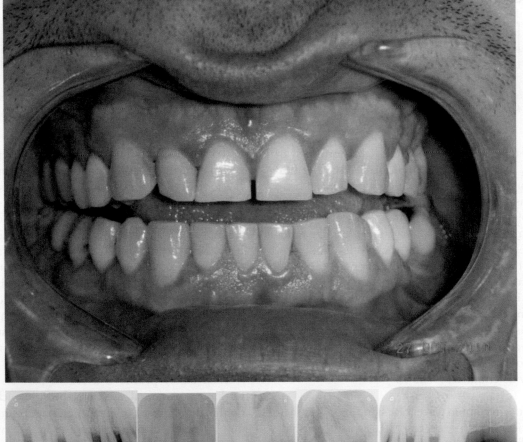

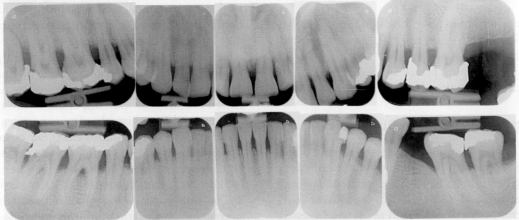

- **Figure 2.1.2** Male patient, aged 42, former heavy smoker but with no other risk factors, widespread pockets of 4–6 mm, most of which display BoP.

An example patient is shown at Figure 2.1.2; this patient is male, age 42, a former heavy smoker but with no other risk factors, with widespread pockets of 4–6 mm, most of which displayed BoP. The full diagnosis for this patient would be:

Distribution – most teeth have some bone loss, so the distribution is generalised.

Classification – the worst affected site is UR7, where there is about 50% bone loss in the middle third of the root, making the stage/grade III/C.

Current status – there is pocketing over 4 mm with BoP so status is unstable.

Risk factor profile – the patient is a former smoker, and this should be recorded in the diagnosis because former smokers often take up the habit again.

In this case the diagnosis that would be recorded in the patient's records would be: generalised periodontitis stage III/grade C, currently unstable, former smoker.

For further examples of periodontal diagnosis using the 2017 classification system (BSP modification), the reader is referred to the online content of this book.

Summary

The classification of periodontal (and peri-implant) diseases represents a crucial first step in the management of patients with periodontal problems, but used alone the classification of periodontal diseases does not provide a thorough enough framework for subsequent treatment planning. It is important when planning the most appropriate therapeutic approach to take other factors into account, namely current status and risk factor profile, in order to arrive at an accurate diagnosis which will then inform the treatment-planning process.

Multiple choice questions on the contents of this chapter are available online at Elsevier eBooks+.

A series of videos demonstrating how to assess the periodontium are also available online.

References

American Academy of Periodontology, 1989. In: *Proceedings of the World Workshop in Clinical Periodontics, American Academy of Periodontology, Chicago*. 1989:1/23–1/24.

Armitage GC. Development of a classification system for periodontal diseases and conditions. *Ann Periodontol*. 1999;4:1–6.

Berglundh T, Armitage G, et al. Peri–implant diseases and conditions: Consensus report of workgroup 4 of the 2017 World Workshop on the Classification of Periodontal and Peri–Implant Diseases and Conditions. *J Clin Periodontol*. 2018;45(Suppl 20):S286–S291.

British Society of periodontology and Implant Dentistry. *The Basic Periodontal Examination*; 2016. http://www.bsperio.org.uk/publications.

Briggs L. Probing deeper into periodontics claims. *DDU Journal*;2014:9-21. https://www.theddu.com/guidance-and-advice/journals/march-2014/probing-deeper-into-periodontics-claims.

Caton JG, Armitage G, Berglundh T, et al. A new classification scheme for periodontal and peri-implant diseases and conditions - introduction and key changes from the 1999 classification. *J Periodontol*. 2018;89(suppl 1):S1S8.

Chapple ILC, Mealey BL, et al. Periodontal health and gingival diseases and conditions on an intact and a reduced periodontium: consensus report of workgroup 1 of the 2017 World Workshop on the Classification of Periodontal and Peri–Implant Diseases and Conditions. *J Clin Periodontol*. 2018;45(Suppl 20):S68–S77.

Dietrich T, Ower P, Tank M, et al. Periodontal diagnosis in the context of the 2017 classification system of periodontal diseases and conditions - implementation in clinical practice. *Br Dent J*. 2019;226(1):1622.

Fauchard P. *Le chirurgien dentiste, ou traite des dents. Ou l'on enseigne les moyens de les entretenir propres & faines, de les embellir, d'en réparer la pette & de remedier à celles des gencives & aux accidens qui peuvent furvenir aux autres parties voilines des dents*. Paris: Jean Mariette; 1728.

Highfield J. Diagnosis and classification of periodontal disease. *Aust Dent J*. 2009;54(suppl 1):S11–S26.

Jepsen S, Caton JG, et al. Periodontal manifestations of systemic diseases and developmental and acquired conditions: consen– sus report of workgroup 3 of the 2017 World Workshop on the Classification of Periodontal and Peri–Implant Diseases and Conditions. *J Clin Periodontol*. 2018;45(Suppl 20):S219–S229.

Papapanou PN, Sanz M, et al. Periodontitis: Consensus report of workgroup 2 of the 2017 World Workshop on the Classification of Periodontal and Peri–Implant Diseases and Conditions. *J Clin Periodontol*. 2018;45(Suppl 20):S162–S170.

Proceedings of the World Workshop on the Classification of Periodontal and Peri-implant Diseases and Conditions. *J Clin Periodontol*. 45(Suppl 20):S1S291.

Ranney RR. 1977. Pathogenesis of periodontal disease. In: *Proceedings of the International Conference on Research in the Biology of Periodontal Disease*. 1977:223–265.

Tonetti MS, Greenwell H, Kornman KS. Staging and grading of periodontitis: framework and proposal of a new classification and case definition. *J Clin Periodontol*. 2018;45(suppl 20):3S149S161.

Tonetti MS, Greenwell H, Kornman KS. Staging and grading of peri–odontitis: Framework and proposal of a new classification and case definition. *J Clin Periodontol*. 2018;45(Suppl 20):S149–S161.

Tonetti MS, Sanz M. Implementation of the new classification of periodontal diseases: decision-making algorithms for clinical practice and education. *J Clin Periodontol*. 2019;46:398405.

Trombelli L, Farina R, Silva CO, Tatakis DN. Plaque–induced gingivitis: Case definition and diagnostic considerations. *J Clin Periodontol*. 2018;45(Suppl 20):S44–S66.

2.2

Periodontal Assessment and Monitoring

PHILIP OWER AND LEO BRIGGS

CHAPTER OUTLINE

OVERVIEW OF THE CHAPTER

This chapter details commonly used clinical assessment techniques for new patients, recalled patients and patients on longer-term monitoring.

By the end of the chapter the reader should:

- Be able to describe how to carry out a full assessment of a periodontal patient
- Be aware of the use and limitations of the basic periodontal examination (BPE)
- Be able to assess and monitor a periodontal patient.

The chapter covers the following topics:

- Introduction
- What should be assessed?
- The Basic Periodontal Examination (BPE)

- Assessment of disease activity
- Assessment of plaque (biofilm)
- Assessment of the gingivae
- Assessment of periodontal pockets
- Assessment of loss of attachment
- Assessment of tooth mobility
- Assessment of furcation involvement
- Assessment of suppuration
- Assessment of bone support
- Radiographs in periodontal assessment
- Monitoring a periodontal patient.

Introduction

Over the years, various methods have been described for assessing the condition of the periodontal tissues of a patient. Each clinician needs to decide which methods they will use to assess a patient and ensure that their assessment is as consistent as possible. An understanding of the advantages and disadvantages of the various assessment methods is vital and detailed records about the methods used should always be kept. It is fundamental that there is an understanding of the differences between health and disease. Past disease activity should be distinguished from current (active) disease. Patients who have been successfully treated can achieve periodontal health although they may have reduced bone support as well as loss of attachment, which is often seen clinically as recession, residual pocketing and tooth mobility. The 2017 World Workshop on Classification (Chapple et al. 2018) described periodontal health on both an intact (no past periodontitis) and reduced (past periodontitis, treated and stable) periodontium, whilst recognising that the latter group of patients are at increased risk of recurrent periodontitis and should be closely monitored throughout life. Periodontal assessment is therefore a vitally important aspect of periodontal management, both at the start of disease control and throughout the life of the periodontal patient.

KEY POINT 1

Full periodontal assessment should include:
- Plaque
- Gingival inflammation
- Calculus
- Probing pocket depths (PPD)
- Recession
- Marginal bleeding (MB)
- Bleeding on probing (BoP)
- Mobility
- Suppuration

What should be Assessed?

The ideal periodontal assessment of a patient should take into consideration all of the following:
- Plaque
- Gingival inflammation

- Calculus and other plaque-retentive factors
- Periodontal pockets
- Recession
- Marginal bleeding
- Bleeding on probing
- Mobility of teeth
- Presence of suppuration (pus)
- Level of alveolar bone support
- Furcation involvements.

These factors must be considered in the broader context of the patient's medical and social histories and the other oral structures.

To do this for every patient would be very time consuming and unnecessary. For this reason, the Basic Periodontal Examination (BPE) was developed as a screening tool for use in general practice in the UK. Similar systems operate in other countries.

The Basic Periodontal Examination

The BPE was developed by the British Society of Periodontology and Implant Dentistry (BSP) from the Community Periodontal Index of Treatment Needs (CPITN) (Ainamo et al. 1982). The CPITN was created to help with workforce planning by assessing treatment need of a population. The BPE was designed as a fast and simple general practice screening system to identify patients with periodontal diseases. The purpose of the BPE is to screen for the presence or absence of periodontal diseases. It should *not* be used for the full assessment of patients with periodontal diseases or for the monitoring of patients who have been treated for periodontal diseases. It is a hierarchical scoring system which means that the higher the score, the greater the level of disease. Appendix 2, which describes how the 2017 classification system can be used to arrive at a diagnosis, also describes how BPE is mapped to the new classification system.

How to Record BPE

1. The dentition is divided into six sextants: The upper right posterior sextant (UR7–UR4); the upper anterior sextant (UR3–UL3); the upper left posterior sextant (UL4–UL7). The lower right posterior sextant (LR7–LR4); the

lower anterior sextant (LR3–LL3); the lower left posterior sextant (LL4–LL7).

2. All teeth in each sextant are examined except for third molars.

3. For a sextant to qualify for recording, it must contain at least two teeth. If only one tooth is present in a sextant, the score for that tooth is included in the recording for the adjoining sextant.

4. A WHO (World Health Organization) probe is used. This has a "ball end" 0.5 mm in diameter and a black band from 3.5 to 5.5 mm. A probing force of 20–25 grams should be used. A picture of this probe is shown earlier in this book (see Figure 1.3.1).

5. The probe should be "walked around" the sulcus or pockets in each sextant, and the highest score recorded. As soon as a code 4 is identified in a sextant, the clinician can then move directly on to the next sextant, though it may be better to continue to examine all sites in the sextant. This will help to gain a fuller understanding of the periodontal condition and will make sure that furcation involvements are not missed. If a code 4 is not detected, then all sites should be examined to ensure that the highest score in the sextant is recorded before moving on to the next sextant.

6. The scores are recorded in a grid (see Figure 1.3.2).

A video showing how the BPE is performed can be viewed in the online section of this book. It should be noted that while the WHO probe used to record BPE has the black band marking from 3.5 mm to 5.5 mm, clinicians and researchers often refer to 4 mm and 6 mm pockets as being thresholds for clinical decision-making. This is not as anomalous as it may seem at first sight; if the black band starts to enter a pocket, then that pocket is at least 4 mm in depth and if the black band just disappears into a pocket, then that pocket is at least 6 mm in depth.

KEY POINT 2

Basic periodontal examination (BPE) codes:
0   Health, pockets less than 3.5 mm
1   Pockets less than 3.5 mm, bleeding on probing
2   Pockets less than 3.5 mm, calculus or other plaque-retentive factor is present
3   Pocket depth between 3.5 and 5.5 mm
4   Pocket deeper than 5.5 mm
*   Furcation involvement.

BPE scores

0 = Health, pockets less than 3.5 mm
1 = Pockets less than 3.5 mm, bleeding on probing
2 = Pockets less than 3.5 mm, calculus or another plaque-retentive factor is present
3 = Pocket depth between 3.5 and 5.5 mm
4 = Pocket deeper than 5.5 mm
* = Furcation involvement.

If an * is recorded, both the number and the * should be recorded for that sextant; for example, 4* would indicate that there is at least one tooth with pocketing deeper than

5.5 mm in the sextant and at least one tooth with a furcation involvement.

Advantages and Disadvantages of BPE

The BPE is a quick and simple method of establishing a provisional diagnosis of periodontal health, gingivitis or periodontitis in patients with or without overt signs of periodontal diseases. In addition, because sextants are scored, it helps to produce a simple map of the healthy and diseased areas of the mouth. However, the hierarchical scoring assumes that a higher score is worse than a lower score. This is not always the case. For example, a patient may have a 6 mm pocket with no recession, which would give a score of 4. However, this pocket may be easily accessible to oral hygiene and debridement so should be relatively simple to treat compared to a tooth which has large calculus deposits in a more inaccessible site in the mouth but with a pocket of 5 mm and 3 mm of recession, which would give a score of 3. Code 2 may also be misleading; it is possible for calculus, or other plaque retention factors, such as restoration overhangs, to be present at sites with no gingivitis or attachment loss. In addition, BPE is of little or no value in established periodontitis patients because BPE is based on bleeding on probing (BoP) and PPD, rather than recording attachment and bone loss. Such patients require regular and full periodontal assessment.

When to Record BPE

The BSP has produced guidelines on the use of the BPE that are updated regularly. These may be viewed at: https://www.bsperio.org.uk/assets/downloads/BSP_BPE_Guidelines_2019.pdf.

Readers are advised to visit the website to check for the latest updates to BPE guidelines.

The guidelines state that:

- All new patients should have the BPE recorded.
- For patients with codes 0, 1 or 2, the BPE should be recorded at least annually.
- For patients with BPE codes of 3 or 4, more detailed periodontal charting is required:
  - Code 3: initial therapy including self-care advice (oral hygiene and risk factor control), then post–initial therapy, record a 6-point pocket chart in that sextant only
  - Code 4: if there is a code 4 in any sextant, then record full probing depths (six sites per tooth) throughout the entire dentition.
- The BPE cannot be used to assess the response to periodontal therapy because it does not provide information about how sites within a sextant change after treatment. To assess the response to treatment, probing depths should be recorded at six sites per tooth pre- and post-treatment.
- For patients who have undergone initial therapy for periodontitis (i.e., who had pre-treatment BPE scores of 3 or 4), and who are now in the maintenance phase of care, full probing depths throughout the entire dentition should be recorded at least annually.

In addition the guidelines state that:

- BPE should not be used around implants (4- or 6-point pocket charting should be used)
- Radiographs should be available for all code 3 and code 4 sextants. The type of radiograph used is a matter of clinical judgement but crestal bone levels should be visible. Many clinicians would regard periapical views as essential for code 4 sextants to allow assessment of bone loss as a percentage of root length and visualisation of the periapical tissues.
- When a 6-point pocket chart is indicated it is only necessary to record sites of 4 mm and above (although six sites per tooth should be measured).
- BoP should always be recorded in conjunction with a 6-point pocket chart.

Assessment of Disease Activity

Disease activity is defined as current loss of connective tissue attachment with apical migration of the junctional epithelium and loss of alveolar bone. There are no validated methods for determining disease activity. It is a common misconception that BoP is an indicator of disease activity. However, inflammation and deviation from health can be detected using surrogate markers of disease activity, such as PPD and BoP. In order to assess a patient fully, it is important to take into consideration the amount of plaque that is present, the condition of the gingivae, the presence of calculus and other plaque-retentive factors, the depth of periodontal pockets and any gingival recession or overgrowth. In addition, bleeding from the gingival margin, bleeding

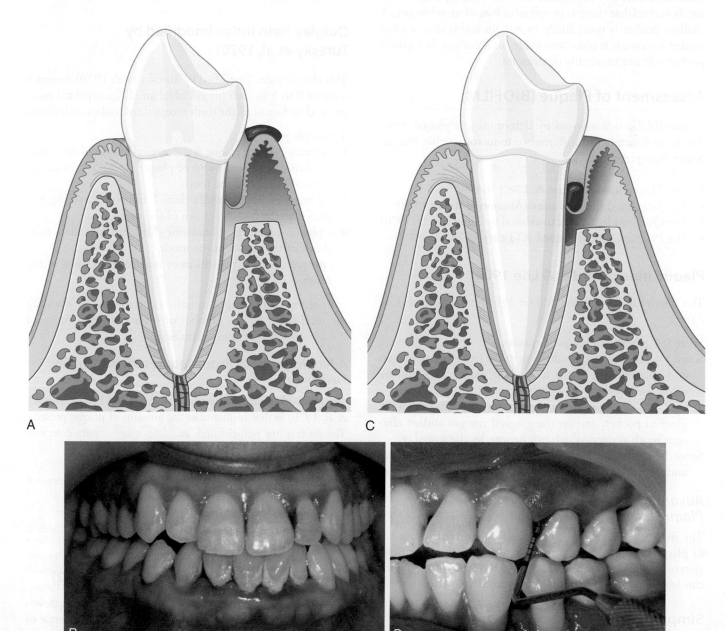

• **Figure 2.2.1** (A) Diagram showing bleeding from the gingival margin. (B) Bleeding from the gingival margin after shallow probing as shown in (A). (C) Diagram showing bleeding from the base of a pocket. (D) Bleeding from the base of a pocket.

on probing, any mobility of teeth, the presence of suppuration (pus), the level of alveolar bone support and any furcation involvements should be noted.

Marginal Bleeding and Bleeding on Probing

Marginal bleeding (MB) and BoP are not the same; MB is bleeding from the gingival margin when the gingivae have been gently touched. MB is thus a reliable indicator of the effectiveness or otherwise of self-performed plaque control. BoP is bleeding from the base of a pocket following probing to the full pocket depth (Figure 2.2.1).

Absence of BoP indicates the likelihood of periodontal stability. Although BoP indicates the presence of inflammation, it does not necessarily indicate that a periodontitis site is active (that there is progressive loss of attachment). A shallow pocket is more likely to remain stable than a deep pocket because it is more accessible for a patient, but a deep pocket will not inevitably deteriorate.

Assessment of Plaque (BIOFILM)

Plaque (biofilm) is assessed by determining a plaque score. There are a number of different systems for scoring plaque. Some examples are:

- The Plaque Index (Silness & Löe 1964)
- The Simplified Plaque Index (Ainamo and Bay 1975)
- The Quigley Hein Index (modified by Turesky et al. 1970)
- The Plaque Control Record (O'Leary 1972).

Plaque Index (Silness & Löe 1964)

The Plaque Index (Silness & Löe 1964) has scores of 0, 1, 2 or 3.

Score 0 – absence of plaque deposits.
Score 1 – a film of plaque adhering to the free gingival margin and adjacent area of the tooth. The plaque may only be recognised by running a probe across the tooth surface.
Score 2 – moderate accumulations of soft deposits within the gingival pocket, and on the gingival margin and/or adjacent tooth surface, which can be seen by the naked eye.
Score 3 – abundance of soft matter within the gingival pocket and/or on the gingival margin and adjacent tooth surface.

Advantages and Disadvantages of the Plaque Index

The main advantage is the attempt to quantify the amount of plaque present. The main disadvantage is the interpretation of the different scores. The criteria are subjective, which can lead to errors in repeatability of measurements.

Simplified Plaque Index (Ainamo & Bay 1975)

Ainamo & Bay (1975) introduced a simplified version of the Plaque Index. This is probably one of the most commonly used and reliable methods of assessing plaque.

In the Simplified Plaque Index, there are two scores, 0 or 1.

Score 0 – no plaque detected.
Score 1 – visible plaque detected.

Advantages and Disadvantages of the Simplified Plaque Index

The main advantage of the Simplified Plaque Index (Ainamo & Bay 1975) is that the criteria are easy to interpret (visible plaque is either present or absent) so repeatability is better. The main disadvantage is that no attempt has been made to quantify the amount of plaque present.

This system can be used to produce a percentage score for sites with plaque present. This system for recording plaque has been incorporated into many dental software packages.

Quigley Hein Index (modified by Turesky et al. 1970)

This plaque index (modified by Turesky et al. 1970) assigns a score of 0 to 5 to each buccal/labial and lingual/palatal non-restored surface of all the teeth except third molars, as follows:

0 – no plaque.
1 – separate flecks of plaque at the cervical margin of the tooth.
2 – a thin continuous band of plaque up to 1 mm at the cervical margin of the tooth.
3 – a band of plaque wider than 1 mm but covering less than one-third of the crown of the tooth.
4 – plaque covering at least one-third but less than two-thirds of the crown of the tooth.
5 – plaque covering two-thirds or more of the crown of the tooth.

A score for the entire mouth is determined by dividing the total score by the number of surfaces (a maximum of $2 \times 2 \times 14 = 56$ surfaces) examined.

Advantages and Disadvantages of the Quigley Hein Index

The main advantage of this plaque index (modified by Turesky et al. 1970) is that it quantifies the amount of plaque present. The criteria are well-defined, enabling more accurate repeatability of measurements. The main disadvantages are:

- interpretation of the different scores may vary between operators leading to inconsistent scoring
- only non-restored surfaces are scored
- no measurement of plaque on the interdental surfaces is recorded.

Plaque Control Record (O'Leary et al. 1972)

The Plaque Control Record (O'Leary et al. 1972) was developed to give a simple method of recording the presence of the plaque on individual tooth surfaces. These surfaces are:

- Mesial
- Distal

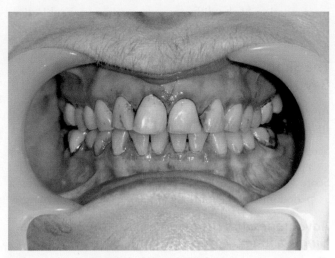

• **Figure 2.2.2** Disclosed dentition.

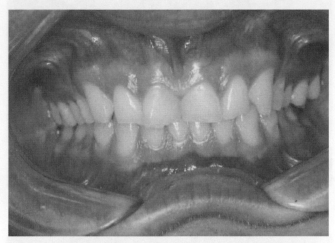

• **Figure 2.2.3** Healthy gingivae.

- Buccal
- Lingual.

A suitable disclosing solution, such as Bismarck Brown or a proprietary brand, is painted on all exposed tooth surfaces (Figure 2.2.2). After the patient has rinsed, the operator, using the tip of a probe, examines each stained surface for soft accumulations at the dento-gingival junction. When found, deposits are recorded as present. The surfaces which do not have soft accumulations at the dento-gingival junction are not recorded. After all teeth are examined and scored, the index is calculated by dividing the number of plaque-containing surfaces by the total number of available surfaces. It is expressed as a percentage.

Advantages and Disadvantages of the Plaque Control Record

The main advantages of this plaque index (O'Leary et al. 1972) are:

- plaque is disclosed to enable easy detection
- criteria are well-defined, which enables more accurate repeatability of measurements.
  The main disadvantages are:
- soft deposits are stained, which can lead to over-recording of plaque if other debris (such as food) is present
- stain needs to be removed.

There is no universally accepted plaque score. However, the Simplified Plaque Index (presence or absence of visible plaque) is one of the most useful systems to use in clinical practice due to the ease with which it can be used as well as the clarity of interpreting the different scores.

It should be appreciated that plaque scoring is one of the least reproducible indices; this is because many patients will improve their usual oral hygiene immediately before a dental appointment so there may be an unusually low score when they visit a dental professional. On the other hand a patient who normally cleans to a high standard may attend having not been able to brush before the visit and would then record an abnormally high plaque score. This can give rise to difficulties in relating

the recorded plaque score with the presence of gingival inflammation. Because of this, marginal bleeding (see later) may be a more reliable indicator of the patient's ability to remove accessible plaque and so control marginal inflammation.

Remember that the presence of plaque does not inevitably lead to gingivitis or periodontitis at that site.

> **KEY POINT 3**
> Plaque scoring is one of the least reliable indices. Marginal bleeding is a more reliable indicator of a patient's plaque removal ability.

Assessment of the Gingivae

The two most common features of the gingivae to assess are the appearance and levels of inflammation.

Appearance

Colour, contour and consistency are assessed.

- Colour – describe the colour of the gingivae. Remember that healthy gingivae (Figure 2.2.3) will be paler in colour than inflamed gingivae. It is important to take into account normal pigmentation of the gingivae when deciding whether or not they are inflamed. Smoking might mask some outward signs of inflammation.
- Contour – healthy gingivae should have a scalloped shape with a knife-edge margin.
- Consistency – gingivae can be inflamed (Figure 2.2.4), in which case they tend to lose the knife-edge margin with the tissues appearing slightly thicker and slightly "spongy".

Some people can have hypertrophic or hyperplastic gingivae which will also appear enlarged, but the gingival colour may be pale due a lack inflammation. Fibrotic gingivae will tend to be larger than normal and appear paler and thicker, as is commonly seen in smokers (Figure 2.2.5).

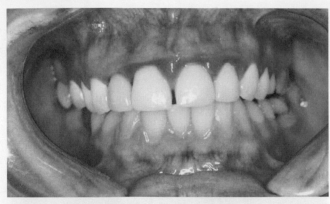

• **Figure 2.2.4** Inflamed gingivae.

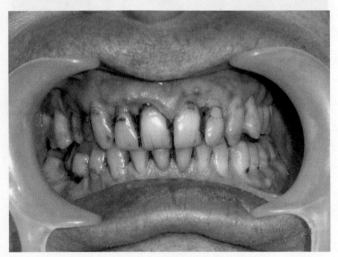

• **Figure 2.2.5** Fibrotic gingivae in a smoker.

Assessment of Gingival Inflammation

Gingival indices are used to assess gingival inflammation by identifying marginal bleeding.

Gingival Indices

A number of gingival indices have been proposed.

The Gingival Index (Löe & Silness 1963)

The Gingival index (Löe & Silness 1963) has scores of 0, 1, 2 or 3.

0 – normal gingiva.
1 – mild inflammation – slight change in colour, slight oedema. No bleeding on probing.
2 – moderate inflammation – redness, oedema and glazing. Bleeding on probing.
3 – severe inflammation – marked redness and oedema. Ulceration. Tendency to spontaneous bleeding.

Advantages and Disadvantages of the Gingival Index

The main advantage is the attempt to quantify the amount of inflammation present. The main disadvantage is the

interpretation of the different scores; criteria are subjective, potentially leading to errors in repeatability of measurements.

The Simplified Gingival Index (Ainamo & Bay 1975)

Ainamo & Bay (1975) developed the Simplified Gingival Index. It has two scores, 0 or 1.

Score 0 – no bleeding from the gingival margin detected after a periodontal probe is briefly run along the gingival margin.
Score 1 – bleeding from the gingival margin detected after a periodontal probe is briefly run along the gingival margin.

Advantages and Disadvantages of the Simplified Gingival Index

The main advantage of the Simplified Gingival Index is that the criteria are easy to interpret (bleeding is either present or absent), so repeatability is better. The main disadvantage is that no attempt has been made to quantify the amount of inflammation present.

This is one of the most widely used systems for assessing gingival inflammation in practice. It is simple and reliable. It can also be expressed as a percentage score. Many of the commercially available dental computer software packages allow this index to be recorded on a computer.

Assessment of Calculus

A number of systems for assessing calculus have been proposed. The main disadvantage of many of these is the difficulty in interpretation of the criteria set down. A simple visual assessment should be made of the presence or absence of both supragingival and subgingival calculus.

Assessment of Periodontal Pockets

Periodontal pockets are assessed by measuring the pocket depth with a periodontal probe. Charts will often be recorded as 4-point pocket charts (mesial and distal measurements on both the buccal/labial and lingual/palatal surfaces), or 6-point pocket charts (measuring a mid-buccal/labial and mid-lingual/palatal point as well as the four "corners" of the tooth measured in a 4-point pocket chart). Although the measurement of PPD is an important indicator of past periodontal disease, it is important to appreciate that PPD is not an indicator of current disease activity and PPD does not correlate with future disease progression – a deeper pocket may stay stable, and a shallow pocket can progress (Lindhe et al. 1983).

Probing Pocket Depths

The probing pocket depth is the distance from the gingival margin to the location of the tip of a periodontal probe, ideally located at the base of the pocket. The probe should be inserted in the pocket with a light probing force of 20–25 g.

The type of probe used affects the measurement. Narrow probes tend to give higher values than wider probes. The force used also affects the measurement.

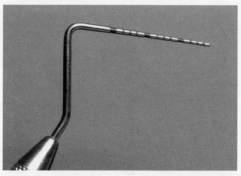

• **Figure 2.2.6** Manual probe (University of North Carolina [UNC] 15).

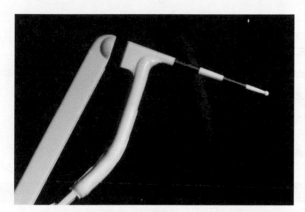

• **Figure 2.2.7** Constant pressure probe.

Measurements can be affected by the use of different probes; it is therefore critical to use the same type of probe whenever a pocket is measured. Clinicians should try always to use the same probing force whenever measuring a pocket. This can sometimes be more difficult than it sounds. If tissues are inflamed, probing can be very uncomfortable for a patient, which leads to a tendency to use lighter pressure and so under-record the true pocket depth. In addition, when tissues are inflamed, if the correct probing force is used there can be a tendency for the probe to penetrate the base of the pocket, which results in over-recording the true pocket depth (and further pain for the patient).

There are three generations of periodontal probes. The first generation are manual probes, the second are manual constant pressure probes and the third are computerised probes (Figures 2.2.6, 2.2.7 and 2.2.8).

Constant pressure and computerised probes can help reduce inappropriate probing force as a possible source of error.

Inter- and Intra-Operator Variability in Probing Measurements

There can be considerable variation in the reproducibility of probing depth measurements; repeat examinations by the same examiner will assess intra-operator variability. Duplicate examinations by two or more examiners will assess inter-operator variability. An experienced operator should be able to reliably record a pocket depth to ± 1 mm when using a manual probe.

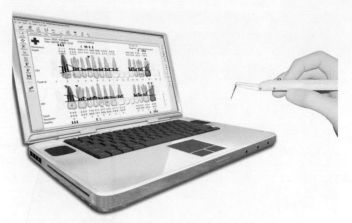

• **Figure 2.2.8** Computerised probe.

Other Probing Errors

It is important to try to angle the probe correctly so that it is kept as parallel as possible to the long axis of the tooth. This is not always straightforward because of crown or root morphology. There can also be obstructions, such as subgingival calculus, which prevent an accurate pocket depth reading. The position of the probe will also affect the measurement because pocket bases have complex shapes due to the highly variable pattern of destruction that is usually seen. As a result, the true pocket depth may be difficult to measure.

There are many different types of probes available. Clinicians should become proficient with using one type of probe so that their measurements are as reproducible as possible. In addition, the same type of probe should always be used (and the type noted in the records) when repeated measurements are taken.

KEY POINT 4

Sources of probing error:
- Pressure
- Position
- Angulation
- Obstacles
- Probe shape
- Probe tip diameter
- Inflammatory status.

Assessment of Attachment Loss

The clinical attachment level is the distance from a fixed point on a tooth, usually the cemento-enamel junction, to the tip of the probe when the probe is inserted into the full depth of the sulcus or pocket.

The Difference between Probing Pocket Depth and Loss of Attachment

The probing pocket depth is the distance from the gingival margin to the depth of the pocket. Loss of attachment (LOA) measures the distance from a fixed point on the tooth to the depth of the pocket (Figure 2.2.9). Measuring any recession and adding it to the pocket depth will record LOA.

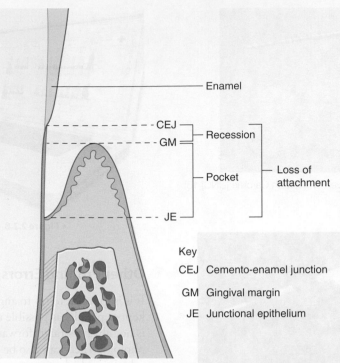

Key
CEJ   Cemento-enamel junction
GM   Gingival margin
JE   Junctional epithelium

• **Figure 2.2.9** Diagram showing the difference between pocket depth and loss of attachment.

The LOA measurement is sometimes referred to as the clinical attachment level. If a patient has active periodontal destruction which involves progressive recession, measuring pocket depths alone may fail to record this, which is why it is useful to note recession as well as pocket depths.

Identifying the cemento-enamel junction can often be difficult; sometimes it has been worn down by tooth surface loss, and if there is gingival enlargement it may be subgingival. As a result, full mouth 6-point clinical attachment level measurements are rarely taken in general practice.

Assessment of Bleeding on Probing

The assessment of BoP is the most important measure of periodontal disease status. It is the only measure that evaluates the inflammatory status of the periodontal tissues. There have been various BoP indices developed over the years. As with the plaque indices, some have tried to quantify the amount of bleeding. The most widely used BoP measure is the simple presence or absence of bleeding following probing to the base of the pocket. As noted above MB is not the same as BoP, and it is sometimes difficult to distinguish between the two. One way around this, however, is to delay BoP measurements until initial therapy (which includes oral hygiene instruction) has reduced marginal inflammation and MB readings. It is then more likely that any bleeding recorded is coming from pocket depths rather than the marginal gingival tissues.

When interpreting a BoP score, it is important to remember that bleeding on probing indicates the presence of inflammation; it does not necessarily indicate that there is active periodontitis.

KEY POINT 5

The assessment of BoP is the most important measure of periodontal disease status. It is the only measure that evaluates the inflammatory status of the periodontal tissues.

Assessment of Tooth Mobility

Most systems for assessing tooth mobility have developed criteria to define mild, moderate or severe tooth mobility. The most commonly used system to record tooth mobility is that devised by Miller (1950), which identifies 4 degrees of movement.

Degree 0 – "physiological" mobility; the tooth can be moved 0.1–0.2 mm in a horizontal direction.

Degree 1 – the tooth can be moved between 0.2 and 1 mm in a horizontal plane (bucco-lingual or mesio-distal direction).

Degree 2 – the tooth can be moved 1–2 mm in a horizontal plane but there is no mobility in a vertical plane (occluso-apical direction).

Degree 3 – the tooth can be moved in excess of 2 mm in a horizontal plane and/or in a vertical direction.

Assessment of Furcation Involvement

There are three basic ways to assess a furcation involvement: probing, radiographic assessment and clinical appearance.

Probing

Furcations are difficult to probe, particularly the distal furcation of an upper molar. The Nabers probe is a curved

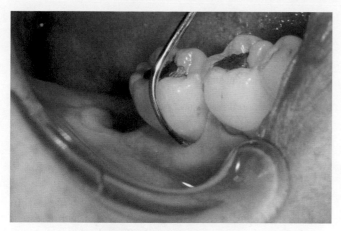

• **Figure 2.2.10** Nabers probe.

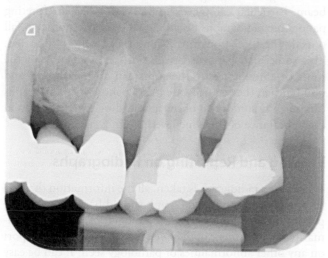

• **Figure 2.2.11** Radiograph showing a furcation involvement at the upper first molar.

probe that has been designed to overcome these difficulties (Figure 2.2.10).

Radiographic Assessment

Furcation involvements should be visible on radiographs. However, it is not always possible to interpret accurately the amount of bone loss in the furcation area. Upper molars are usually the most difficult teeth to assess on radiographs (Figure 2.2.11).

Clinical Assessment

The difficulty with relying on the visible appearance of a furcation is that there needs to have been enough recession for the furcation to be visible (Figure 2.2.12).

In common with the classification systems for tooth mobility, most systems for the assessment of furcation involvement have developed criteria to define mild, moderate or severe furcation involvements. One example is the system described by Lindhe & Nyman (1975) using a Nabers probe graduated at 3 mm:

Degree I – horizontal penetration into furcation <3 mm.
Degree II – horizontal penetration into furcation >3 mm but not encompassing the total width of the furcation area.

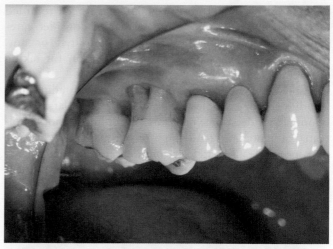

• **Figure 2.2.12** Clinically visible furcation involvement at the upper first molar.

Degree III – a "through-and-through" furcation defect.

A similar system devised by Hamp et al. (1975) uses the width of the tooth as the measure of furcation involvement and is more commonly used:

Degree 1 – loss of horizontal periodontal support not exceeding one-third of the width of the tooth.
Degree 2 – loss of horizontal periodontal support exceeding one-third of the width of the tooth but not encompassing the total width of the furcation.
Degree 3 – a "through-and-through" furcation defect.

Assessment of Suppuration

Suppuration is assessed by noting the presence or absence of suppuration (pus). Pus can sometimes be mixed with blood and can be under-recorded.

Assessment of Bone Support

The only practical way of assessing bone levels is by radiography. Choice of radiographic technique should be made after a thorough clinical examination. The overall dental needs of the patient, not just the periodontal needs, should be considered. For further guidance, see the Faculty of General Dental Practice (UK) *Selection Criteria for Dental Radiography*, 3rd edition (2013, updated 2018).

If a patient has uniform loss of attachment less than 6 mm, horizontal bitewing radiographs of the posterior teeth should capture the bone levels of the posterior teeth (Figure 2.2.13).

If a patient has loss of attachment of 6 mm or more, consider taking vertical bitewing radiographs rather than horizontal bitewing radiographs. However, vertical bitewings are rarely used in general practice and most clinicians would prefer periapical views, using a paralleling technique (Figure 2.2.14), which have a number of advantages:

• The periapical tissues can be assessed for pathological change.
• The entire root system can be assessed for other pathology.
• Bone loss can be assessed in percentage terms.

If detailed clinical measurements have been recorded and previous radiographs are available, consider carefully whether new radiographs are required or not. There should always be clinical justification for taking radiographs.

If there are concurrent problems for which radiography is indicated, for example, symptomatic third molars or orthodontic considerations, or if intra-oral films cannot be tolerated, a panoramic radiograph of optimal quality may be an appropriate alternative to consider. However, in general, periapical radiographs have better diagnostic value than panoramic radiographs.

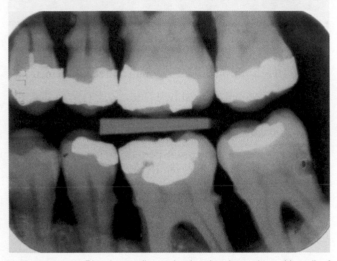

• **Figure 2.2.13** Bitewing radiograph showing bone loss. Not all of the bone margins are visible on this bitewing radiograph. This is an example of which it might have been better to take vertical bitewing radiographs.

Radiographs in Periodontal Assessment

Interpretation of Radiographs

Radiographs tend to underestimate the level of bone loss. In addition, changes in the settings of an X-ray machine, such as voltage and exposure time, will affect the image seen as will changes in the angulation of the film and/or the X-ray beam. Particular care needs to be taken when interpreting panoramic radiographs because if teeth or parts of teeth fall outside the focal trough, the appearance will be distorted. This sometimes happens because of the angulation of the roots of anterior teeth. The roots can appear shorter and blunter than they actually are. Also, panoramic radiographs can magnify some areas of the jaw, leading to a distortion in the appearance of the bone levels.

Viewing and Reporting on Radiographs

Whenever a radiograph is taken, all the information that can be obtained from the radiograph should be reported in the patient records. For example, if radiographs were taken primarily for assessment of the bone levels, remember to report on any other abnormalities or pathology seen. It can be easy to forget to note a carious lesion when the primary reason for taking the radiograph was for a periodontal assessment.

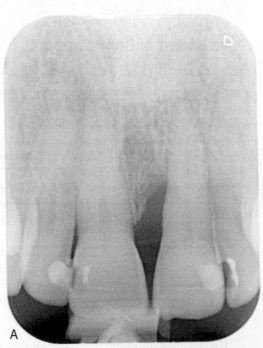
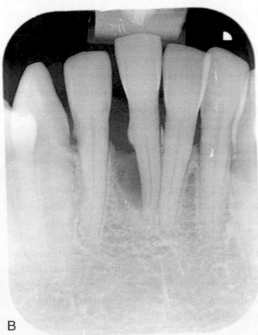

A   B

• **Figure 2.2.14** Periapical radiographs of anterior teeth with bone loss.

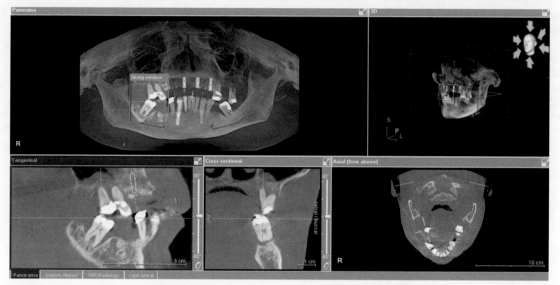

• **Figure 2.2.15** CBCT image, including periodontal defects.

When assessing the periodontium on a radiograph, always note the amount of bone present as a percentage of the total that should be present. Take into account the age of the patient. Always compare older radiographs with recently taken ones. It is then possible to monitor the amount of bone loss that has occurred since the last radiographs were taken. It might be possible to obtain copies of older radiographs from a colleague so consider asking for these before deciding whether or not new radiographs need to be taken.

New Radiographic Techniques

Cone beam computerised tomography (CBCT) is starting to gain wider acceptance. It has the advantage of providing a very detailed image of the site under investigation. It is possible to view the full three-dimensional appearance of a periodontal bony defect (Figure 2.2.15). The main disadvantage of CBCT is the amount of radiation required to obtain the image. If a CBCT image is taken, as with any radiographic image, it is vital that everything detected on the image is fully reported. It may therefore be necessary to obtain a report from a colleague who has additional training in this form of dental radiography.

Monitoring a Periodontal Patient

Once a patient has been assessed, a diagnosis can be reached and a treatment plan can be formulated. Following treatment, it is essential that the patient is reassessed to see if the treatment has been successful or not. Once periodontal stability has been achieved, it is important to monitor the patient to ensure there is no recurrence of disease.

Monitoring for life will be important to check that the patient remains stable.

All assessments and reassessments should be accurately recorded in the dental records. There are a number of computerised record management systems and various paper record charts. It does not matter which system is used as long as the information is recorded accurately and can be retrieved at a later date so that any record can be compared with previous records to monitor patient progress.

KEY POINT 7

To assess and monitor the periodontal condition of an individual patient:
- Take a complete set of measurements.
- Compare with previous sets of measurements.
- Decide if any radiographs are required.
- Interpret all the information gathered.
- Draw up an appropriate treatment plan which should include how frequently to reassess the patient.
- Monitor the patient by repeated reassessments to check the condition of the patient.

Multiple choice questions on the contents of this chapter are available online at Elsevier eBooks+.

A series of videos demonstrating how to assess the periodontium are also available online.

References

Ainamo J, Bay I. Problems and proposals for recording gingivitis and plaque. *Int Dent J.* 1975;25:229–235.

Ainamo J, Barmes D, Beagrie G, Cutress T, Martin J, Sardo-Infiri J. Development of the World Health Organisation (WHO) Community Periodontal Index of Treatment Needs (CPITN). *Int Dent J.* 1982;32:281–291.

Chapple ILC, Mealey BL, et al. Periodontal health and gingival diseases and conditions on an intact and a reduced periodontium: consensus report of workgroup 1 of the 2017 World Workshop on the Classification of Periodontal and Peri-Implant Diseases and Conditions. *J Clin Periodontol.* 2018;45(suppl 20):S68–S77.

Hamp SE, Nyman S, Lindhe J. Periodontal treatment of multirooted teeth. Results after 5 years. *J Clin Periodontol.* 1975;2:126–135.

Lindhe J, Nyman S. The effect of plaque control and surgical pocket elimination on the establishment and maintenance of periodontal health. A longitudinal study of periodontal therapy in cases of advanced disease. *J Clin Periodontol.* 1975;2:67–79.

Lindhe J, Haffajee AD, Socransky SS. Progression of periodontal disease in adult subjects in the absence of periodontal therapy. *J Clin Periodontol.* 1983;10:433–442.

Löe H, Silness J. Periodontal disease in pregnancy. Prevalence and severity. *Acta Odontol Scand.* 1963;21:533–551.

Miller SC. *Textbook of Periodontia.* 3rd ed. Philadelphia: The Blakeston Co; 1950.

O'Leary TJ, Drake RB, Naylor JE. The plaque control record. *J Periodontol.* 1972;43:38.

Silness J, Löe H. Periodontal disease in pregnancy. II. Correlation between oral hygiene and periodontal condition. *Acta Odontol Scand.* 1964;22:121–135.

Turesky S, Gilmore ND, Glickman I. Reduced plaque formation by the chloromethyl analogue of vitamine C. *J Periodontol.* 1970;41:41–43.

2.3

Gingival Enlargement

ALAN WOODMAN

CHAPTER OUTLINE

OVERVIEW OF THE CHAPTER

This chapter explains the varied aetiology, descriptive terminology, clinical significance and practical management of gingival enlargement.

By the end of the chapter the reader should:

*   Appreciate the practical difficulties which gingival enlargement presents in periodontal treatment
*   Understand the varied origins of gingival enlargement
*   Recognize the potential interactions with associated medications
*   Understand the options for reduction of gingival enlargement
*   Be able to discuss with patients the implications of gingival enlargement.

The chapter covers the following topics:

*   Introduction
*   The aetiology of gingival enlargement
*   The mechanisms of gingival enlargement
*   Common causes of gingival enlargement
*   Drug-induced gingival enlargement
*   Hormonal gingival enlargement
*   Other causes of gingival enlargement
*   Conclusion (reaching a diagnosis)

Introduction

Gingival enlargement may, in very rare circumstances, be associated with serious disease such as leukaemia but, in the vast majority of cases, the condition has a less sinister origin and causes problems of a more practical nature. From the patient's perspective, gingival enlargement may reach disfiguring proportions and be a cause of cosmetic distress, whereas the clinician's cause for concern lies with the obstruction of good oral hygiene practice and its probable consequences: the development of gingivitis or periodontitis and dental caries.

In the past, the terms "gingival hyperplasia" and "gingival hypertrophy" have been used, often inappropriately,

in the description of this condition. However, without histological examination of the affected tissues these terms are unsuitable and are best avoided unless a firm histopathological diagnosis is made. Thus the use of the term "gingival enlargement" is considered more appropriate, as recommended by the 2017 World Workshop on Classification in Periodontology, than the formerly used "gingival overgrowth", to which historical references will be frequently found (Caton et al. 2018).

The Aetiology of Gingival Enlargement

There are many causes of enlargement of the gingival tissues, the most common and obvious being the presence of

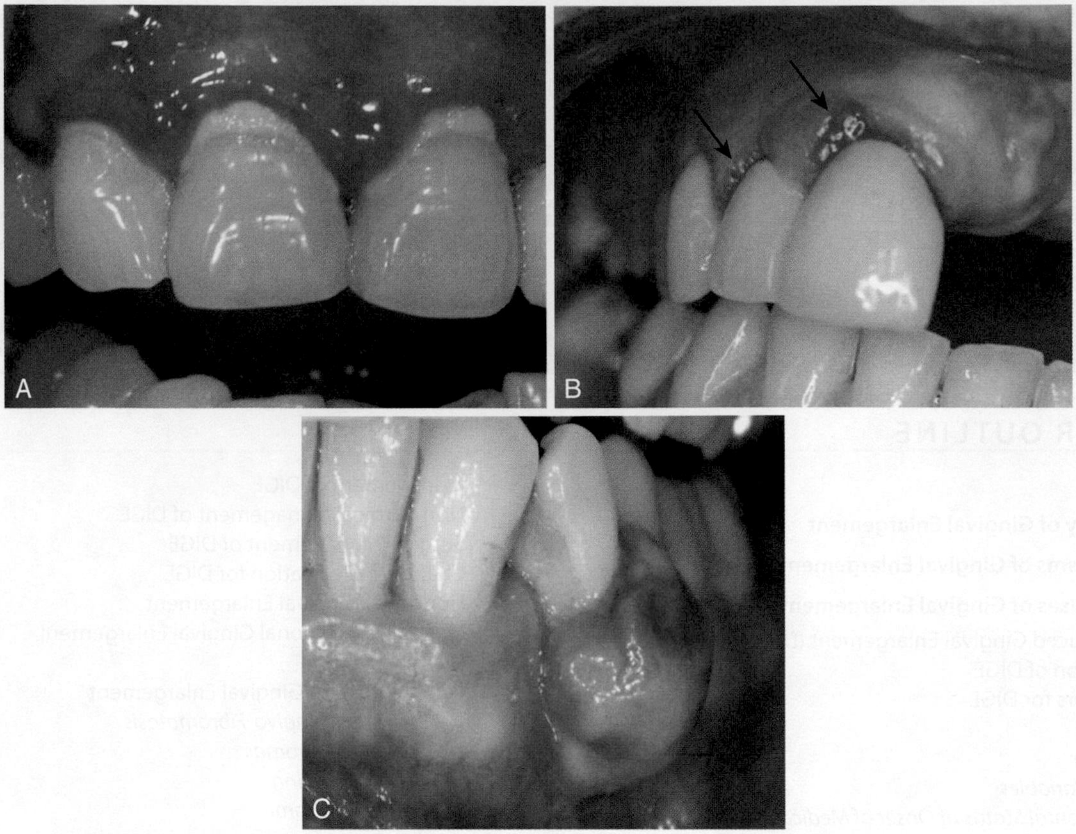

• **Figure 2.3.1** Examples of inflammatory, oedematous, plaque-induced gingival enlargements: (A) poor plaque control in the presence of a desquamative gingivitis; (B) poorly designed crowns prohibiting effective oral hygiene; (C) a pyogenic granuloma.

inflammatory oedema associated with gingivitis (Figure 2.3.1). However, the term "gingival enlargement" is generally regarded as being related to an altered production of the cellular components of the tissue, in particular gingival fibroblasts.

This chapter concentrates on the non-inflammatory components of the process, although inflammation of the disordered tissue may well accompany the cellular irregularities.

To achieve such changes in cell activity, a stimulus is required, which may be in the form of:
• Drugs
• Hormones
• Developmental aberrations
• Genetic influences
• Neoplasms.

Types of tissue enlargement may be determined histologically as:
• Hypertrophic
• Hyperplastic.

However, the clinical appearance of enlarged tissues alone cannot distinguish between these descriptors.

Hypertrophy means that the tissue is enlarged due to the presence of enlarged cells.

Definition: "A non-tumorous enlargement of an organ or a tissue as a result of an increase in the size rather than the number of constituent cells".

Any cell type can become hypertrophic:
• epithelium
• fibroblasts

• myoblasts.

Histologically, the cell type that is affected will have a normal appearance in all aspects except for the fact that it is abnormally large.

Hyperplasia means that the tissue contains an abnormal number of or "too many" cells.

Definition: "An abnormal increase in the number of cells in an organ or a tissue with consequent enlargement".

Any cell type can become hyperplastic:
• epithelium
• fibroblasts
• myoblasts.

Histologically, the cell type that is affected will have a normal appearance but there is simply an excessive number of cells.

The Mechanisms of Gingival Enlargement

Although extensively studied, the actual mechanism for the over-production of gingival tissues remains unproven. The most common cell involved in the development of gingival enlargement appears to be the fibroblast, but the development is only rarely found without some influence of plaque biofilm (Seymour et al. 1996).

Studies of drug-induced gingival enlargement (DIGE) have implicated the fibroblast in three possible ways (Seymour et al. 1996).
• An over-production of cells (hyperplasia)

- An over-production of collagenous matrix, associated with the actions of known inflammatory mediators such as matrix metalloproteinases (MMPs) and tissue inhibitors of MMPs (TIMPs)
- An over-production of non-collagenous matrix (glycosaminoglycans and proteoglycans), as shown by in vitro studies
- An alteration in connective tissue metabolism, resulting in reduced degradation of collagen.

In drug-induced enlargement, which has been most extensively studied, it is proposed that the fibroblasts in those subjects who show gingival enlargement are more susceptible to the presenting stimuli, especially medication, having been shown to exhibit increased protein synthesis (of collagen). However, there is no evidence of such fibrotic change in other parts of the body, thus allowing for speculation that the local presence of the dental plaque biofilm and the attendant inflammatory pathogenic pathways and subsequent inflammatory mediators conspire to produce an enhanced response to the plaque (Seymour et al. 1996).

A common finding of many histochemical studies of such tissues is that there is a shift in the normal calcium/sodium flux within the fibroblasts, irrespective of the particular drug used, which may provide the common link between the different groups of drugs associated with gingival enlargement (Seymour et al. 1996).

More recently it has been proposed that, under the influence of certain medications, decreased cation influx of folic acid active transport within gingival fibroblasts leads to decreased cellular folate uptake, which in turn leads to changes in matrix metalloproteinase metabolism and the failure to activate collagenase. Decreased availability of activated collagenase results in decreased degradation of accumulated connective tissue, which presents as DIGE (Brown & Arany 2014, Ramirez-Ramiz et al. 2017).

As gingival enlargement develops, the epithelial layer deepens and the rete pegs become more pronounced into the connective tissue layer, where the majority of the changes take place. The increasing density of collagen gives the tissue a pitted or fissured appearance and increased surface keratinization is common (American Academy of Periodontology [AAP] 2004).

Common Causes of Gingival Enlargement

Drug-Induced Gingival Enlargement (DIGE)

For many years, the drug most commonly encountered in patients presenting with gingival enlargement was that associated with anti-epileptic therapy, phenytoin (brand names Dilantin, Epanutin) (Figure 2.3.2). However, with the development of medical techniques for organ transplantation, several "anti-rejection" drugs have also been associated with DIGE. In more recent years, the increasing use of "calcium channel blocking" medication in the control of hypertension, a very common complaint in the middle aged and elderly, has led to the development of a much more

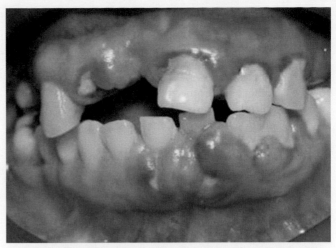

• **Figure 2.3.2** DIGE associated with phenytoin.

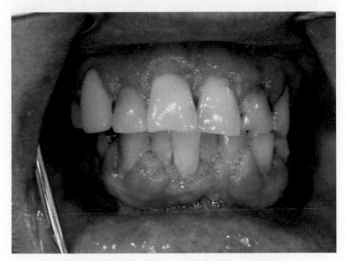

• **Figure 2.3.3** DIGE associated with amlodipine.

widespread "at risk" population and such enlargement is presenting in the dental surgery more frequently as a result (Figure 2.3.3). Fortunately such effects are now more widely recognized within the specialty of cardiology in particular, and the need for an inter-disciplinary approach to patient management is clear (Bajkovec et al. 2021).

> ### KEY POINT 1
> Check the patient's medical history for drugs such as:
> - Anticonvulsants
> - Immunosuppressants (calcineurin inhibitors)
> - Calcium channel blockers.

Commonly used drugs that can cause gingival enlargement include:
- Phenytoin (Dilantin, Epanutin)
  - for treatment of epileptic conditions
  - use has declined in recent years, as other medication has been introduced (e.g. phenobarbitone and carbamazepine), but when used in combination with these other anti-convulsants the overgrowth is likely to be greater
  - also used prophylactically in the prevention of post-neurosurgical seizures.

- Cyclosporin
  - immunosuppressant used in anti-rejection treatment for transplant patients that
    may also be used in the treatment of:
    - diabetes
    - Bechet's syndrome
    - multiple sclerosis
    - systemic lupus erythematosus
    - erosive lichen planus.
- Calcium channel blockers (e.g. nifedipine, amlodipine, diltiazem) used as
  - blood pressure regulators and as vasodilators in angina and hypertension.

Several other drugs have reportedly been *associated* with gingival enlargement, but there is insufficient evidence to prove their involvement:

- Tacrolimus: a relatively new anti-rejection drug; however, it may be that patients who are changed from cyclosporin to tacrolimus have a residual effect from the cyclosporin
- Sodium valproate and erythromycin, but these are both case reports only.

Distribution of DIGE

Findings from various studies, mainly based on patients seen in referral centres, show that:

- DIGE is more prevalent in the anterior labial gingiva
- the interdental areas predominate
- the enlargement is dense, firm and characteristically lobulated
- there is a minimal tendency to bleed, unless plaque levels are high
- gingival changes usually occur within 3 months of starting medication
- growth is most rapid in the first year
- histologically, enlargement shows an increase in the connective tissue component of the gingiva, rather than a cellular hyperplasia
- thus fibroblasts are the cells usually deemed responsible for the over-reaction or proliferation.

Risk Factors for DIGE

Age

Children and teenagers are more susceptible; this may be a hormonal factor as androgens stimulate fibroblast activity.

Gender

Males are more susceptible than females. However, there have been more males in the relevant studies, and the studies may have been influenced by related periodontal, genetic or hormonal factors.

Drug Variables

Drug dosage does not appear to be related to severity or prevalence.

Drugs used in combination, e.g. cyclosporin with nifedipine or amlodipine, may increase the severity and prevalence

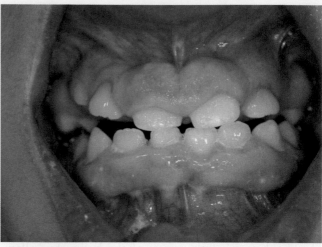

- **Figure 2.3.4** Gingival enlargement and delayed maturation in a 13-year-old affected by heroin *in utero*.

of enlargement, whereas transplant patients also receiving prednisolone and azathioprine show reduced severity (King et al. 1993, Wilson et al. 1998, Montebugnoli et al. 2000). Drug abuse may have an effect on the development of the gingival tissues in utero, producing "thick" tissues obstructive to normal eruption (Figure 2.3.4).

Periodontal Status at Onset of Medication

It is logical to assume that poor plaque control plays a major role in predisposing the tissues in the susceptible patient; however, it is uncertain whether the plaque initiates the enlargement or accumulates subsequently. It is agreed that the re-growth of tissue can be reduced by meticulous plaque control (Seymour et al. 2000).

Incidence of DIGE

The incidence of clinically significant gingival enlargement in patients receiving the three main drugs has been estimated as (Thomason et al. 1993):

- Phenytoin 50%
- Cyclosporin 27%
- Nifedipine 20%
- Cyclosporin and nifedipine 48%.

Management of DIGE

Mavrogiannis et al. (2006) have suggested that the management of the enlargement will depend upon the underlying cause and the clinical significance, considering the following:

- How obstructive or disfiguring are the tissues?
- Is there restriction of normal function by gross enlargement?
- Is a change in medication realistic or possible?
- Could a simple change to oral hygiene activity control the plaque component?
- Would the patient accept a surgical approach?

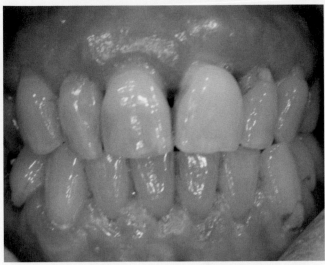

• **Figure 2.3.5** Patient on long-term nifedipine, managed by good plaque control alone and regular dental hygienist supportive care.

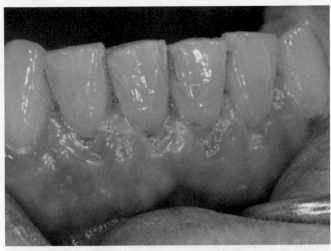

• **Figure 2.3.6** The same patient on long-term nifedipine; note the gingival enlargement is not unsightly, nor a problem for function.

Therefore, three approaches may be taken, either singly or in combination.
- Conventional, non-surgical periodontal therapy
  - With meticulous personal and professional plaque control
- Surgical reduction of the enlargement
  - Accompanied by meticulous personal and professional plaque control
- Change in medication
  - With meticulous personal and professional plaque control.

Non-Surgical Management of DIGE

The main aim is to reduce the inflammatory component in the tissues (Seymour et al. 1996, Montebugnoli et al. 2000, AAP 2004).

Case reports show that the conventional non-surgical management and subsequent plaque control can result in complete resolution of DIGE, especially from calcium channel blockers (Thomason et al. 1993, Montebugnoli et al. 2000) (Figures 2.3.5 and 2.3.6).

All patients at risk will benefit from a course of non-surgical periodontal treatment and extensive follow up. They should ideally receive such treatment before they start medication, but this is often impractical especially for organ transplant patients.

Antiseptic mouthwash, such as chlorhexidine gluconate, may be used as an adjunct to the non-surgical management and, in animal studies, it has been shown that chlorhexidine alone can reduce the cyclosporin DIGE.

Systemic antibiotics have also been studied and it is postulated that antibiotics reduce the bacterial infection and hence inflammation and also reduce the activity of the fibroblasts.

Phenytoin is known to inhibit folic acid metabolism, so a folic acid mouthwash may be of use in patients who are low in folate.

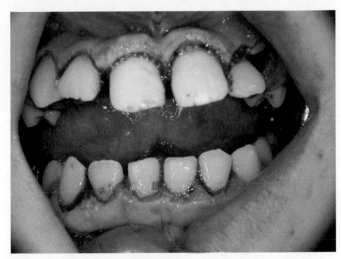

• **Figure 2.3.7** Gingivectomy approach using radiowave frequency surgery to the upper and lower gingiva for the child in Figure 2.3.4 at age 13, recurrence of the enlargement having taken place.

Surgical Management of DIGE

Surgical management of DIGE also applies to other causes of gingival enlargement. The objective is to remove the excess tissue for improvement in plaque control and aesthetics.

This can be done as a gingivectomy, using:

- Incisional surgery
- Electrosurgery (diathermy) or
- Radiowave frequency surgery (Figure 2.3.7).
- These approaches leave a painful raw surface, and a protective periodontal dressing may be required for 7–10 days. The final shape of the healed tissue may prove unpredictable, especially if the medication remains unchanged.
- Alternatively an inverse bevel ("filleting") flap procedure may be used. This leaves a less exposed, more comfortable surface and more control can be exercised over the final shape (Figure 2.3.8) but
- the technique is more difficult to carry out, especially on grossly enlarged, fibrous tissues.

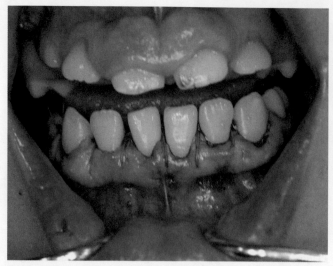

• **Figure 2.3.8** Flap approach to the lower gingiva for the same child at age 16.

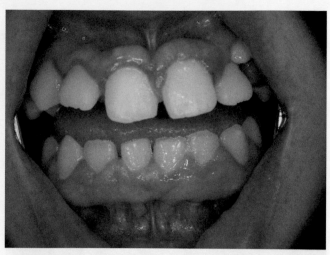

• **Figure 2.3.9** Healing 10 months after the radiowave frequency surgery shown in 2.3.7. Note the tissues are again showing a tendency for enlargement to recur.

Whichever approach is undertaken, it is essential that the patient's personal and professional plaque control is meticulous to avoid recurrence of the enlargement, *especially if their medication does not change.*

Should the patient's medication not change they must be warned that re-growth of the tissues may still occur despite the preventive approaches described previously (Figure 2.3.9). Studies have reported as many as 34% of patients requiring repeated surgical intervention (Mavrogiannis et al. 2006).

> **KEY POINT 2**
> Regular dental hygiene supportive care is an integral part of the management process, usually at 3 to 4 monthly intervals.

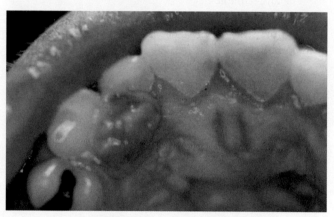

• **Figure 2.3.10** A pregnancy "epulis".

Changing Medication for DIGE

This is the ideal long-term solution but, while it may seem appealing to the dentist simply to ask the patient's medical practitioner to change the medication, this is not always practical. The underlying health reasons for the continuing prescription of these important drugs will carry more weight than the dental complications. It may be that alternative medications have already been tried and found less effective, but patients should always be made aware that either they or their dentist should approach the medical practitioner to explore their options. The major difficulty lies in convincing the treating physician that reducing the effects on their patient's "gums" will be worthwhile.

Hormonal Gingival Enlargement

This is plaque related, and the female hormones during pregnancy, oestrogen in particular, can be responsible for inducing:

- An altered microcirculation (from increased progesterone) and an altered sub-gingival microflora from the second to eighth months of pregnancy, allowing gingival fragility, increased bleeding and an enhanced reaction

to the plaque – "pregnancy gingivitis" (Carrillo-de-Albornoz et al. 2012).
- Specific localized gingival enlargement, in combination with plaque-induced inflammatory processes:
  - Pregnancy epulis (tumour) (Figures 2.3.10 and 2.3.11).
- Generalized plaque-related enlargement and similar gingival fragility can be associated with:
  - Puberty
  - Oral contraception (OC)
  - Hormone replacement therapy (HRT)
  - Any situation where disturbed levels of progesterone/oestrogen is found, such as ovarian disease.

Usually, the gingiva returns to normal when plaque control is achieved and the hormone levels are stable but, in some cases, fibrotic scarring may remain and distort the gingival contour.

Managing Hormonal Gingival Enlargement

A pregnancy epulis may need surgical resection (in the same manner as DIGE) (see Figure 2.3.11) if it becomes unsightly or obstructive to oral hygiene or occlusal function. Lesser lesions usually resolve with the end of pregnancy.

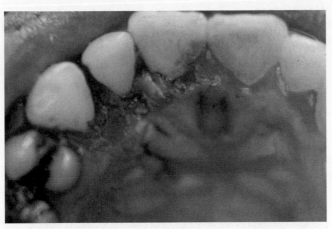

• **Figure 2.3.11** Pregnancy "epulis" removed with electrosurgery.

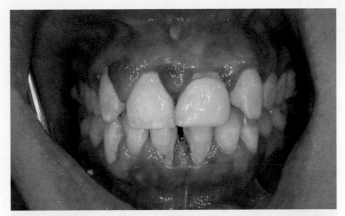

• **Figure 2.3.12** A 26-year-old woman after 8 years with poor diabetic control.

In the majority of cases, when the pregnancy ends, any fragility of the gingival tissue will resolve with good oral hygiene and suitable dental hygiene support.

Varying the type or dosage of OC or HRT medication may reduce the problem. Many patients receive HRT without having a true titre of their oestrogen or progesterone levels taken. Thus the oestrogen level achieved by the medication may be too high or too low and a degree of trial and error is often required to find the acceptable level to cope with the symptoms and effects of menopause. It is during this period that any gingival effects are most likely.

Good personal oral hygiene and continued regular professional hygiene support are the most important factors to minimize the risk of continuing gingival enlargement, or re-growth after surgical reduction.

Diabetes

Periodontal diseases in the presence of unstable diabetes may be associated with an exaggerated response to the plaque, resulting in an enlargement of inflammatory origin, which is often referred to as "hyperplastic gingivitis", as illustrated in Figure 2.3.12. With conventional nonsurgical care, this will resolve and, in many cases (such as this 26-year-old patient), the reduction in inflammatory mediators may facilitate an improvement in diabetic stability (Figure 2.3.13).

Other Causes of Gingival Enlargement

Hereditary Gingivo-Fibromatosis

This is a rare condition of unexplained origin where multiple enlargements occur within the oral environment.

- These may be obstructive to oral hygiene, or disfiguring.
- Surgical resection may be carried out but there is a strong tendency to recur.

Individual Fibromas

Such localized enlargements of the gingival margin are uncommon but, when they do occur (Figure 2.3.14), provide a cosmetic challenge to the clinician. These are best treated with an incisional approach, allowing for maximum

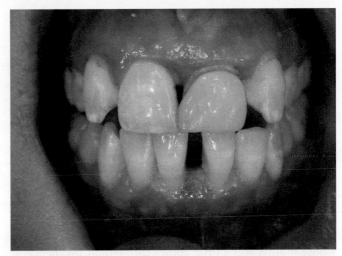

• **Figure 2.3.13** The same patient as seen in Figure 2.3.12, 3 months after non-surgical periodontal care and stabilisation of her diabetic control, showing an improvement in the gingival condition.

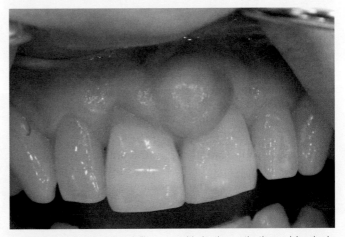

• **Figure 2.3.14** A localized fibroma with both aesthetic and hygienic compromises.

removal of the base of the fibrous tissue, thus minimizing the chance of recurrence (Figure 2.3.15).

Other unusual conditions that have been associated with gingival enlargement include:

- Wegner's granulomatosis, described as "strawberry gingivae"

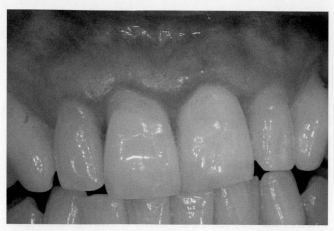

• **Figure 2.3.15** The same patient as seen in Figure 2.3.14 after fibroma excision to improve tissue contour.

- Neuro-fibromatosis
- Sarcoidosis
- Crohn's disease
- Scurvy – vitamin C deficiency
- Acromegaly.

These may have effects on the development of the gingival and dental tissues, presenting with delayed eruption – very thick gingival tissues resulting in failure of maturation of the normal gingival margin:crown relationship and a reduced clinical crown height. Surgical treatment may be indicated to achieve an improvement in aesthetics, to remove the tissues obstructing eruption or to facilitate orthodontic treatment. The previous illustrations in Figures 2.3.4, 2.3.7, 2.3.8 and 2.3.9 provide an example of a 13-year-old girl, whose mother was a drug abuser throughout pregnancy, at presentation and subsequently following gingival corrective surgery with an incisional approach and using radiowave frequency surgery.

Mouth Breathing

Patients who persistently mouth breathe, with poor lip seal, often show enlargement of the upper labial gingiva in the presence of minimal plaque and may present with an established enlargement of inflammatory origin. If fibrous scarring occurs within the gingiva, this condition can be very stubborn and may be difficult to suppress unless some protection from the drying effect of the mouth breathing can be achieved by lubrication or physical protection. Unless the mouth breathing can be addressed, a surgical solution is not appropriate. However, the periodic use of botulinum toxin to produce some immobilization of the upper lip over the revealed gingiva may prove beneficial.

Down's Syndrome

Patients with Down's syndrome have characteristically thick and fibrous gingiva. Although not usually considered as "gingival enlargement", the tissue may be similarly obstructive to oral hygiene measures, and, in some extreme circumstances, reshaping of the tissue may be deemed necessary to manage periodontal problems.

Neoplasms

Among the many sites and varieties of neoplastic disease identified within the oral cavity, tumours of the gingival tissues are fortunately rare, but squamous cell carcinoma may present as enlargement, with or without ulceration, and be confused with the other causes of gingival enlargement discussed previously. *Thus the presentation of unexplained enlargements should always be considered suspicious,* particularly as leukaemias may present in this way and do not always follow the characteristic bluish appearance generally described.

> ### KEY POINT 3
> Should excisional surgery be performed for localized lesions without a definitive drug- or hormone-related aetiology, *histological analysis should always be undertaken* to rule out a neoplasm.

- The enlargement in leukaemic patients is associated with both the dense infiltration of white blood cells into the tissues and an inability of the affected white blood cells to control the gingival infection associated with plaque. Although the management of neoplasms lies outside the scope of this chapter, the reader is strongly recommended to refer to the case report of gingival infiltration in acute monoblastic leukaemia in the *British Dental Journal* (Gallipoli & Leach 2007). This reminds clinicians that the acute onset of gingival enlargement is an unusual physical sign with a narrow differential diagnosis.

Conclusion – Reaching a Diagnosis

Determining the cause of the visible enlargement can usually be achieved by careful observation and history taking, without the need for histological analysis, in the case of:
- Prescription drugs: always establish the name of the drug the patient is prescribed
- Non-prescription drugs: is there a history of admitted abuse?
- Hormones: pregnancy is usually admitted or identifiable!
- Hormones: OC or HRT should be known as part of the medical history, but has this changed?
- Hormones: is the patient a diabetic and, if so, stable?
- Genetics: a family history may be obvious or admitted. The practitioner should also establish:
- How long has the enlargement been present?
- Are there any systemic or local modifying factors?
- Is there a known medical factor which might be implicated, e.g. diabetes?
- Has the patient recently been hospitalized or received a transplant?
- Is a detailed drug history available? (the most common cause of recent onset gingival enlargement is drug therapy)
- Are there any other unusual signs or symptoms?

Multiple choice questions on the contents of this chapter are available online at Elsevier eBooks+.

References

American Academy of Periodontology. Report on drug-associated gingival enlargement. *J Periodontol.* 2004;75:1424–1431.

Bajkovec L, Mrzljak A, Likic R, Alajbeg I. Drug-induced gingival overgrowth in cardiovascular patients. *World J Cardiol.* 2021;13(4):6875.

Brown RS, Arany PR. Mechanism of drug-induced overgrowth revisited: a unifying hypothesis. *Oral Diseases.* 2014;21(1):5161.

Carrillo-de-Albornoz A, Figuero E, Herrera D, Cuesta P, Bascones-Martínez A. Gingival changes during pregnancy: III. Impact of clinical, microbiological, immunological and socio-demographic factors on gingival inflammation. *J Clin Periodontol.* 2012;39:272–283.

Caton JG, Armitage G, Berglundh T, et al. A new classification scheme for periodontal and peri-implant diseases and conditions – Introduction and key changes from the 1999 classification. *J Clin Periodontol.* 2018;45(suppl 20):S1–S8.

Gallipoli P, Leach M. Gingival infiltration in acute monoblastic leukaemia. *Br Dent J.* 2007;205:507–509.

King GN, Fullinfaw R, Higgins TJ, Walker RG, Francis DMA, Wiesenfeld D. Gingival hyperplasia in renal allograft recipients receiving cyclosporin-A and calcium antagonists. *J Clin Periodontol.* 1993;20:286–293.

Mavrogiannis M, Ellis JM, Thomason JM, Seymour RA. The management of drug-induced gingival overgrowth. *J Clin Periodontol.* 2006;33:434–439.

Montebugnoli L, Servidio D, Bernardi F. The role of time in reducing gingival overgrowth in heart-transplanted patients following cyclosporin therapy. *J Clin Periodontol.* 2000;27:611–614.

Ramirez-Ramiz A, Brunet-Llobet L, Lahor-Soler E, Miranda-Ruis J. On the cellular and molecular mechanism of drug-induced gingival overgrowth. *Open Dent J.* 2017;11:420534.

Seymour RA, Thomason JM, Ellis JS. The pathogenesis of drug-induced gingival overgrowth. *J Clin Periodontol.* 1996;23:165–175.

Seymour RA, Ellis JS, Thomason JM. Risk factors for drug-induced gingival overgrowth. *J Clin Periodontol.* 2000;27:217–223.

Thomason JM, Seymour RA, Rice N. The prevalence and severity of cyclosporin and nifedipine-induced gingival overgrowth. *J Clin Periodontol.* 1993;20:37–40.

Wilson RF, Morel A, Smith D, Koffman CG, Ogg CS, Rigden SPA, Ashley FP. Contribution of individual drugs to gingival overgrowth in adult and juvenile renal transplant patients treated with multiple therapy. *J Clin Periodontol.* 1998;25:457–464.

2.4

PERIODONTITIS AND SYSTEMIC DISEASES

MARILOU CIANTAR AND KENNETH EATON

CHAPTER OUTLINE

OVERVIEW OF THE CHAPTER

This chapter covers the possible inter-relationship between periodontal and systemic diseases. It will examine how this may occur at a molecular level with a view to preventing and managing the respective diseases and their potential interactions.

By the end of this chapter the reader should be able to:

- Understand the possible interactions between periodontitis and certain systemic diseases
- View the management of periodontitis in the wider (systemic) context
- Offer better advice to patients suffering from periodontitis and concurrent systemic diseases which seem to have a possible interaction with periodontitis
- Consider the importance of liaising with physicians in managing such patients
- Recognise systemic conditions affecting the periodontium
- Be aware of the effect of medication on the periodontium.

This chapter will cover the following topics:

- Periodontitis and diabetes mellitus
- Periodontitis and cardiovascular disease
- Periodontitis and adverse pregnancy outcomes
- Periodontitis and respiratory diseases
- Periodontitis and dementia
- Periodontitis and other systemic diseases, including COVID-19
- Systemic conditions affecting the periodontium
- Systemic medication affecting the periodontium.

Introduction

Although the oral cavity is an integral part of the human body, it tends to be perceived, both by the general public and by dentists and doctors, as a separate entity from the rest of the body. This might be because the oral cavity and diseases associated with it fall within the remit of dentistry, whereas the diseases afflicting the rest of the body are encompassed in medicine often with little interaction taking place between the two disciplines. However, the perception that an interactive link between oral infections and systemic diseases might exist has long been established (Figure 2.4.1).

In the latter part of the last century, there was renewed interest in the focal infection concept, especially with respect

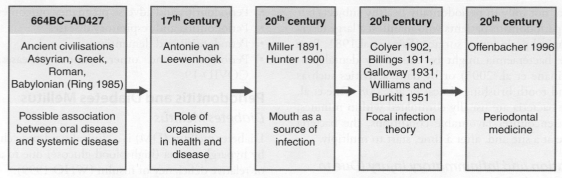

664BC–AD427	17th century	20th century	20th century	20th century
Ancient civilisations Assyrian, Greek, Roman, Babylonian (Ring 1985)	Antonie van Leewenhoek	Miller 1891, Hunter 1900	Colyer 1902, Billings 1911, Galloway 1931, Williams and Burkitt 1951	Offenbacher 1996
Possible association between oral disease and systemic disease	Role of organisms in health and disease	Mouth as a source of infection	Focal infection theory	Periodontal medicine

• **Figure 2.4.1** Periodontal–systemic interactions: chronological development.

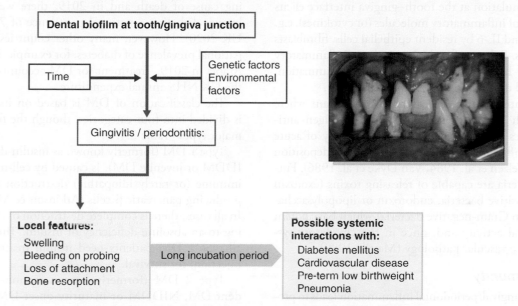

• **Figure 2.4.2** Possible link between periodontal diseases and systemic diseases.

to the field of periodontology. Within dentistry, periodontal diseases are a distinct entity in that they are more akin to medicine rather than the rest of dentistry in terms of disease aetiology, pathobiology and treatment. This has led to the development of periodontal medicine (Offenbacher 1996) – a two-way relationship in which periodontitis may influence the individual's systemic health and systemic disease may influence periodontal health.

In the last two decades there has been increasing interest and research in the topic, and new knowledge of the links between periodontitis and systemic diseases is being uncovered. For example in the last 6 years there have been several studies which have confirmed a link between periodontitis and dementia. Most recently, links between the severity of COVID-19 and periodontitis have been investigated.

Periodontitis and Systemic Disease

A clinical feature of periodontitis is inflammation leading to swelling of the gingiva and destruction of the periodontium. Histologically, this is confirmed not only by alveolar bone resorption and breakdown of the periodontal ligament but also by extensive ulceration of the pocket epithelium. It is estimated that in a patient with generalized moderate periodontitis

(probing depths averaging 5–6 mm per pocket), the total surface area of the pocket epithelium coming into contact with the subgingival bacterial biofilm is 25 cm² (Page 1998). This presents a large, ulcerated surface area in close approximation to the periodontal biofilm leading to potential transmigration of bacteria or their toxic products into the circulatory system. This, in addition to the severity and chronic nature of periodontitis, initiates a host-mediated immune response forming a reservoir of cytokines (interleukin-1 or IL-1, tumour necrosis factor-α or TNF-α, prostaglandin E₂ or PGE₂, thromboxane) in the periodontium which can induce and perpetuate both local and systemic effects (Figure 2.4.2) (Page 1998).

Potential Mechanisms Linking Oral Disease to Secondary Non-Oral Disease

Three mechanisms have been suggested which could potentially link oral and systemic disease (Thoden van Velzen et al. 1984, Van Dyke & Winkelhoff 2013).

Metastatic Infection (Due to Transient Bacteraemia)

Oral bacteria at the tooth/gingiva interface are capable of entering the periodontal tissues and eliciting a transient bacteraemia, not only in periodontally healthy subjects but more so in periodontitis patients who manifest a large ulcerated subgingival periodontal surface (Saito et al.1981, Page 1998). The bacteraemia might be caused by dental procedures (Kinane et al. 2005) or by daily activities such as chewing and tooth brushing (Lucas et al. 2008, Fine et al. 2010). The bacteria are usually eliminated within minutes, but if they encounter favourable conditions, the bacteria might settle at a site and, after a time, start to multiply.

Inflammation and Inflammatory Injury (Due to Innate Immunity)

Bacterial accumulation at the tooth–gingiva interface elicits cellular release of inflammatory molecules (or cytokines), e.g. TNF-α, IL-1 and IL-6 by resident epithelial cells, fibroblasts and phagocytes. Release of such chemical pro-inflammatory mediators may have an impact on systemic inflammation, e.g. endothelial dysfunction (D'Aiuto et al. 2004).

Bacterial antigens may enter the blood stream where they react with host antibodies to produce antigen–antibody complexes which may give rise to a variety of acute and chronic inflammatory reactions at sites of deposition (Thoden van Velzen et al. 1984, Van Dyke et al. 1986). Furthermore, bacteria are capable of releasing toxins (exotoxin from Gram-positive bacteria, endotoxin or lipopolysaccharide (LPS) from Gram-negative bacteria) which have potent pharmacological activity and, once in the circulatory system, can induce vascular pathology (Mattila 1989).

Adaptive Immunity

Persistence of gingival/periodontal inflammation leads to processing of bacterial antigens by the adaptive immune system, i.e. T-cell and B-cell activation. The B cells release antibodies (Ab), a soluble form of immunoglobulin, the aim of which is to eliminate invading bacterial antigens. T cells release a host of cytokines including IL and TNF-α which can contribute to periodontal tissue destruction and to other inflammatory conditions such as diabetes and cardiovascular disease.

Periodontal Diseases Contributing to Systemic Disease Susceptibility

Periodontitis may affect the patient's susceptibility to disease in three ways (Page 1998):
1. shared risk factors, e.g. smoking, ageing, stress and ethnicity are risk factors for both periodontitis and cardiovascular disease
2. subgingival biofilm – acts as a reservoir for bacterial toxins
3. a persistently inflamed periodontium acts as a reservoir for inflammatory mediators (cytokines).

Recent advances and research into periodontal medicine have shown that there is a possible relationship (correlation not causation) between periodontitis and the following systemic diseases (Van Dyke & van Winklehoff 2013, Linden et al. 2013):
- Periodontitis and diabetes mellitus
- Periodontitis and cardiovascular disease
- Periodontitis and adverse pregnancy outcomes
- Periodontitis and respiratory diseases
- Periodontitis and dementia
- Periodontitis and other systemic diseases, such as COVID-19.

Periodontitis and Diabetes Mellitus
Diabetes Mellitus

Diabetes mellitus (DM) is a clinical syndrome characterized by hyperglycaemia (high blood glucose) due to an absolute or relative deficiency of insulin (WHO 1999).

In the UK, DM complications are the seventh leading cause of death and in 2019, there were 4.9 million known diabetics, a national prevalence of 7.4% (Diabetes UK 2020). However, many other countries have a higher national prevalence of diabetes, for example 32.8% in Saudi Arabia in 2019. Treatment for DM accounts for 5–10% of the UK NHS annual expenditure.

The classification of DM is based on its aetiology and is divided into four categories, though the first two are the major types (Table 2.4.1).

Type 1 DM (formerly known as insulin-dependent DM, IDDM or juvenile DM), is caused by cell-medicated autoimmune (or rarely idiopathic) destruction of the insulin-producing pancreatic β cells (Atkinson & Maclaren 1994). In all cases, there is complete destruction of the β cells, leading to an absolute deficiency of insulin. This explains why all type 1 DM patients need insulin treatment (given by injection) for survival.

Type 2 DM (formerly known as non-insulin-dependent DM, NIDDM or maturity-onset DM) results from the interplay between genetic factors, obesity, increasing age and lack of physical exercise (Yki-Jarvinen 1994). Although the specific aetiologies of this type of DM are not known, autoimmune destruction of the β cells does not occur. Type 2 DM is characterized by impaired insulin secretion, peripheral resistance to insulin and hepatic insulin insensitivity. Impaired insulin secretion is due to reduced cell mass and altered insulin release (Crawford & Cotran 1994). Thus the pulsating release of insulin in response to a high glucose load seen in non-DM subjects is lost in type 2 DM patients. The hyperglycaemia seen in type 2 DM subjects can be controlled by dietary restriction and exercise. If it does not respond to such measures, additional treatment may include oral hypoglycaemic tablets and insulin.

Diagnosis

The primary methods used to diagnose and monitor blood glucose levels have traditionally been fasting blood glucose, a combination of fasting blood glucose and a 2-hour post-prandial glucose loading and oral glucose tolerance tests (American Diabetes Association 2015; Box 2.4.1). DM may be diagnosed by any one of the three methods; whichever method is used, it must be confirmed on a subsequent day using one of the three methods.

TABLE 2.4.1	Classification of diabetes mellitus (DM) based on the American Diabetes Association Classification	
Type of DM	**Aetiology**	
Type 1 DM	Autoimmune Idiopathic	
Type 2 DM	Obese type 2 DM Non-obese type 2 DM Maturity onset diabetes of the young (MODY)	
Gestational DM	Pregnancy	
DM secondary to systemic disease	Genetic defects in β-cell function Genetic defects in insulin function Pancreatic diseases or injury Infections Drug/chemical induced Endocrinopathies Other genetic syndromes associated with DM	

American Diabetes Association 2015

Pathobiology of diabetes mellitus

Prolonged hyperglycaemia leads to the formation of irreversible proteins known as AGEs (advanced glycation end products). The AGEs are widely deposited in cells and tissues and are responsible for the pathological features of DM, namely ophthalmic, neurological, cardiovascular, renal and vascular dysfunction and damage (WHO 1999). The altered vascular function and permeability, the altered cellular function (including migration and phagocytic activity of mononuclear and polymorphonuclear cells) and higher cytokine production increase the patient's susceptibility to infection, including periodontitis (Figure 2.4.3).

The Relationship Between Periodontitis and Diabetes Mellitus

The relationship between DM and periodontitis has long been established (Seiffert 1962). DM per se does not cause periodontitis. However, it is known to be a risk factor for periodontal breakdown (Taylor 2001). DM patients manifest an increased susceptibility in terms of periodontitis prevalence, severity and progression (Cianciola et al. 1992, Löe 1993, Collin et al. 1998), particularly in those with poorly controlled DM (Ainamo et al. 1990, Seppälä & Ainamo 1994) and DM of long duration (Firatli 1997). Periodontitis has been implicated as the sixth complication of DM (Löe 1993).

The clinical features of periodontitis in DM subjects are no different to those seen in non-DM subjects. However, the extent and severity of periodontitis may be more pronounced in patients with undiagnosed or poorly controlled diabetes. This holds true for both type 1 and type 2 DM. Patients who manifest advanced periodontitis should be questioned as to the possibility of having undiagnosed DM especially if they have a positive family history; a referral to the patient's doctor should be encouraged. In young

1. Symptoms of DM plus casual (non-fasting) plasma glucose of ≥11.1 mmol/L (≥200 mg/dL) Casual: any time of day or night without regard to time since last meal Symptoms of DM: polyuria, polydipsia, polyphagia
2. Fasting plasma glucose of ≥7 mmol/L (≥126 mg/dL); fasting: no caloric intake for 8 hours
3. Two-hour post-prandial glucose ≥11.1 mmol/L (≥200 mg/dL) after an oral glucose tolerance test (as per WHO, using a glucose load containing the equivalent of 75 g anhydrous glucose dissolved in water).
4. Glycated haemoglobin (HbA1c) ≥6.5% (test should be performed in a laboratory using an NGSP-certified method and standardized to DCCT assay).

DCCT: diabetes control and complications trial; NGSP: national glycohaemoglobin standardization programme

patients, recurrent periodontal abscesses might indicate the possibility of undiagnosed type 1 DM.

For a long time, the association between periodontitis and DM was considered unidirectional, i.e. DM predisposing to periodontitis. Recent research has shown that the relationship is most likely to be bi directional (see Figure 2.4.3 and Chapter 1.6) in that DM predisposes to periodontitis while periodontitis might exacerbate DM complications in a dose-dependent manner and is associated with an increased risk of developing type 2 diabetes (Taylor 2001, Mealey 2006, Lalla & Papapanou 2011, Lakschevitz et al. 2011, Borgnakke et al. 2013).

The cytokine reservoir produced as a result of periodontitis not only leads to periodontal destruction, but it also interferes with glucose metabolism leading to hyperglycaemia, therefore exacerbating the pathology associated with diabetes. Chronic hyperglycaemia undermines macrophage and neutrophil function, reducing their antibacterial activity, and alters vascular function, increasing the patient's susceptibility to periodontitis. The inflammatory cell phenotype consequent to hyperglycaemia leads to a burst of inflammatory cytokines (TNF-α, IL-1, IL-6) which contribute to periodontal destruction and interfere with wound healing. In addition, alterations in gingival crevicular fluid, collagen metabolism and altered subgingival microflora (McNamara et al. 1982, Ciantar 2002) contribute to periodontitis.

Periodontal Treatment in Diabetes Patients

Effective antimicrobial (plaque control) therapy is the mainstay of periodontal treatment. In DM–periodontitis subjects, diabetes needs to be controlled in order to achieve satisfactory outcomes after periodontal treatment. Where diabetes control is established, the periodontal outcome is the same as for non-diabetics (Tervonen & Karjalainen 1997). In addition, recent evidence has shown that periodontal treatment seems to improve glucose control in both type 1 and type 2 diabetic subjects (Grossi et al. 1997, Iwamoto et al. 2001, Engebretson & Kocher 2013, Sgolastra

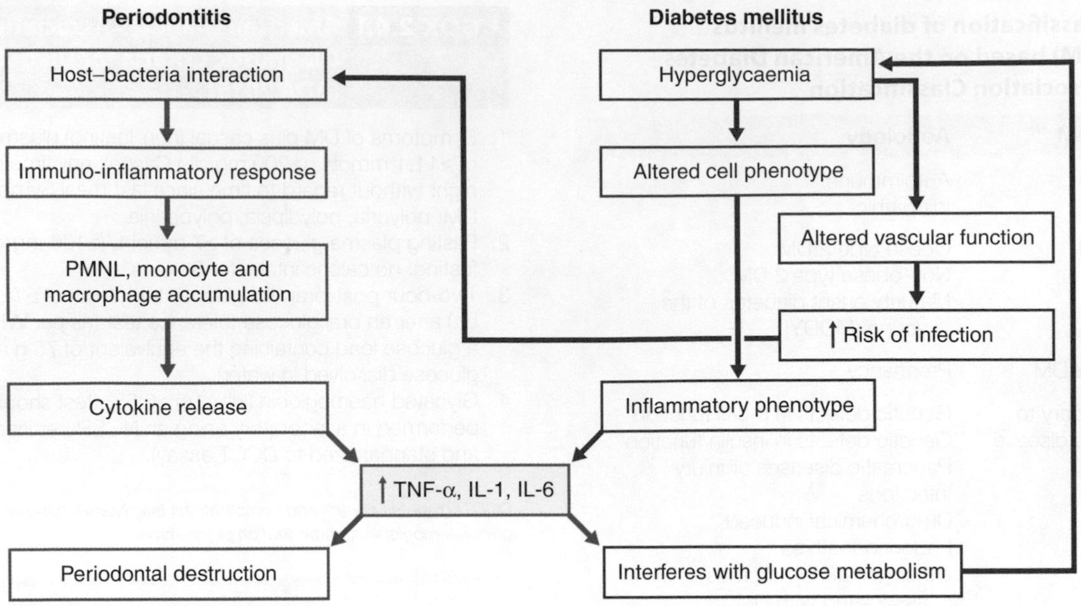

Periodontitis

Diabetes mellitus

```
Host–bacteria interaction                 Hyperglycaemia
         │                                      │
         ▼                                      ▼
Immuno-inflammatory response          Altered cell phenotype
         │                                      │
         ▼                                      ▼
PMNL, monocyte and                    Altered vascular function
macrophage accumulation                      │
         │                                      ▼
         ▼                              ↑ Risk of infection
Cytokine release                      Inflammatory phenotype
```

↑ TNF-α, IL-1, IL-6

```
Periodontal destruction          Interferes with glucose metabolism
```

• **Figure 2.4.3** Bi-directional relationship between periodontitis and diabetes mellitus.

et al. 2013). The most plausible explanation is that periodontal treatment reduces circulating levels of TNF-α, increased levels of which suppress insulin action thereby leading to elevated blood glucose (Kanety et al. 1995). Thus control of periodontal inflammation is crucial to eliminate periodontal disease and seems to benefit diabetes control.

Robust and consistent evidence showing that severe periodontitis undermines glycaemic control in DM subjects and that it contributes to DM complications in a dose-dependent manner has led to guidelines being issued highlighting the importance of periodontal care in such patients (Chapple & Genco 2013). The guidelines provide patient management recommendations to dentists, physicians and other healthcare professionals and educational information to DM patients regarding the need for periodontal care. DM patients should also be made aware of other oral complications of diabetes, e.g. burning mouth, xerostomia, increased risk of infections (bacterial and fungal) and delayed wound healing.

KEY POINT 1

- Periodontitis and DM have a bi-directional relationship
- DM does not cause periodontitis
- DM is a risk factor for periodontitis
- Uncontrolled DM of long duration exacerbates periodontitis
- Treatment of periodontitis seems to lead to some improvement in diabetes control
- Dentists should ask patients about the possibility of undiagnosed DM
- For all recently diagnosed type 1 & 2 DM patients, periodontal examination is recommended as part of their diabetes management
- Dentists and physicians should collaborate in the management of DM patients
- Patients should be made aware of the importance of periodontal care especially if they are diagnosed with DM
- Oral health care education should be provided to all DM patients

---

Periodontitis and Cardiovascular Diseases

Cardiovascular diseases comprise high blood pressure, coronary heart disease, angina pectoris and myocardial infarction, peripheral arterial disease and stroke (cerebrovascular accident). These diseases are consequent to narrowing of blood vessels or atherosclerosis. Atherosclerosis can lead to significant morbidity and mortality; atherosclerosis and the ensuing cardiovascular complications are the leading cause of death in the Western world. Although the main cause of atherosclerosis is fat deposition in the arterial wall possibly due to a high fat diet and lack of exercise, increasing evidence suggests that chronic infections may cause atherosclerosis (Syrjanen et al. 1998, Leinonen et al. 2002).

Periodontitis, because of its chronic nature, has been implicated as a potential risk factor leading to atherosclerosis (Beck & Offenbacher 2001, Desvarieux et al. 2003).

The hypothesis linking periodontitis and cardiovascular disease was first proposed in the late 1980s (Mattila et al. 1989). This research was initiated as the traditional risk factors for cardiovascular disease (hypertension, smoking, diabetes, high serum cholesterol concentration, low high-density lipoprotein cholesterol concentration and low socio-economic status) could not fully account for the clinical and epidemiological features of atherosclerotic cardiovascular disease.

The original hypothesis implicating periodontitis as a contributory factor to atherosclerosis was that periodontal pathogens (such as *Porphyromonas gingivalis*) were isolated from atheromatous plaques (Haraszthy et al. 2000). In vitro studies have shown that this organism is capable of invading endothelial cells (Deshpande et al. 1998, Dorn et al. 1999, Kuramitsu et al. 2002). The subsequent abundant release of biochemical mediators consequent to *P. gingivalis* invasion is thought to be an important contributor to the development of atherosclerosis (Yumoto et al. 2005). Furthermore, oral bacteria are also capable of inducing platelet aggregation

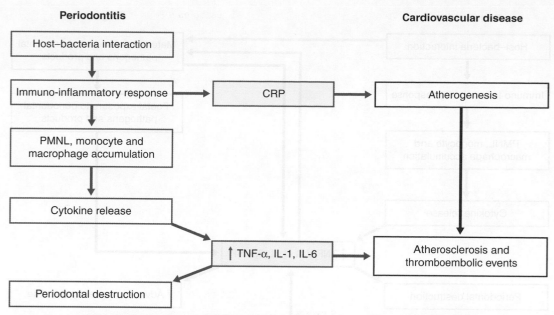

Periodontitis

Cardiovascular disease

• **Figure 2.4.4** Possible mechanisms between periodontitis and cardiovascular disease.

and thrombus formation, thereby contributing to the progression of the atherosclerotic lesion (Herzberg et al. 1994). However, while oral bacteria might become nested within atherosclerotic lesions and contribute to their progression, this might not always be the case.

An indirect plausible hypothesis linking periodontitis to atherosclerosis and, therefore, cardiovascular disease is based on the systemic increase of inflammatory cytokines (TNF-α, CRP, IL-1, IL-6) triggered by bacterial components, such as lipopolysaccharide, subsequent to periodontitis-induced bacteraemia and endotoxaemia (Figure 2.4.4). C-reactive protein (CRP) is an acute phase protein produced by the liver in response to an infection or inflammatory process. Most importantly, CRP is positively associated with cardiovascular disease (Danesh et al. 1998). Therefore, periodontitis-induced systemic bacteraemia, endotoxaemia and cytokine release seem to contribute to the inflammatory aetiology of atherosclerosis. Other factors, which either singularly or in combination could contribute to the link between periodontitis and cardiovascular disease, include an exaggerated host hyper-inflammatory immune response, increased pro-thrombotic state and increased cholesterol biosynthesis (Schenkein & Loos 2013).

Some clinical human studies have shown that patients manifesting cardiovascular disease tend to experience higher levels of periodontitis (Mattila et al. 1989, Paiuno et al. 1993, Deliargyris et al. 2004, Dietrich et al. 2013). However, it is important to remember that the two conditions share common risk factors. Although there is biological plausibility linking cardiovascular disease and periodontitis, further investigations are required (Schenkein & Loos 2013).

Periodontal Treatment and Cardiovascular Diseases

There is currently no evidence to indicate that treatment of periodontitis will prevent or treat atherosclerosis (D'Aiuto et al. 2013). However, conventional periodontal therapy is effective both locally, by reducing the microbial burden

(Löe et al. 1965, Axelsson & Lindhe 1981) and systemically, by improving endothelial function (Tonetti et al. 2007) and by reducing systemic cytokine levels (D'Aiuto et al. 2004, 2005), all of which might deter atherosclerosis disease initiation and progression.

Stroke: A stroke occurs when cerebral blood vessels supplying blood to the brain are blocked; it can also occur after a cerebral aneurysm. Some studies suggest that poor oral health is more common in patients with cerebrovascular disease (Syrjanen et al. 1989, Loesche & Lopatin 1998).

> **KEY POINT 2**
> - A direct causal relationship between periodontitis and cardiovascular disease is not established.
> - Periodontitis is a risk factor or risk marker for coronary heart disease.
> - The two conditions have many common risk factors.
> - Periodontitis seems to potentiate systemic elevation of cytokines associated with atherosclerosis.
> - Atherosclerosis seems to have an inflammatory aetiology.
> - The host's inflammatory response is a significant determining factor.
> - Periodontal treatment reduces the oral microbial burden.
> - Periodontal treatment reduces systemic inflammatory response.
> - Patients should be encouraged to maintain good periodontal health especially if they have an increased risk of atherosclerotic heart disease.
> - Dentists, physicians and healthcare workers should work together and encourage patients to adopt a healthy lifestyle.

Periodontal Disease and Adverse Pregnancy Outcomes

Oral infections seem to increase the risk for, or contribute to, adverse pregnancy outcomes (Offenbacher et al. 1998).

Adverse pregnancy outcomes include preterm low birthweight (PTLBW), miscarriage or early pregnancy loss and pre-eclampsia (elevated blood pressure in a pregnant mother

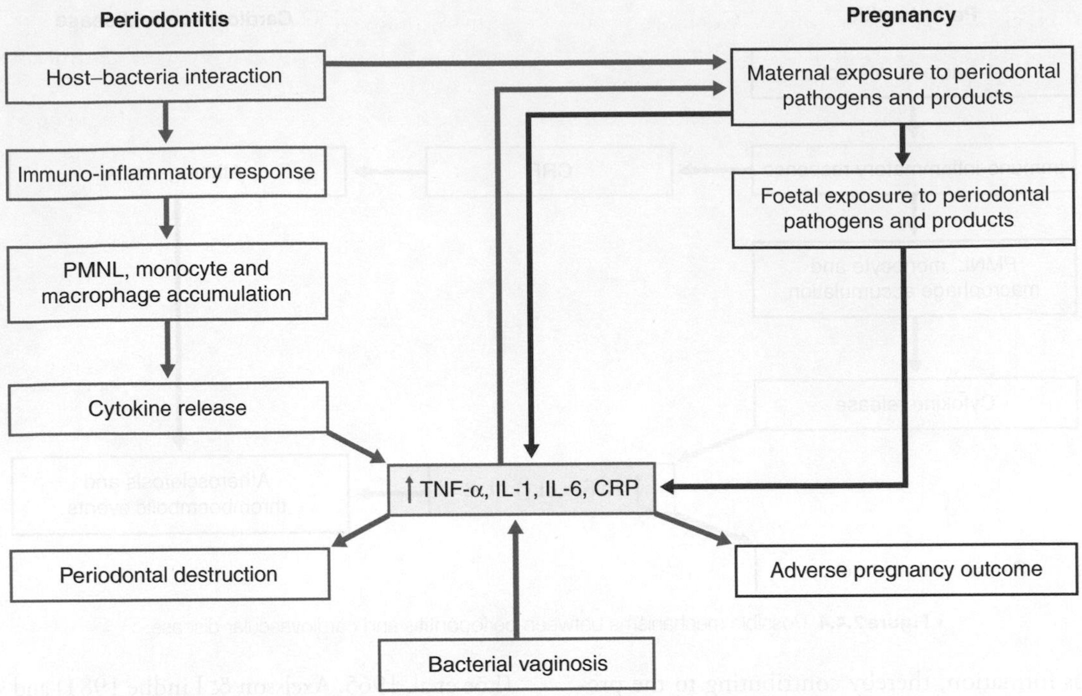

• **Figure 2.4.5** Possible mechanisms between periodontitis and adverse pregnancy outcomes.

which can have significant morbidity and mortality outcomes for both mother and child). Preterm birth is defined as birth prior to 37 weeks' gestation; low birthweight is defined as birthweight less than 2500 g. Such adverse pregnancy outcomes lead to significant infant mortality or morbidity, which is often associated with lifelong consequences, e.g. neurodevelopmental disturbances (Offenbacher et al. 1996a, Williams et al. 2000), respiratory disturbances, congenital malformations and developmental delays (Hack et al. 1983); this has substantial social and public health implications.

Known risk factors for PTLBW include: maternal age (younger than 17 years or older than 34 years), ethnic origin (increased prevalence in Hispanics, African-Americans and those with low socio-economic status), drug, alcohol and tobacco use, maternal stress, inadequate prenatal care, diabetes and genitourinary infections. An acute example of the latter is bacterial vaginosis which is an infection caused by Gram-negative bacteria (similar to periodontitis). The infection can affect the maternal foetal membranes, leading to an increased production of inflammatory cytokines which can in turn lead to premature rupture of membranes and hence preterm low birthweight.

Childbirth is a normal physiological process which is effected by a steady increase of cytokines (prostaglandin E_2 [PGE2] and TNF-α) until a critical threshold is reached that induces delivery of the neonate (Offenbacher et al. 1996b). Distant sites of infection can contribute to the build-up of these cytokines in the maternal circulation either directly due to the host response or indirectly due to lipopolysaccharide (LPS), a known potent inducer of cytokines such as IL-1, IL-6, TNF-α and PGE_2 (Darveau et al. 1997).

In the mid-1990s, it was hypothesized that oral Gram-negative infections such as periodontitis might contribute to adverse pregnancy outcomes (Offenbacher et al. 1996a). The subgingival microflora in pregnant females tends to become

predominantly Gram negative during the second trimester of pregnancy (Kornman & Loesche 1980). Pregnant females manifesting an increased susceptibility to periodontitis have an elevated inflammatory response. Therefore, the rationale behind the hypothesis is that the resulting elevated bacteraemia, endotoxaemia and increased cytokines (IL-1β, TNF-α, IL-6, CRP), all of which are potent inducers of labour, flowing through the maternal circulation could augment the levels of these same cytokines produced physiologically and collectively. These can affect the foetal–placental unit, leading to premature rupture of membranes and therefore premature birth (Figure 2.4.5). Although periodontal pathogens are important inducers of the maternal inflammatory response, the scale of the response is dependent on the host's immuno-inflammatory trait. If the maternal infection is contained, the foetus is spared; if not, then local foetal cytokine release may lead to premature rupture of the membranes and uterine contractions, which could lead to miscarriage or preterm birth (Madianos et al. 2013). Although there is some evidence to show a modest association between periodontitis and adverse pregnancy outcomes (Ide & Papapanou 2013), and that periodontitis is more severe in subjects giving birth to PTLBW infants (Offenbacher et al. 1996b, 1998), the results are inconclusive. The association between the two conditions might be due to the patient's elevated inflammatory response making periodontitis a risk marker, rather than a risk factor, for PTLBW.

Periodontal Treatment and Adverse Pregnancy Outcomes

A number of studies have investigated the effect of treatment of periodontitis on adverse pregnancy outcomes. The results are conflicting, with some studies suggesting that periodontitis is a significant risk factor for PTLBW

(Offenbacher et al. 1996a, 2001, 2006, Goepfert et al. 2004, Lieff et al. 2004, Boggess et al. 2006, Bosnjak et al. 2006), whereas others found no association (Davenport et al. 2002, Holbrook et al. 2004, Moore et al. 2005, Meurmann et al. 2006). The conflicting results could be due to population/ethnic differences. A common feature of all studies showed that periodontal treatment delivered during pregnancy was safe. All pregnant females should be encouraged to maintain good oral health before, during and after pregnancy. Currently, there is no evidence to support the notion that non-surgical periodontal therapy improves adverse pregnancy outcomes (Polyzos et al. 2010, Weidlich et al. 2013).

KEY POINT 3

- A direct causal relationship between periodontitis and preterm delivery is not established.
- Increased susceptibility to periodontitis seems to result in an increased susceptibility to premature births.
- Periodontitis might increase the cytokine burden, precipitating adverse pregnancy outcomes.
- The host's inflammatory response is a significant determining factor.
- Dentists should work in close collaboration with physicians, obstetricians and midwives to encourage good oral health in pregnant females before, during and after pregnancy.
- It is safe for pregnant females to undergo periodontal therapy.
- Non-surgical periodontal therapy does not reduce the risk of adverse pregnancy outcomes.
- Elective procedures should be avoided during the first trimester due to possible foetal stress; these are preferably delayed or carried out during the second trimester.
- Pregnant females should be educated regarding the possible interaction between periodontal disease and pregnancy; they should be made aware of possible physiological periodontal changes occurring during pregnancy such as higher incidence of gingival bleeding and gingival enlargement.

Periodontitis and Respiratory Diseases

Pneumonia and chronic obstructive pulmonary disease (COPD) are two respiratory conditions which have been associated with periodontitis.

Pneumonia is an infection of the lower respiratory tract (alveoli) most often caused by bacteria or viruses and, less commonly, by other microorganisms, certain drugs and other conditions such as autoimmune diseases. Typical symptoms include a cough, chest pain, fever and difficulty breathing. Pneumonia can be classified as community acquired or hospital acquired (nosocomial).

COPD is a condition characterised by chronic obstruction to airflow caused by excessive sputum production resulting from chronic bronchitis and/or emphysema. Clinical symptoms include cough, difficulty breathing, dyspnoea and fatigue, all of which become more pronounced during a period of exacerbation. It is not known what causes an exacerbation, though it is thought to be provoked in part by a bacterial infection.

Both of these respiratory conditions cause significant morbidity and mortality especially in the elderly and the infirm, more so in those in intensive care units or subjects residing in nursing homes. This has significant social, medical and financial implications.

The lower respiratory tract beneath the oropharynx is usually sterile. Infection may result from a defect in host defences, infection with a particularly virulent organism or aspiration of oral/oropharyngeal fluids. The crucial factor is colonisation beneath the oropharynx, as this will in turn lead to microbial colonisation of the lower respiratory tree (Finegold 1991). Obligate anaerobes constitute the predominant microflora in the oropharynx and in the oral cavity of periodontitis patients. An increasing number of reports (Terpenning et al. 2001, Scannapieco et al. 2003, Scannapieco 2006) show that pneumonia is more common in patients with poor oral hygiene, dental caries and periodontal diseases and especially in those who are prone to aspiration of oral fluids (intubated intensive care patients and elderly/infirm patients who have trouble swallowing). Oral bacteria, such as *Aggregatibacter actinomycetemcomitans*, *Eikenella corrodens*, *Fusobacterium nucleatum*, *Porphyromonas* and *Prevotella* species, have been isolated from lung fluid specimens (Suwanagool et al. 1983, Brook & Frazier 1993, Chen et al. 1995, Verma 2000, Van decandelaere et al. 2012).

Potential mechanisms (Figure 2.4.6) by which oral bacteria could be implicated in the pathogenesis of respiratory diseases (Scannpieco et al. 1999) are:

- Bacterial aspiration: poor oral hygiene manifesting as excessive dental plaque (biofilm) accumulation (whether on teeth, mucosal surfaces or dentures), periodontitis and dental caries can act as a source/reservoir of potential respiratory pathogens (PRPs) which initially colonise the oral cavity and can subsequently be aspirated into the lower respiratory tract, leading to pneumonia or COPD (Scannapieco et al. 1992, 2003, Russel et al. 1999, Terpenning et al. 2001)
- Periodontitis-induced enzyme modification of the oral mucosa: periodontitis-related bacteria produce enzymes which are released into saliva and can enhance adhesion and colonisation of the oral mucosa with PRPs (Woods et al. 1981)
- Periodontitis-induced salivary pellicle destruction: hydrolytic enzyme activity in saliva is related to periodontal and oral hygiene status (Gibbons & Ethereden 1986). Elevated levels of such enzymes may destroy protective host mechanisms which would otherwise protect against colonisation with respiratory pathogens
- Periodontitis-induced cytokine alteration of the respiratory epithelium: cytokines released in response to periodontitis can upregulate the expression of receptors on the mucosal surfaces, encouraging colonisation with PRPs (Svandborg et al. 1996).

Periodontal Treatment and Respiratory Diseases

Although the precise contribution of periodontitis to the development of pneumonia is unknown, poor oral health has been linked to increased levels of hospital-acquired pneumonia (Mehndiratta et al 2016), and studies have shown that interventions improving oral hygiene can reduce the incidence of nosocomial pneumonia quite significantly – between 40% (Scannapieco et al. 2003, Scannapieco 2006)

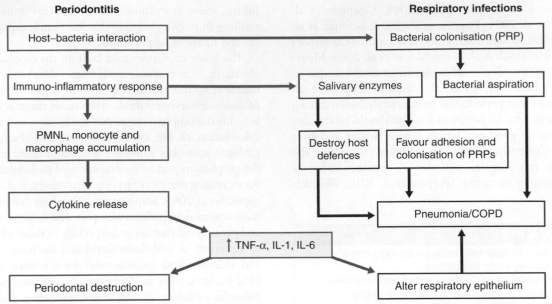

Periodontitis   **Respiratory infections**

• **Figure 2.4.6** Potential mechanisms by which oral bacteria could be implicated in the pathogenesis of respiratory diseases. PRP, Potential respiratory pathogens.

and 83% (Azarpazhooh & Leake 2006) – and of pneumonia in institutionalised elderly subjects (Yoneyama et al. 2002). There is increasing evidence that better oral health-care improves the outcome of patients in intensive care units (Rabello et al. 2018) and of those in nursing homes (Terpenning et al. 2001, Okuda et al. 2005, Terpenning 2005).

The importance of maintaining the oral hygiene of patients on mechanical ventilation has been recognised (Wainer 2020). This is becoming more important as patients are living longer and are undergoing more complex medical care, and because they are tending to retain their teeth for longer. In some medical intensive care units, it is becoming standard practice to implement oral hygiene care to intubated patients on a daily basis.

KEY POINT 4

- A direct causal relationship between periodontitis and pneumonia has not been firmly established.
- However, it appears that periodontitis increases the risk of pneumonia in immune-compromised and frail patients.
- Poor oral hygiene seems to be associated with a higher incidence of respiratory diseases.
- Dental biofilms seem to harbour potential respiratory pathogens.
- Oral colonisation of such bacteria could contribute to pulmonary infections.
- Some studies have shown reduced risk of pneumonia and COPD with improved oral hygiene.
- The importance of good oral hygiene especially in subjects who are at high risk of respiratory infections (intensive care patients and elderly/infirm patients with feeding problems, especially those in nursing homes) should be emphasized.
- Dentists, dental hygienists and therapists as well as physicians and staff working in intensive care units and nursing homes should emphasize the importance of oral hygiene in these vulnerable patients.
- Dental and oral hygiene can potentially have cost-saving and life-saving implications.

Periodontitis and Dementia

At least three systematic reviews published between 2017 and 2020 have investigated the relationship between periodontitis and Alzheimer's disease. One review (Leira et al. 2017) concluded that there was "a significant association between periodontitis and Alzheimer's disease and that further studies should be carried out in order to investigate the direction of the association and factors that may confound it". Liccardo et al. (2020) concluded that periodontitis and Alzheimer's disease often coexist. Dioguardi et al. (2020) concluded that bacteria involved in, and inflammatory products arising from, periodontitis can intensify inflammation in the central nervous system but that as yet there is no definitive evidence to consider periodontitis a risk factor for Alzheimer's disease. Nevertheless, they considered that the oral hygiene of older people with dementia should be improved and that this should be achieved by educating care assistants to carry out daily oral hygiene of the residents in their care homes and regular monitoring of these patients' oral health by dental professionals (Dioguardi et al. 2020).

Research into periodontitis and dementia continues.

Periodontitis and Other Systemic Diseases

A number of other systemic diseases have been associated with periodontitis (Box 2.4.2). Apart from COVID-19, the evidence to date is tenuous. However, with more studies underway and improved scientific techniques, it is anticipated that clearer and more convincing scientifically based data will be obtained.

By August 2021, a number of studies and case reports which investigated oral health and severity of COVID-19 complications had been published. One found that after adjusting for potential confounders, "Periodontitis was associated with higher risk of ICU admission, need for assisted ventilation and death and with increased blood levels of bio-markers linked to worse disease outcomes" (Marouf et al. 2021). There is considerable interest, and further research into this topic is taking place.

Systemic Conditions Affecting the Periodontium

A number of systemic conditions (acquired or genetic) affect the periodontium. The clinical picture will vary depending on the aetiology; however, in most cases, severe periodontitis seems to be a common feature. Although these conditions are rare, they should be included in the differential diagnosis, especially when the severity of peri-odontitis is not commensurate with the presenting clinical picture (e.g. young child presenting with advanced peri-odontitis) (Table 2.4.2).

Systemic Medication Affecting the Periodontium

Systemic medication may affect the periodontium. Drug-influenced gingival enlargement is seen in patients

---

• BOX 2.4.2 Possible Associations between Periodontitis and Other Systemic Conditions

COVID-19
Obesity
Osteoporosis
Rheumatoid arthritis
Head and neck squamous cell carcinoma
Inflammatory bowel disease
Erectile dysfunction

TABLE 2.4.2 Systemic conditions affecting the periodontium

Condition	Underlying pathology	Clinical features
Haematological conditions		
Neutropenia	Reduced levels of PMNLs	Severe periodontitis leading to premature loss of both deciduous and permanent dentition
Leukaemia	Bone marrow malignancy	Oral mucosal ulceration, gingival hyperplasia/hypertrophy, gingival haemorrhage, gingival pallor, periodontitis
Genetic conditions		
Down's syndrome	Defective PMNLs	Excessive plaque and calculus accumulation leading to rapid and severe periodontitis before 30 years of age; noted also in deciduous dentition
Papillon–Lefèvre syndrome	Defective PMNLs	Severe periodontitis noted in deciduous dentition, may affect permanent dentition
Chronic granulomatous disease	Defective PMNLs and macrophages	Oral ulceration but may also manifest gingivitis, periodontitis
Chediak–Higashi syndrome	Defective phagocytes	Severe childhood periodontitis
Ehlers–Danlos syndrome	Defective collagen synthesis	Childhood periodontitis
Hypophosphatasia	Defective formation/mineralization of cementum	Premature loss of deciduous teeth
Job's syndrome	Excessive IgE and histamine release by mast cells and IgE immune complex formation	Painful, bleeding gingivae, aggressive periodontitis
Histiocytosis X	Proliferation and dissemination of Langerhans cells	Gingivitis, severe periodontitis
Leucocyte adhesion deficiency syndrome	Defective PMN diapedesis	Acute inflammation, proliferation of gingival tissues, rapid bone loss, reduced wound healing
Cohen syndrome	Neutropenia	Periodontitis
Marfan's syndrome	Connective tissue disorder	Severe periodontitis
Diabetes mellitus	Increased risk of infection, reduced wound healing	Recurrent periodontal abscesses, advanced periodontitis

Adapted from Chapple & Gilbert 2002. IgE: immunoglobulin E; PMNLs: polymorphonuclear leucocytes.

taking cyclosporin, phenytoin and calcium channel blockers. Patients on anti-resorptive medication (bisphosphonates) prescribed orally for the treatment of osteoporosis can receive periodontal treatment if necessary. Prior to treatment, patients should be warned of the low risk of developing anti-resorptive agent-induced osteonecrosis of the jaw (ARONJ). Oral anti-resorptive medication is not a contraindication to non-surgical or surgical periodontal treatment. The importance of good oral hygiene and periodontal supportive therapy should be emphasised as this reduces or eliminates the need for dental extractions and/or periodontal treatment. Patients undergoing periodontal treatment should be advised to rinse with 0.2% chlorhexidine gluconate prior to dental treatment and to continue rinsing twice a day for 7 days after treatment.

Intravenous administration of anti-resorptive medication poses a high risk of development of ARONJ. The patient should be warned of this and, if at all possible, elective oral or periodontal surgery be deferred. If treatment is necessary, the patient is best managed by being referred to a multidisciplinary team who is experienced in the management of ARONJ.

Summary

Scientific advances have enriched our understanding of the pathobiology of periodontal diseases and the relationships between periodontal health and systemic health. The oral cavity is an integral part of the human body and therefore management of periodontal diseases should be seen as contributing towards general, as well as oral, health and wellbeing. Periodontal medicine should be at the forefront of each clinician's mind when treating periodontitis.

The potential associations between periodontitis and systemic disease have been under intense investigation and has been brought to the forefront in a joint publication issued by the European Federation of Periodontology and the American Academy of Periodontology (Tonetti & Kornman 2013).

Future advances in periodontology in general and in periodontal medicine in particular will lead to an improved understanding of potential interactions between periodontitis and systemic diseases. As clinicians we will then be able to provide even better care for patients.

Multiple choice questions on the contents of this chapter are available online at Elsevier eBooks+.

References

Ainamo J, Lahtinen A, Uitto VJ. Rapid periodontal destruction in adult humans with poorly controlled diabetes. *J Clin Periodontol.* 1990;17:22–28.

American Diabetes Association. Classification and diagnosis of diabetes. *Sec* 2. *In* Standards of medical care in diabetes. *Diabetes Care.* 2015;38(Suppl. 1):S8–S16.

Atkinson MA, Maclaren NK. The pathogenesis of insulin dependent diabetes. *NEJM.* 1994;331:1428–1436.

Axelsson P, Lindhe J. Effect of controlled oral hygiene procedures on caries and periodontal disease in adults. Results after 6 years. *J Clin Periodontol.* 1981;8:239–248.

Azarpazhooh A, Leake JL. Systematic review of the association between respiratory diseases and oral health. *J Periodontol.* 2006;77:1465–1482.

Beck JD, Offenbacher S. The association between periodontal disease and cardiovascular disease: a state-of-the-science review. *Ann Periodontol.* 2001;6:9–15.

Billings F. Chronic focal infections and their etiologic relations to arthritis and nephritis. *Arch Intern Med.* 1911;9:484–498.

Boggess KA, Beck JD, Murtha AP, Moss K, Offenbacher S. Maternal periodontal disease in early pregnancy and risk for a small-for-gestational-age infant. *Am J Obstet Gynecol.* 2006;194:1316–1322.

Borgnakke WS, Ylöstalo PV, Taylor GW, Genco RJ. Effect of periodontal disease in diabetes: systematic review of epidemiologic observational evidence. *J Clin Periodontol.* 2013;40(Suppl. 14):S135–S142.

Bosnjak A, Relja T, Vucićević-Boras V, Plasaj H, Plancak D. Pre-term delivery and periodontal disease: a case-control study from Croatia. *J Clin Periodontol.* 2006;33:710–716.

Brook I, Frazier EH. Aerobic and anaerobic microbiology of empyema. A retrospective review in two military hospitals. *Chest.* 1993;103:1502–1507.

Chapple IL, Genco R. Diabetes and periodontal disease: consensus report of the Joint EFP/AAP workshop on periodontitis and systemic disease. *J Clin Periodontol.* 2013;40(Suppl. 14):S106–S112.

Chapple IL, Gilbert A. Understanding periodontal diseases: assessment and diagnostic procedures in practice. *QuintEssentials of dental practice.* 2002;1. Quintessence 97–131.

Chen AC, Liu CC, Yao WJ, Chen CT, Wang JY. Actinobacillus actinomycetemcomitans pneumonia with chest wall and subphrenic abscess. *Scand J Infect Dis.* 1995;27:289–290.

Cianciola LJ, Park BH, Bruck E, Mosovich L, Genco RJ. Prevalence of periodontal disease in insulin-dependent diabetes mellitus (juvenile diabetes). *J Am Dent Assoc.* 1992;104:653–660.

Ciantar M. *Capnocytophaga Species and Diabetes-Mellitus Periodontitis.* University of London; 2002. PhD Thesis.

Collin HL, Uusitupa M, Niskanen L, Kontturi-Närhi V, Markkanen H, Koivisto AM, et al. Periodontal findings in elderly patients with non-insulin dependent diabetes mellitus. *J Periodontol.* 1998;69:962–966.

Colyer S. Oral sepsis and some of its effects. *Dental Record.* 1902;20:200–206.

Crawford JM, Cotran RS. The pancreas. In: Schoen FJ, Cotran RS, Kumar V, Robbins SL, eds. *Robbins Pathogenic Basis of Disease.* Philadelphia: WB Saunders; 1994:897–926.

D'Aiuto F, Parkar M, Andreou G, et al. Periodontitis and systemic inflammation: control of the local infection is associated with a reduction in serum inflammatory markers. *J Dent Res.* 2004;83:156–160.

D'Aiuto F, Nibali L, Parkar M, Suvan J, Tonetti MS. Short-term effects of intensive periodontal therapy on serum inflammatory markers and cholesterol. *J Dent Res.* 2005;84:269–273.

D'Aiuto F, Orlandi M, Gunsolley JC. Evidence that periodontal treatment improves biomarkers and CVD outcomes. *J Clin Periodontol.* 2013;40(Suppl. 14):S85–S105.

Danesh J, Collins R, Appleby P, Peto R. Association of fibrinogen, C-reactive protein, albumin or leukocyte count with coronary heart disease. Meta analyses of prospective studies. *J Am Med Assoc.* 1998;279:1477–1482.

Darveau RP, Tanner A, Page RC. The microbial challenge in periodontitis. *Periodontol.* 1997;14:12–32. 2000.

Davenport ES, Williams CE, Sterne JA, Murad S, Sivapathasundram V, Curtis MA. Maternal periodontal disease and preterm low birthweight: case-control study. *J Dent Res.* 2002;81:313–318.

Deliargyris EN, Madianos PN, Kadoma W, et al. Periodontal disease in patients with acute myocardial infarction: prevalence and contribution to elevated C-reactive protein levels. *Am Heart J.* 2004;147:1005–1009.

Deshpande RG, Khan MB, Genco CA. Invasion of aortic and heart endothelial cells by Porphyromonas gingivalis. *Infect Immun.* 1998;66:5337–5343.

Desvarieux M, Demmer RT, Rundek T, et al. Relationship between periodontal disease, tooth loss, and carotid artery plaque: the oral infections and vascular disease epidemiology study (INVEST). *Stroke.* 2003;34:2120–2125.

Diabetes U K. Diabetes prevalence in 2019. Diabetes UK 2020. www.diabetes.org.uk. accessed on 9 August 2021.

Dietrich T, Sharma P, Walter C, Weston P, Back J. The epidemiological evidence behind the association between periodontitis and incident cardiovascular disease. *J Clin Periodontol.* 2013;40(Suppl. 14):S70–S84.

Dioguardi M, Crincoli V, Laino L, et al. The role of periodontitis and Periodontal bacteria in the onset and progression of Alzheimer's disease: a systematic review. *J Clin Med.* 2020;9(2):495. https://doi.org/10.3309/jcm9020495.

Dorn BR, Dunn WA, Porgulske-Fox A. Invasion of human coronary artery cells by periodontal pathogens. *Infect Immun.* 1999;67:5792–5798.

Engebretson S, Kocher T. Evidence that periodontal treatment improves diabetes outcomes: a systematic review and meta analysis. *J Clin Periodontol.* 2013;40(Suppl. 14):S153–S163.

Fine DH, Furgang D, McKiernan M, et al. An investigation of the effect of an essential oil mouthrinse on induced bacteraemia: a pilot study. *J Clin Periodontol.* 2010;37:840–847.

Finegold SM. Aspiration pneumonia. *Rev Infect Dis.* 1991;13:S737–S742.

Firatli E. The relationship between clinical periodontal status and insulin dependent diabetes mellitus. Results after 5 years. *J Periodontol.* 1997;68:136–140.

Galloway CE. Focal infection. *Am J Surg.* 1931;14:643–645.

Gibbons RJ, Ethereden I. Fibronectin-degrading enzymes in saliva and their relationship to oral cleanliness. *J Dent Res.* 1986;21:386–395.

Goepfert AR, Jeffcoat MK, Andrews WW, et al. Periodontal disease and upper genital tract inflammation in early spontaneous preterm birth. *Obstet Gynecol.* 2004;104:777–783.

Grossi S, Skrepcinski FB, DeCaro T, et al. Treatment of periodontal disease in diabetics reduces glycated hemoglobin. *J Periodontol.* 1997;68:713–719.

Hack M, Caron B, Rivers A, Fanaroff AA. The very low birth weight infant: the broader spectrum of morbidity during infancy and early childhood. *J Dev Behav Pediatr.* 1983;4:243–249.

Haraszthy VI, Zambon JJ, Trevisan M, Zeid M, Genco RJ. Identification of periodontal pathogens in atheromatous plaques. *J Periodontol.* 2000;17:1554–1560.

Herzberg MC, Macfarlane GD, Liu P-X, Erickson PR. The platelet as an inflammatory cell in periodontal diseases: Interactions with Porphyromonas gingivalis. In: Genco RJ, Mergenhagen S, McGhee J, Lehner T, Hamada S, eds. *Molecular Basis for Pathogenesis and Molecular Targeting in Periodontal Diseases.* Washington DC: American Society for Microbiology; 1994:247–255.

Holbrook WP, Oskarsdóttir A, Fridjónsson T, Einarsson H, Hauksson A, Geirsson RT. No link between low-grade periodontal disease and preterm birth: a pilot study in a healthy Caucasian population. *Acta Odontol Scand.* 2004;62:177–179.

Hunter W. Oral sepsis as a cause of disease. *Br Med J.* 1900;1:215–216.

Ide M, Papapanou PN. Epidemiology of association between maternal periodontal disease and adverse pregnancy outcomes – systematic review. *J Clin Periodontol.* 2013;40(Suppl. 14):S181–S194.

Iwamoto Y, Nishimura F, Nakagawa M, et al. The effect of antimicrobial periodontal treatment on circulating tumor necrosis factor-alpha and glycated haemoglobin levels in patients with type 2 diabetes. *J Periodontol.* 2001;72:774–778.

Kanety H, Feistein R, Papa MZ, Hemi R, Karasiki A. Tumor necrosis factor α-induced phosphorylation of insulin receptor substrate-1 (IRS-1). Possible mechanism for suppression of the insulin-stimulation tyrosine phosphorylation of IRS-1. *J Biol Chem.* 1995;270:23780–23784.

Kinane DF, Riggio MP, Walker KF, MacKenzie D, Shearer B. Bacteraemia following periodontal procedures. *J Clin Periodontol.* 2005;32:708–713.

Kornman KS, Loesche WJ. The subgingival microflora during pregnancy. *J Periodontal Res.* 1980;15:111–122.

Kuramitsu HK, Miyawaka H, Qi M, Kang IC. Cellular response to oral pathogens. *Ann Periodontol.* 2002;7:90–94.

Lakschevitz F, Aboodi G, Tenenbaum H, Glogauer M. Diabetes and periodontal diseases: interplay and links. *Curr Diabetes Rev.* 2011;7:433–439.

Lalla E, Papapanou PN. Diabetes mellitus and periodontitis: a tale of two common interrelated diseases. *Nat Rev Endocrinol.* 2011;7:738–748.

Leinonen M, Saikku P. Evidence for infectious agents in cardiovascular disease and atherosclerosis. *Lancet Infect Dis.* 2002;2:11–17.

Leira Y, Dominguez C, Seoane J, et al. Is periodontal disease associated with Alzheimer's disease? A systematic review with meta-analysis. *Neuroepidemiology.* 2017;48:2131.

Lieff S, Boggess KA, Murtha AP, et al. The oral conditions and pregnancy study: periodontal status of a cohort of pregnant women. *J Periodontol.* 2004;75:116–126.

Liccardo D, Marzano F, Carraturo F, et al. Potential bidirectional relationship between periodontitis and Alzheimer's disease. *Front Physiol.* 2020;11:683. 10.3389/phys.2020.00683. eCollection 2020.

Linden GJ, Lyons A, Scannpieco FA. Periodontal systemic associations: review of the evidence. *J Clin Periodontol.* 2013;40(Suppl. 14):S8–S19.

Löe H. Periodontal disease. The sixth complication of diabetes mellitus. *Diabetes Care.* 1993;16:329–334.

Löe H, Theilade E, Jensen SB. Experimental gingivitis in man. *J Periodontol.* 1965;36:177–187.

Loesche WJ, Lopatin DE. Interactions between periodontal disease, medical diseases and immunity in the older individual. *Periodontol.* 1998;16:80–105.

Lucas VS, Gafan G, Dewhurst S, Roberts GJ. Prevalence, intensity and nature of bacteraemia after tooth brushing. *J Dent.* 2008;36:481–487.

Madianos PN, Bobetsis YA, Offenbacher S. Adverse pregnancy outcomes (APOs) and periodontal disease: pathogenic mechanisms. *J Clin Periodontol.* 2013;40(Suppl. 14):S170–S180.

Marouf N, Cai W, Said KN, et al. Association between periodontitis and severity of COVID-19 infection: A case-control study. *J Clin Periodontol.* 2021;48:483–491.

Mattila KJ. Viral and bacterial infections in patients with acute myocardial infarction. *J Intern Med.* 1989;225:293–296.

Mattila KJ, Nieminen MS, Valtonen VV, et al. Association between dental health and acute myocardial infarction. *Br Med J.* 1989;298:779–781.

McNamara TF, Ramamurthy NS, Mulvihill JE, Golub LM. The development of an altered gingival crevicular microflora in the alloxan-diabetic rat. *Arch Oral Biol.* 1982;27:217–223.

Mealey BL. Periodontal disease and diabetes. A two-way street. *J Am Dent Assoc.* 2006;137(Suppl.):26S–31S.

Mehndiratta M, Nayak R, Ali S, Sharma A, Gulati N. Ventilators in ICU: a boon or a burden. *Ann Indian Acad Neurol.* 2016;19:69–73.

Meurmann JH, Furuholm J, Kaaja R, Rintamaki H, Tikkanen U. Oral health in women with pregnancy and delivery complications. *Clin Oral Investig.* 2006;10:96–100.

Miller WD. The human mouth as a focus of infection. *Dental Cosmos.* 1891;33:689–713.

Moore S, Randhawa M, Ide M. A case-control study to investigate an association between adverse pregnancy outcome and periodontal disease. *J Clin Periodontol.* 2005;32:622–627.

Offenbacher S. Periodontal diseases. Pathogenesis. *Ann Periodontol.* 1996;1:821–878.

Offenbacher S, Jared HL, O'Reilly PG, et al. Potential pathogenic mechanisms of periodontitis associated pregnancy complications. *Ann Periodontol.* 1996a;3:233–250.

Offenbacher S, Katz V, Fertik G, et al. Periodontal infection as a possible risk factor for preterm low birth weight. *J Periodontol.* 1996b;67(Suppl. 10):1103–1113.

Offenbacher S, Beck JD, Lieff S, Slade G. Role of periodontitis in systemic health: spontaneous preterm birth. *J Dent Educ.* 1998;62:852–858.

Offenbacher S, Boggess KA, Murtha AP, et al. Progressive periodontal disease and risk of very preterm delivery. *Obstet Gynecol.* 2006;107:29–36.

Offenbacher S, Lieff S, Boggess KA, et al. Maternal periodontitis and prematurity, Part 1: obstetric outcome of prematurity and growth restriction. *Ann Periodontol.* 2001;6:164–174.

Okuda K, Kimizuka R, Abe S, Kato T, Ishihara K. Involvement of periodontopathic anaerobes in aspiration pneumonia. *J Periodontol.* 2005;76:2154–2160.

Page RC. The pathobiology of periodontal diseases may affect systemic disease: inversion of a paradigm. *Ann Periodontol.* 1998;3:108–120.

Paiuno K, Impivaara O, Tiesko J, Mäki J. Missing teeth and ischemic heart disease in men aged 45–64 years. *Eur Heart J.* 1993;14(Suppl. K):54–56.

Polyzos NP, Polyzos IP, Zavos A, et al. Obstetric outcomes after treatment of periodontal disease during pregnancy: systematic review and meta-analysis. *Br Med J.* 2010;341:c7017.

Rabello F, Araujo VV, Magalhães S. Effectiveness of oral chlorhexidine for the prevention of nosocomial pneumonia and ventilator-associated pneumonia in intensive care units: overview of systematic reviews. *Int J Dent Hyg.* 2018;16:441–449.

Ring ME. *An Illustrated History of Dentistry.* Abradale Press; 1985.

Russel SL, Boylan RJ, Kaslick RS, Scannapieco FA, Katz RV. Respiratory pathogen colonisation of the dental plaque of institutionalised elders. *Spec Care Dentist.* 1999;19:128–134.

Saito I, Watanabe O, Kawahara H, Igarashi Y, Yamamura T, Shimono M. Intercellular junctions and the permeability barrier in the junctional epithelium. *J Periodontal Res.* 1981;16:467–480.

Scannapieco FA. Role of oral bacteria in respiratory infection. *J Periodontol.* 1999;70:793–802.

Scannapieco FA. Pneumonia in non-ambulatory patients. The role of oral bacteria and oral hygiene. *J Am Dent Assoc.* 2006;137:21S–25S.

Scannapieco FA, Stewart EM, Mylotte JM. Colonisation of dental plaque by respiratory pathogens in medical intensive care patients. *Crit Care Med.* 1992;20:740–745.

Scannapieco FA, Bush RB, Paju S. Associations between periodontal disease and risk for nosocomial bacterial pneumonia and chronic obstructive pulmonary disease. A systematic review. *Ann Periodontol.* 2003;8:54–69.

Schenkein HA, Loos BG. Inflammatory mechanisms linking periodontal diseases to cardiovascular diseases. *J Clin Periodontol.* 2013;40(Suppl. 14):S51–S69.

Seiffert A. Der zahnaszt als diagnositker. *Deutsche Wehn Zahnheil.* 1962;3:153.

Seppälä B, Ainamo J. A site by site follow-up study on the effect of controlled versus poorly controlled insulin-dependent diabetes mellitus. *J Clin Periodontol.* 1994;21:161–165.

Sgolastra F, Severino M, Pietropaoli D, Gatto R, Monaco A. Effectiveness of periodontal treatment to improve metabolic control in patients with chronic periodontitis and Type 2 diabetes: a meta-analysis of randomized clinical trials. *J Periodontol.* 2013;84:958–973.

Suwanagool S, Rothkopf MM, Smith SM, LeBlanc D, Eng D. Pathogenicity of Eikenella corrodens in humans. *Arch Intern Med.* 1983;143:2265–2268.

Svandborg C, Hedlund M, Connell H, et al. Bacterial adherence and mucosal cytokine responses. Receptors and transmembrane signalling. *Ann N. Y. Acad Sci.* 1996;797:177–190.

Syrjanen J, Peltola J, Valtonen V, Iivanainen M, Kaste M, Huttunen JK. Dental infections in association with cerebral infraction in young and middle-aged men. *J Intern Med.* 1989;225:179–184.

Syrjanen J, Valtonen VV, Iivanainen M, Kaste M, Huttunen JK. Preceding infection as an important risk factor for ischemia brain infarction in young middle aged patients. *Br Med J.* 1998;296:1156–1160.

Taylor GW. Bidirectional interrelationships between diabetes and periodontal diseases: an epidemiologic perspective. *Ann Periodontol.* 2001;6:99–112.

Terpenning M. Geriatric oral health and pneumonia risk. *Clin Infect Dis.* 2005;40:1807–1810.

Terpenning MS, Taylor GW, Lopatin DE, et al. Aspiration pneumonia: dental and oral risk factors in an older veteran population. *J Am Geriatr Soc.* 2001;49:557–563.

Tervonen T, Karjalainen K. Periodontal disease related to diabetic status. A pilot study of the response to periodontal therapy in Type 1 diabetes. *J Clin Periodontol.* 1997;24:505–510.

Thoden van Velzen SK, Abraham-Inpijn I, Moorer WR. Plaque and systemic disease: a reappraisal of the focal infection concept. *J Clin Periodontol.* 1984;11:209–220.

Tonetti M, D'Aiuto F, Nibali L, et al. Treatment of periodontitis and endothelial function. *NEJM.* 2007;356:911–920.

Tonetti MS, Kornman K. Periodontitis and systemic diseases. Proceedings of a workshop jointly held by the European Federation of Periodontology and the American Academy of Periodontology. *J Clin Periodontol.* 2013;40(Suppl. 14):S1–S208.

Van decandelaere I, Matthijs N, Van Nieuwerburgh F, et al. Assessment of microbial diversity in biofilms recovered from endotracheal tubes using culture dependent and independent approaches. *PLoS ONE.* 2012;7(e3840):1–8.

Van Dyke TE, Winkelhoff AJ. Infection and inflammatory mechanisms. *J Clin Periodontol.* 2013;40(Suppl. 14):S1–S7.

Van Dyke TE, Dowell Jr VR, Offenbacher S, Snyder W, Hersh T. Potential role of micro-organisms isolated from periodontal lesions in the pathogenesis of inflammatory bowel disease. *Infect Immun.* 1986;53:671–677.

Verma P. Laboratory diagnosis of anaerobic pulmonary infections. *Semin Respir Infect.* 2000;15:114–118.

Wainer C. The importance of oral hygiene for patients on mechanical ventilation. *Br J Nursing.* 2020;29:23.

Weidlich P, Moreira CH, Fiorini T, et al. Effect of nonsurgical periodontal therapy and strict plaque control on preterm/low birth weight: a randomized controlled clinical trial. *Clin Oral Investig.* 2013;17:37–44.

WHO. *Definition, diagnosis and classification of diabetes mellitus and its complications. Report of a WHO consultation. Part 1: diagnosis and classification of diabetes mellitus*; 1999. WHO/NCD/NCS/99.2.

Williams NB, Burkett LW. Focal infection – a review. *Phila Med.* 1951;46:1509.

Williams CE, Davenport ES, Sterne JA, Sivapathasundaram V, Fearne JM, Curtis MA. Mechanisms of risk in preterm low-birthweight infants. *Periodontol.* 2000;23:142–150.

Woods DE, Straus DC, Johanson WG, Bass JA. Role of fibronectin in the prevention of adherence of Pseudomonas aeruginosa to buccal cells. *J Infect Dis.* 1981;143:784–790.

Yki-Jarvinen H. Pathogenesis of non-insulin-dependent diabetes mellitus. *Lancet.* 1994;343:91–95.

Yoneyama T, Yoshida M, Ohuri T, et al. Oral care reduces pneumonia in older patients in nursing homes. *J Am Geriatr Soc.* 2002;50:430–433.

Yumoto H, Chou HH, Takahashi Y, Davey M, Gibson FC, Genco CA. Sensitisation of human aortic endothelial cells to lipopolysaccharide via regulation of Toll-like receptor 4 by bacteria fimbria-dependent invasion. *Infect Immun.* 2005;73:8050–8059.

2.5

DETERMINING PERIODONTAL PROGNOSIS

MONICA LEE

CHAPTER OUTLINE

OVERVIEW OF THE CHAPTER

Sound periodontal health provides a foundation for overall dental health and should be established before any other form of dental treatment, such as restorative reconstruction or orthodontic realignment, can be considered. However, a patient with periodontitis may be at risk of tooth loss, and it can be helpful when treatment planning to estimate the life expectancy of individual teeth in order to improve the predictability of any proposed treatment. This chapter will examine the reliability of trying to determine the likely future of periodontally involved teeth.

By the end of this chapter the reader should:

- Understand the principles of prognosis
- Recognise which factors affect prognosis and their weighting
- Be aware of the different prognostic classification schemes
- Understand how the determination of prognosis can be improved.

This chapter covers the following topics:

- Introduction
- What is a prognosis?
- Factors affecting prognosis
- Assigning a prognosis
- When to determine prognosis
- Weighting prognostic factors
- Improving the determination of prognosis.

Introduction

One of the hardest tasks for a dentist is to determine the prognosis of an individual tooth predictably. Sometimes, it is necessary to try to predict the future without having any knowledge of what has happened in the past. This chapter will explore what information is required in order to determine the prognosis of a tooth or teeth for periodontal patients. The aim is always to make clinical decisions based on good sound scientific research. However, the determination of periodontal prognosis is an inexact science. This is because multiple factors (local, systemic, psychological amongst others) can influence the prognoses of teeth. Nevertheless, estimating prognosis is a useful component of periodontal treatment planning. It can only be achieved by gathering as much information as possible about the patient and individual teeth.

What is a Prognosis?

The definition of prognosis is the forecasting of the course and outcome of a specific disease, and the chances of recovery. When a prognosis is suggested, it is an attempt to predict how a tooth or teeth will respond to treatment in the long term, taking into account all the factors which may affect the outcome. Inflammatory periodontal diseases are complex and are among the most prevalent chronic diseases of humans. As described in previous chapters of this book, patients vary greatly in their risk for developing disease as a result of the interaction of microbial, genetic and environmental factors. The factors that determine the initiation and progression of disease are referred to as risk factors (see Chapter 1.6). Risk factors for a disease have been defined as certain characteristics of a person or their environment which, when present, directly result in an increased likelihood of that person getting the disease and, when absent, directly result in a decreased likelihood (Beck 1995). They are causally associated with a disease. Examples for periodontal diseases are genetics, smoking, stress and some systemic diseases.

> ### KEY POINT 1
> Risk factors are characteristics of a person or their environment which, when present, directly result in an increased likelihood of that person getting the disease, and when absent directly result in a decreased likelihood.

Many risk factors are also prognostic factors since they are characteristics that help the clinician to predict outcome (tooth survival) once the disease process has been initiated. Such factors include smoking, diabetes and poor oral hygiene.

Determining the prognosis of individual teeth can be difficult because of the multiple factors that influence treatment outcome. In order to evaluate the prognosis of a tooth, sufficient information is required with regards to patient factors and local factors. This means that in an individual, each tooth will have a different prognosis because of differing local factors, despite the same patient factors occurring.

Factors Affecting Prognosis

Any factor that contributes to the way a disease progresses can be defined as a prognostic factor. Both general and local factors need to be considered.

General Factors

1. Patient Adherence

- Bacterial plaque is the major aetiological factor for periodontal diseases. It follows therefore that effective plaque removal by the patient and adherence to regular

supportive periodontal therapy (SPT) are essential to maintain a stable periodontium and improve prognosis.
- Several studies have shown that a lack of regular SPT will adversely affect prognosis even if the periodontal disease process has been stabilised (Nyman et al. 1975, Axelsson & Lindhe 1981, Hujoel et al. 2000, Eickholz et al. 2008, Rahim-Wöstefeld et al. 2020).
- Patients attending for SPT irregularly were shown to have nearly three times more tooth loss (17.6%) compared with patients attending regularly for SPT (6%) over a period of 20 years (Rahim-Wöstefeld et al. 2020), with similar findings seen in shorter studies.
- Other studies and reviews have demonstrated similar findings in teeth with hopeless prognosis, showing teeth can be maintained and even improve their prognosis with appropriate treatment and regular SPT (Lindhe & Nyman 1984, Cortellini et al. 2011, Carvalho et al. 2021).

> ### KEY POINT 2
> Poor compliance with oral hygiene and irregular supportive periodontal therapy have a negative effect on the prognosis, with greater risk of tooth loss.

2. Smoking

- Smoking is a significant risk factor and prognostic factor in periodontal diseases and tooth loss (Fardal et al. 2004, Eickholz et al. 2008).
- Even in patients undergoing regular SPT, smokers are almost five times more susceptible to periodontal tooth loss (Chambrone et al. 2010).
- Smoking is strongly associated with worsening prognosis and has been shown to double the likelihood of worsening prognosis at 5 years (McGuire & Nunn 1996).
- The effects of smoking after cessation are dose related, and heavy smokers continue to have a significant risk of tooth loss compared with non-smokers for up to 15 years (Dietrich et al. 2015, Ravidà et al. 2020).

> ### KEY POINT 3
> There is a dose-related effect between the number of cigarettes smoked and severity of the disease/response to treatment, which significantly affects prognosis.

3. Diabetes

- Diabetic control is an important factor in periodontal prognosis, with poor glycaemic control associated with worse periodontal outcomes (Sanz et al. 2017).
- The bi-directional relationship between diabetes and periodontitis is well established, and an increased risk of periodontitis and severity of disease is associated with hyperglycaemia. Poorer periodontal outcomes have been shown following periodontal treatment in hyperglycaemic patients, therefore affecting prognosis (Mealey & Oates 2006).

> ### KEY POINT 4
> Uncontrolled diabetics have a poorer periodontal prognosis than well-controlled diabetics.

4. Other Systemic Conditions

Some systemic disorders have been shown to be associated with poorer periodontal prognosis; these are beyond the scope of this chapter but conditions include:

- Neutrophil disorders such as Down's syndrome, Chediak–Higashi syndrome, Papillon–Lefèvre syndrome and chronic neutropaenias
- Osteoporosis: Increased periodontal attachment loss in post-menopausal women with osteoporosis has been shown in a small cohort of patients, and higher levels of tooth loss are reported (Nicopoulou-Karavianni et al. 2009, Penoni et al. 2017)

5. Interleukin 1 (IL-1) Genotype

- IL-1-positive genotype has been reported to have an increased effect on tooth loss with a risk ratio (RR) of 2.66 over a period of 5–16 years. The combined effect with heavy smoking increases this effect to RR 7.7 (McGuire & Nunn 1999). A positive IL-1 genotype can be detected by genetic testing, but it seems to influence the severity of disease rather than initiation of the disease (Kornman et al. 1997). Other studies have shown that the presence of the IL-1 polymorphism has been a significant factor when assessing tooth loss; however, when including tooth-related logistic multilevel regression analysis the IL-1 positive genotype failed to show significance (Eickholz et al. 2008, Pretzl et al. 2008).

6. Age

- Age has been shown to be associated with greater tooth loss. Age over 60 years has been correlated with the number of teeth lost for periodontal reasons with various odds ratios (OR) between 1.1–7.1 reported (Fardal et al. 2004, Chambrone & Chambrone 2006). When considering tooth loss in the older cohorts >80 years of age, higher risk of losing ≥3 teeth has been shown with an OR of 3.3 (1.6–6.8) compared with younger old categories (Nilsson et al. 2019).
- Prevalence and severity of periodontitis does not seem to be affected by age (Needleman et al. 2018).
- Greater exposure over time, rather than increased susceptibility and altered immune function, may play a role in the increased tooth loss seen in older patients. Other factors to consider are access to dental care and ability to perform effective oral health measures, which will also affect the prognosis of the teeth.

7. Gender

- Male gender has been described as a prognostic indicator for tooth loss (Fardal et al. 2004), but the gender differences have been low, with less than 10% difference in disease prevalence between men and women (Shiau & Reynolds 2010). Gender has been shown to have little significance in tooth loss rates in many studies (Needleman et al. 2018).

Local Factors

1. Bacterial Biofilm

- It is widely accepted that patient compliance is a key element in improving long-term tooth survival rates.
- Good patient oral hygiene and compliance have been major factors in maintaining teeth, even for teeth with questionable/hopeless prognoses (Chace & Low 1993, McGuire & Nunn 1996, Graetz et al. 2011).

2. Bone Loss

- Advanced bone loss has been reported to be associated with greater future bone loss and reduced tooth survival rates when bone loss is over 75% (McGuire & Nunn 1996). The type of bone loss (vertical or horizontal) appears to have little impact on tooth survival. Baseline interproximal bone loss is associated with increased risk of tooth loss. However with regular SPT 93% of teeth with 60–80% bone loss at baseline survived 10 years (Pretzl et al. 2008).

3. Furcation Involvement

- Less favourable outcomes in treatment have been shown for furcation-involved teeth; McFall (1982) showed that, over 15 years, 57% of furcation-involved teeth were lost, whereas Hirshfeld & Wassermann (1978) showed over 22 years that 19.3% of furcation-involved teeth were lost, even in well-maintained individuals. Higher rates of tooth loss in furcation-involved teeth have been shown in longitudinal studies (Helal et al. 2019).
- More recent studies have shown better outcomes of furcation-involved teeth, with only 15–30% tooth loss over 15–20 years (Dannewitz et al. 2006, Rahim-Wöstefeld et al. 2020).

4. Pocket Probing Depth (PPD)

- Higher initial probing depths have been suggested to be associated with a poorer prognosis than shallower pockets (McGuire & Nunn 1996, Nieri et al. 2002), although other studies have shown no correlation between pocket depth and further attachment loss, suggesting that PPD may be less helpful to consider as a prognostic factor (Goodson et al.1982, Lindhe et al. 1983).

5. Tooth Type

- Inferior survival rates for molars (78.9%) compared to premolars (86.2%) or anterior teeth (93.1%) have been found (Rahim-Wöstefeld et al. 2020).
- Similar findings have been observed in other studies and shown maxillary molars to have a worse prognosis than mandibular molars, especially when furcation involvement is present (Ramfjord et al. 1980, Graetz et al. 2017).
- Tooth type and location has been found to be a factor associated with tooth loss in periodontal maintenance (Chambrone et al. 2010). Significant differences have been shown for retention of single-rooted teeth (91%) compared with multi-rooted teeth with furcations (76.5%) over 20 years (Rahim-Wöstefeld et al. 2020).

6.   Anatomical Defects

- Cervical enamel projections, enamel pearls and developmental grooves in maxillary incisors are all local factors associated with disease progression (Shiloah & Kopczyk 1979).
- Maxillary premolars with pronounced root concavities or "v"-shaped grooves have a worse prognosis because of an inability to access the concavities for treatment and maintenance (Badersten et al. 1987).

7.   Mobility

- The relationship between tooth mobility and periodontal prognosis is still unclear.
- Some studies have shown a poorer long-term prognosis for mobile teeth (Miller classification 2/3) with greater risk of loss of attachment (Wang et al. 1994, McGuire & Nunn 1996, Martinez-Canut 2015).
- Other studies have shown reduced mobility following various modalities of treatment and an improvement in prognosis (Persson 1980, 1981). Similar results over a 5-year period were shown when good plaque control was maintained (Nyman et al. 1975).

8.   Crown-to-Root Ratio

- Unsatisfactory crown-to-root ratio has been reported to worsen periodontal prognosis (McGuire & Nunn 1996, Martinez-Canut 2015). Percentage bone loss-to-root length also influences prognosis.

9.   Abutment Tooth

- Increased loss of teeth used as abutments has been shown, particularly abutment teeth for removable prosthesis with three times the rate of tooth loss (18%) compared to non-abutment teeth (6%), and twice the rate on fixed abutments (12%) compared with the non-abutment group over 10 years (Pretzl et al. 2008).
- Reduced loss of abutment teeth in periodontally compromised patients with cross-arch bridgework has been reported (5%) with regular periodontal maintenance over 10 years (Lulic et al. 2007).

10.   Other Pathology

- Perio-endo lesions – if the correct diagnosis is made and appropriate treatment carried out, prognosis is not affected.
- Non-vital teeth or pulpal lesions which are undetected and left untreated will have a negative impact on overall prognosis.

Assigning Prognosis

There have been many attempts to devise prognostic classification schemes and criteria but none has been validated or widely adopted.

McGuire & Nunn (1996) devised a prognostic system which took certain factors from the initial clinical data to try to correctly assign a prognosis to each tooth. Using these factors they found they could correctly assign a prognosis 81% of the time. However, they found that if the teeth which had been assigned a prognosis of "good" were not included then the predictability level dropped to 50% (i.e. the same level of predictability as tossing a coin). The following are some other studies that have attempted to devise a prognosis classification system:

- Kwok & Caton (2007) described a system to determine prognosis based on future stability rather than an end-point of tooth loss
- Fardal et al. (2004) studied prognosis and actual outcome and found 75% of teeth lost had been given an initial prognosis of questionable or poor, whereas the other 25% of teeth lost had been given an initial prognosis of "good".

Thus it would seem that the predictive accuracy is poor for the "questionable" prognosis teeth and only moderate even for "good" prognosis teeth. This is partly due to the multifactorial nature of the disease, which makes it difficult to know, in individual patients, which factors are having the greatest effects and which may most influence future disease progression.

- Martinez-Canut & Llobell (2018) designed a comprehensive approach to assigning periodontal prognosis. This involved first assessing the risk of tooth loss due to periodontal disease and second estimating the survival time of periodontally involved teeth. A long-term outcome index was used to assess tooth loss due to periodontitis, and a tooth loss prediction model was used to ascertain survival time of the periodontally involved tooth. The prediction model failed to accurately assign survival times in patients with an initial low risk of tooth loss due to periodontal disease. It highlights the difficulties such prediction models have in accurately assigning prognosis. This model considered both patient-related factors and tooth-related factors.

Future prognostic models may try to target the most "at-risk" groups of patients, which may be useful in identifying those patients at risk of higher rates of tooth loss (>3 teeth) at an earlier stage.

Although there is no universal accepted system for determining prognosis, and it is recognised that a high level of subjective clinical judgement is involved in the determination of prognosis, there are some common terms that are used. This allows some comparison in retrospective studies and systematic reviews. Some of the criteria that have been used to determine a good, questionable or hopeless prognosis are described below to give the reader an understanding of the terms.

Good Prognosis

- tooth projected to be retained as a functional unit with little or no treatment
- no evidence of disease
- no significant periodontal risk factors
  Patient prognostic factors:
- no systemic conditions
- no local factors
- good oral hygiene (OH) and good compliance

Questionable Prognosis

- tooth projected to be retained as a functional unit after treatment has been completed but may still be lost >2 years following treatment
- evidence of disease
- presence of periodontal risk factors
  Patient prognostic factors:
- Controlled systemic disease
- Smoker <20 cigarettes/day
- Moderate OH and variable compliance
  Individual tooth prognostic factors have also been used (McGuire & Nunn 1996):
- Greater than 50% attachment loss
- Poor root form/length and poor crown-to-root ratio
- Class 3 or class 2 furcation involvement accessible to maintenance
- Mobility 2 or greater

Hopeless Prognosis

- Tooth projected to be extracted during the course of treatment
  Patient prognostic factors:
- Uncontrolled systemic disease
- Smoker >20 cigarettes/day
- Poor OH and poor compliance
  Individual tooth prognostic factors (Becker et al. 1984):
- 75% bone loss
- Pocket depths 8 mm or more
- Hypermobility
- Class 2 furcations not easily accessible to maintenance
- Poor crown-to-root ratio
- Close root proximity
- Repeated abscesses

Most clinicians do agree when a tooth is beyond treatment, although there is still a "grey area" when some clinicians categorise a dubious prognosis tooth as "hopeless" and others as "questionable".

The reason this grey area exists is many research papers have shown good responses to treatment even from previously hopeless prognosis teeth, with 88% survival rates of hopeless prognosis teeth over 10 years with regeneration (Cortellini et al. 2020).

Hopeless prognosis teeth have also been retained for many years without adversely affecting the adjacent teeth (De Core et al. 1988). Questionable or hopeless prognosis teeth which have undergone treatment and long-term maintenance have shown only 8% tooth loss over 5 years (Cortellini et al. 2011) and 12% tooth loss over 40 years (Chace & Low 1993).

Many clinicians therefore opt to retain teeth, even those considered questionable or hopeless, until initial periodontal treatment has been carried out. This will of course also depend on the wishes of the patient.

When to Determine Prognosis

1. Initial Prognosis (Baseline)

- Tooth-by-tooth prognosis is common practice when first seeing a periodontal patient.
- This relies on effective history taking to determine patient factors such as diabetes and smoking history, sound clinical examination and relevant special tests (vitality testing/radiographs).
- Often no information is available on previous disease progression but as mentioned this would be helpful when determining initial prognosis.

> ### KEY POINT 5
> Initial prognosis is a helpful guide to plan treatment but usually is altered at the reassessment phase when the individual's healing potential, compliance and susceptibility are determined.

2. Revising Prognosis

Lifestyle factors, immune status, behaviour and local factors change with time, and these factors can be expected to have some influence on the prognosis, both overall and on individual teeth. Treatment plans and supportive care have to adapt to these changes over time. Determining prognosis should therefore be thought of as a "dynamic" process (Kwok & Caton 2007) and that prognosis should be re-evaluated periodically as treatment and maintenance progress.

This supports the rationale for regular supportive care, as it allows clinicians to reassess risk and, if appropriate, provide intervention at each visit. Supportive care is thus crucial in the maintenance of periodontal health, because it allows an assessment of patient compliance to supportive care, the monitoring of changes in health (i.e. control of systemic conditions) and the identification of early signs of disease recurrence (i.e. bleeding on probing, increasing in pocket depths and increasing bone loss).

Weighting Prognostic Factors

Certain factors seem to have a greater impact on prognosis – "valuable prognostic factors". Some have a synergistic effect, worsening prognosis if present together, e.g. smoking and hyperglycaemia are believed to have a greater effect together than the sum of the individual factors alone.

The difficulty is "weighting" the prognostic factors and deciding which factor(s) will have the greatest effect in any given individual.

Worsening prognosis has been associated with:
- Smoking – dose related
- Uncontrolled systemic factors, e.g hyperglycaemia
- Advanced initial probing depths with increasing attachment loss
- Advanced initial bone loss with increasing bone loss
- Increasing mobility

BOX 2.5.1 Example Of Criteria Used To Determine Prognosis (Checchi et al. 2002)

Tooth prognosis was determined as follows:
- hopeless: teeth with bone loss greater than 75% or teeth that had at least two characteristics of "questionable" category;
- questionable: bone loss between 50% and 75%, or the presence of an angular defect or furcation involvement;
- good: teeth with less than 50% bone loss or not fitting one of the two previous categories.

(Reprinted from Journal of Clinical Periodontology, 29(7):7, Trombelli et al. (2002), with permission from John Wiley & Sons.)

- Increasing furcation involvement.
  Improving prognosis has been associated with:
- Good oral hygiene (patient compliance)
- Reduction and cessation of modifiable risk factors
- Regular SPT provided
- No initial furcation involvement.

Improving the Determination of Prognosis

The ability to provide a more realistic determination of prognosis will depend on:
- An understanding of an individual's disease progression
  - This will only be possible when our knowledge of disease progression improves. Currently it is still impossible to predict, with certainty, which sites are likely to worsen. Not all sites with inflammation go on to lose attachment, although sites without signs of inflammation remain stable, so the absence of inflammation is a better indicator of health than is the presence of disease (Haffajee et al. 1991).
- Increased use of the World Workshop Classification of Periodontal and Peri-implant Diseases and Conditions (Papapanou et al. 2018), which includes a prognostic determination system by incorporating the concept of risk at the time of diagnosis. This involves the assessment of stability (in terms of bleeding) and risk factors (smoking and diabetes) to arrive at an initial evaluation of prognosis.
- Understanding periodontitis as a multifactorial disease with the ability to identify the factors affecting an individual. This will improve our ability to determine which are more "valuable" as prognostic indicators by collecting more individual data.
  - Detailed smoking histories – quantity, duration, type (nicotine level) and time since cessation
  - Monitoring control of systemic conditions such as regular HbA1c levels
  - Better reporting/monitoring of the individual's daily oral hygiene compliance

The assigning of overall and individual tooth prognosis simultaneously is a major challenge in periodontal management, and so our efforts must be to focus on the individual patient and the reduction of risk factors.

KEY POINT 6

Determining prognosis is a dynamic process. A good history and examination are essential to determine prognosis.
To improve the long-term prognosis it is important to ensure:
- Good patient compliance
- Regular supportive periodontal therapy
- Early smoking cessation to reduce risks to level of a non-smoker
- Encouragement of better general health and well being

Multiple choice questions on the contents of this chapter are available online at Elsevier eBooks+.

References

Axelsson P, Lindhe J. The significance of maintenance care in the treatment of periodontal disease. *J Clin Periodontol.* 1981;8:281–294.

Badersten A, Nilveus R, Egelberg J. Effect of nonsurgical periodontal therapy (VIII). Probing attachment changes related to clinical characteristics. *J Clin Periodontol.* 1987;14:425–432.

Beck JD. Issues in assessment of diagnostic tests and risk for periodontal diseases. *Periodontol 2000.* 1995;7:100–108.

Becker W, Berg L, Becker BE. The long term evaluation of periodontal treatment and maintenance in 95 patients. *Int J Periodontics Restorative Dent.* 1984;4:54–71.

Carvalho R, Botelho J, Machado V, et al. Predictors of tooth loss during long–term periodontal maintenance: an updated systematic review. *J Clin Periodontol.* 2021;1-18.

Chace Sr R, Low SB. Survival characteristics of periodontally-involved teeth: a 40-year study. *J Periodontol.* 1993;64:701–705.

Chambrone LA, Chambrone L. Tooth loss in well-maintained patients with chronic periodontitis during long-term supportive therapy in Brazil. *J Clin Periodontol.* 2006;33:759–764.

Chambrone L, Chambrone D, Lima LA, Chambrone LA. Predictors of tooth loss during long-term periodontal maintenance: a systematic review of observational studies. *J Clin Periodontol.* 2010;37:675–684.

Checchi L, Montevecchi M, Gatto MRA, Trombelli L. Retrospective study of tooth loss in 92 treated periodontal patients. *J Clin Periodontol.* 2002;29(7):651–656.

Cortellini P, Stalpers G, Mollo A, Tonetti MS. Periodontal regeneration versus extraction and prosthetic replacement of teeth severely compromised by attachment loss to the apex: 5-year results of an ongoing randomized clinical trial. *J Clin Periodontol.* 2011;38:915–924.

Cortellini P, Stalpers G, Mollo A, Tonetti MS. Periodontal regeneration versus extraction and dental implant or prosthetic replacement of teeth severely compromised by attachment loss to the apex: a randomized controlled clinical trial reporting 10–year outcomes, survival analysis and mean cumulative cost of recurrence. *J Clin Periodontol.* 2020;47(6):768–776.

Dannewitz B, Krieger JK, Husing J, Eickholz P. Loss of molars in periodontally treated patients: a retrospective analysis five years or more after active periodontal treatment. *J Clin Periodontol.* 2006;33:53–61.

DeCore CH, Beck FM, Horton JE. Retained "hopeless" teeth. Effects on the proximal periodontium of adjacent teeth. *J Periodontol.* 1988;59:647–651.

Dietrich T, Walter C, Oluwagbemigun K, et al. Smoking, smoking cessation, and risk of tooth loss. *J Dent Res.* 2015;94(10):1369–1375.

Eickholz P, Kaltschmitt J, Berbig J, Reitmeir P, Pretzl B. Tooth loss after active periodontal therapy. 1: patient-related factors for risk, prognosis, and quality of outcome. *J Clin Periodontol.* 2008;35:165–174.

Fardal O, Johannessen AC, Linden GJ. Tooth loss during maintenance following periodontal treatment in a periodontal practice in Norway. *J Clin Periodontol.* 2004;31:550–555.

Goodson JM, Tanner AC, Haffajee AD, Sornberger GC, Socransky SS. Patterns of progression and regression of advanced destructive periodontal disease. *J Clin Periodontol.* 1982;9:472–481.

Graetz C, Dorfer CE, Kahl M, Kocher T, Fawzy El-Sayed K, Wiebe JF, et al. Retention of questionable and hopeless teeth in compliant patients treated for aggressive periodontitis. *J Clin Periodontol.* 2011;38:707–714.

Graetz C, Sälzer S, Plaumann A, et al. Tooth loss in generalized aggressive periodontitis: prognostic factors after 17 years of supportive periodontal treatment. *J Clin Periodontol.* 2017;44(6):612–619.

Haffajee AD, Socransky SS, Lindhe J, Kent RL, Okamoto H, Yoneyama T. Clinical risk indicators for periodontal attachment loss. *J Clin Periodontol.* 1991;18:117–125.

Helal O, Göstemeyer G, Krois J, Fawzy El Sayed K, Graetz C, Schwendicke F. Predictors for tooth loss in periodontitis patients: Systematic review and meta–analysis. *J Clin Periodontol.* 2019;46:699–712.

Hirschfeld L, Wasserman B. A long-term survey of tooth loss in 600 treated periodontal patients. *J Periodontol.* 1978;49:225–237.

Hujoel PP, Leroux BG, Selipsky H, White BA. Non-surgical periodontal therapy and tooth loss. A cohort study. *J Periodontol.* 2000;71:736–742.

Kornman KS, Crane A, Wang HY, et al. The interleukin-1 genotype as a severity factor in adult periodontal disease. *J Clin Periodontol.* 1997;24:72–77.

Kwok V, Caton JG. Commentary: prognosis revisited: a system for assigning periodontal prognosis. *J Periodontol.* 2007;78:2063–2071.

Lindhe J, Haffajee AD, Socransky SS. Progression of periodontal disease in adult subjects in the absence of periodontal therapy. *J Clin Periodontol.* 1983;10:433–442.

Lindhe J, Nyman S. Long-term maintenance of patients treated for advanced periodontal disease. *J Clin Periodontol.* 1984;11:504–514.

Lulic M, Brägger U, Lang NP, Zwahlen M, Salvi GE. Ante's (1926) law revisited: a systematic review on survival rates and complications of fixed dental prostheses (FDPs) on severely reduced periodontal tissue support. *Clin Oral Implants Res.* 2007;18:63–72.

Martinez-Canut P. Predictors of tooth loss due to periodontal disease in patients following long-term periodontal maintenance. *J Clin Periodontol.* 2015;42(12):1115–1125.

Martinez-Canut P, Llobell A. A comprehensive approach to assigning periodontal prognosis. *J Clin Periodontol.* 2018;45(4):431–439.

McFall Jr WT. Tooth loss in 100 treated patients with periodontal disease. A long-term study. *J Periodontol.* 1982;53:539–549.

McGuire MK, Nunn ME. Prognosis versus actual outcome. II. The effectiveness of clinical parameters in developing an accurate prognosis. *J Periodontol.* 1996;67:658–665.

McGuire MK, Nunn ME. Prognosis versus actual outcome. IV. The effectiveness of clinical parameters and IL-1 genotype in accurately predicting prognoses and tooth survival. *J Periodontol.* 1999;70:49–56.

Mealey BL, Oates TW. Diabetes mellitus and periodontal diseases. *J Periodontol.* 2006;77(8):1289–1303.

Needleman I, Garcia R, Gkranias N, et al. Mean annual attachment, bone level, and tooth loss: a systematic review. *J Periodontol.* 2018;89:S120–S139.

Nicopoulou-Karayianni K, Tzoutzoukos P, Mitsea A, et al. Tooth loss and osteoporosis: the OSTEODENT Study. *J Clin Periodontol.* 2009;36:190–197.

Nieri M, Muzzi L, Cattabriga M, Rotundo R, Cairo F, Pini Prato GP. The prognostic value of several periodontal factors measured as radiographic bone level variation: a 10-year retrospective multilevel analysis of treated and maintained periodontal patients. *J Periodontol.* 2002;73:1485–1493.

Nilsson H, Sanmartin Berglund J, Renvert S. Longitudinal evaluation of periodontitis and tooth loss among older adults. *J Clin Periodontol.* 2019;46(10):1041–1049.

Nyman S, Rosling B, Lindhe J. Effect of professional tooth cleaning on healing after periodontal surgery. *J Clin Periodontol.* 1975;2:80–86.

Papapanou PN, Sanz M, Buduneli N, et al. Periodontitis: consensus report of workgroup 2 of the 2017 World Workshop on the Classification of Periodontal and Peri-Implant Diseases and Conditions. *J Periodontol.* 2018;89:S173–S182.

Penoni DC, Fidalgo TK, Torres SR, et al. Bone density and clinical periodontal attachment in postmenopausal women: a systematic review and meta-analysis. *J Dent Res.* 2017;96:261–269.

Persson R. Assessment of tooth mobility using small loads. II. Effect of oral hygiene procedures. *J Clin Periodontol.* 1980;7:506–515.

Persson R. Assessment of tooth mobility using small loads. IV. The effect of periodontal treatment including gingivectomy and flap procedures. *J Clin Periodontol.* 1981;8:88–97.

Pretzl B, Kaltschmitt J, Kim T-S, Reitmeir P, Eickholz P. Tooth loss after active periodontal therapy. 2: tooth-related factors. *J Clin Periodontol.* 2008;35(2):175–182.

Rahim–Wöstefeld S, El Sayed N, Weber D, et al. Tooth–related factors for tooth loss 20 years after active periodontal therapy–A partially prospective study. *J Clin Periodontol.* 2020;47(10):1227–1236.

Ramfjord SP, Knowles JW, Morrison EC, Burgett FG, Nissle RR. Results of periodontal therapy related to tooth type. *J Periodontol.* 1980;51:270–273.

Ravidà A, Troiano G, Qazi M, et al. Dose–dependent effect of smoking and smoking cessation on periodontitis–related tooth loss during 10 - 47 years periodontal maintenance—A retrospective study in compliant cohort. *J Clin Periodontol.* 2020;47(9):1132–1143.

Sanz M, Ceriello A, Buysschaert M, et al. Scientific evidence on the links between periodontal diseases and diabetes: consensus report and guidelines of the joint workshop on periodontal diseases and diabetes by the International Diabetes Federation and the European Federation of Periodontology. *J Clin Periodontol.* 2017;45(2):138–149.

Shiau HJ, Reynolds MA. Sex differences in destructive periodontal disease: a systematic review. *J Periodontol.* 2010;81:1379–1389.

Shiloah J, Kopczyk RA. Developmental variations of tooth morphology and periodontal disease. *J Am Dent Assoc.* 1979;99:627–630.

Wang HL, Burgett FG, Shyr Y, Ramfjord S. The influence of molar furcation involvement and mobility on future clinical periodontal attachment loss. *J. Periodontol.* 1994;65:25–29.

Periodontal Treatment Planning

3.1

TREATMENT PLANNING – GINGIVITIS AND PERIODONTITIS

PAUL BAKER

CHAPTER OUTLINE

OVERVIEW OF THE CHAPTER

This chapter outlines treatment planning for gingivitis, acute gingival conditions, periodontitis and the management of furcation-involved teeth.

By the end of the chapter the reader should:

- Understand the aims of periodontal treatment and how these fit into the overall dental treatment plan
- Be familiar with the stepwise approach to periodontal care and how this is reflected in periodontal treatment planning
- Be able to formulate a treatment plan for the management of gingivitis and periodontitis
- Recognise the presentation of acute gingival conditions and outline their management
- Describe the treatment options for furcation-involved multi-rooted teeth.

The chapter covers the following topics:

- Introduction
- Management of simple plaque-induced gingivitis
- Acute gingival conditions and their management
- Outcomes of periodontal treatment
- The stepwise approach to periodontal treatment
- Structuring periodontal treatment
- Achieving the ideal end points of treatment
- Periodontal reassessment
- Management of furcations
- Summary

Introduction

This chapter looks at the treatment of acute periodontal conditions and considers the treatment planning of gingivitis and periodontitis. Chronic periodontal diseases provide a particular challenge in treatment planning in that clinicians do not

"cure" patients with a course of treatment; rather, the aim is to control disease. The short-term responses to active treatment may not entirely resolve the patient's clinical signs of the disease. Also, long-term stability relies heavily on the patient's own efforts with home care. As a result, the management of periodontitis often relies on a staged approach where patients undergo a course of treatment, and the response to each stage of treatment is assessed before decisions about the next stage can be made. It is essential that adequate time is given for the tissues to respond to therapy before a reassessment is made and worth remembering that the supporting tissues include epithelium, connective tissue and bone.

> ### KEY POINT 1
> Periodontal diseases provide a particular challenge in their treatment planning in that clinicians do not "cure" patients with a course of treatment; instead the aim is to control disease. Long-term stability relies heavily on the patient's own efforts with home care.

Management of Simple Plaque-Induced Gingivitis

Gingivitis is an inflammatory response of the marginal gingiva. Dental plaque as the primary cause is supported by overwhelming evidence from clinical, microbiological and epidemiological studies. Management involves the consistent and effective removal of the plaque biofilm at the gingival margin. A classic experimental gingivitis study by Löe et al. (1965) showed that effective oral hygiene will resolve gingivitis in as little as 7–10 days.

As explained in Chapter 2.2, the basic periodontal examination (BPE) identifies gingivitis in BPE codes 1 and 2. Code 1 is defined as bleeding after probing, with no probing depths over 3.5 mm. As such, this common condition should respond to improvements in oral hygiene to remove plaque biofilm from the critical gingival marginal area.

Code 2 describes the presence of plaque-retentive factors in areas that may reduce the effectiveness of oral hygiene techniques by the patient. Plaque-retentive factors are local conditions in the mouth that increase the amount of biofilm that forms in an area or inhibits self-performed plaque control, promoting biofilm accumulation.

Such plaque-retentive factors include calculus, which may interfere with a patient's ability to clean inter-proximally (Figure 3.1.1) and which also presents as a rough surface that may be more difficult to clean. Other plaque-retentive factors include anything that creates an area inaccessible to clean or a surface that is harder to render plaque-free, such as a poor restoration margin, an overhang, a marginal discrepancy, a rough restorative surface or a carious lesion.

> ### KEY POINT 2
> Although a BPE score of 2 indicates the presence of a plaque-retentive factor, sufficient plaque to cause gingival bleeding may not be present at up to a third of sites with this score.

Where plaque-retentive factors are present, they need to be corrected as part of the management of plaque-induced gingivitis. Clinicians must do what they can to ensure that the mouth is more easily cleansable for the patient. This means removing any plaque-retentive factors where possible,

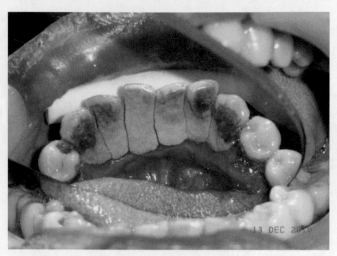

• **Figure 3.1.1** Interproximal calculus hampering plaque control.

including easily accessible calculus, in conjunction with oral hygiene instruction. Poor restoration margins should be corrected, where possible, by reducing and polishing of overhangs (Figure 3.1.2) or the placement of temporary or permanent restorations. The patient then needs to be given the tools they require to achieve an adequate level of plaque control (see Chapter 4.1). It is essential that the patient is reviewed to ensure that they have managed to improve their home care in accordance with the instructions given and that the gingivitis has resolved as a result.

To assess the response to this treatment, a reassessment should be scheduled after an appropriate time to allow the gingivitis to resolve, or for the plaque to re-establish if the patient's oral hygiene is still not adequate. This normally takes at least 2 weeks.

Acute Gingival Conditions and Their Management

- Periodontal abscess
- Necrotising gingivitis
- Acute herpetic gingivostomatitis

Periodontal Abscess

In this context, the periodontal abscess (Figure 3.1.3) is one that originates in a pre-existing periodontal pocket as opposed to one originating primarily from a necrotic pulp, which can, on occasion, track coronally to drain via the gingival crevice or present laterally due to the presence of a lateral canal (the so-called perio-endo lesion).

A periodontal abscess may occur when the coronal margin of a periodontal pocket becomes blocked, preventing drainage of a pre-existing chronic lesion. This can result from the impaction of a foreign body or food debris becoming lodged in the pocket. Alternatively, improved gingival health after periodontal treatment may result in the marginal tissue around the neck of the tooth becoming tighter, preventing drainage from the pocket and, if plaque-retentive factors persist at the base of the pocket, an acute response can occur.

There may also be an increased tendency towards the formation of periodontal abscesses in patients who are immunocompromised, especially in poorly controlled diabetic patients (Herrera et al. 2000). The aetiology and management of periodontal abscesses is shown in Box 3.1.1.

> ### KEY POINT 3
> A periodontal abscess is one that originates in a pre-existing periodontal pocket, as opposed to one originating primarily from a necrotic pulp.

Necrotising Gingivitis

Necrotising gingivitis (Figure 3.1.4 and Box 3.1.2) is an acute infection affecting the marginal gingival tissues around the teeth. It has a very particular clinical picture that is

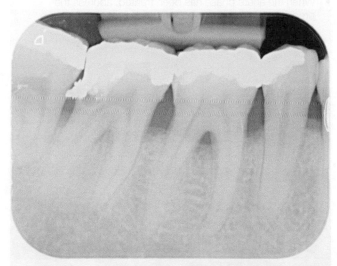

• **Figure 3.1.2** A restoration overhang at LR7 distally which acts as a plaque-retention factor.

characterised by a white slough of necrotic tissue superficially adjacent to the teeth and an adjacent zone of red inflamed tissue. The necrotic area tends to start at the papillae tips. Patients with necrotising gingivitis frequently exhibit an offensive oral odour. The causal organisms for necrotising gingivitis have been described as made up of a "constant flora" and a "variable flora". The constant flora includes spirochaetes such as *Borrelia vincentii* and bacteria such as *B. intermedius* and *Fusobacterium* spp., and the variable flora consists of other species of micro-organisms, the exact mix of which varies from patient to patient and site to site (Loesche et al. 1982).

There are particular predisposing factors that render a patient more susceptible to necrotising gingivitis. These include stress and smoking. In the First World War, over 50% of troops serving in the trenches developed the infection, and in the Second World War, it was very prevalent among submariners. There is also an increased incidence of necrotising gingivitis in patients who are HIV positive.

The management of necrotising gingivitis should include the treatment of acute infection and of the underlying predisposing factors to reduce the risk of recurrence. Recurrent episodes of necrotising gingivitis can lead to interdental cratering where the interdental tissues have been lost (Figure 3.1.5).

Treatment involves gentle cleaning and the use of mouthwashes, such as hydrogen peroxide or chlorhexidine (see Box 3.1.2). Necrotising gingivitis responds well to antibiotics, particularly the penicillins and metronidazole. However, these should be considered an adjunct to mechanical debridement (Hartnett & Shiloah 1991). It is worth noting that although necrotising gingivitis is associated with specific bacteria, it is not a contagious condition and cannot be passed between individuals.

> ### KEY POINT 4
> Although necrotising gingivitis is associated with specific bacteria, it is not thought to be a contagious condition and cannot be passed between individuals.

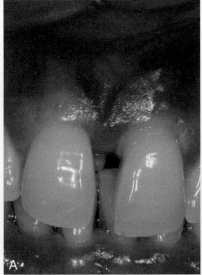
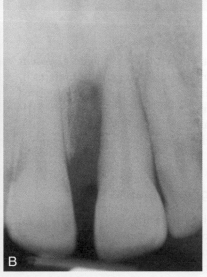

• **Figure 3.1.3** A periodontal abscess.

• BOX 3.1.1   Aetiology of Periodontal Abscesses

Causes of Periodontal Abscess

- Pre-existing periodontal pocket
- Foreign body impaction, including food, in periodontal pocket
- Response to incomplete periodontal therapy
  - Improvement in marginal tissue health before pockets fully debrided
  - Plaque or calculus pushed into tissues during instrumentation
- Compromised immune system
  - Poorly controlled diabetes

Signs and Symptoms of Periodontal Abscess

- Pain
- Localised swelling over the tooth
- Pus may come from the gingival margin on probing or pressure on local soft tissues
- There may be an increase in mobility
- Deep periodontal probing depth
- Evidence of a susceptibility to periodontal disease

Treatment of Periodontal Abscess

- Drainage of the abscess is usually achieved by periodontal instrumentation
- Local anaesthesia and thorough root-surface debridement
- Antibiotics should not routinely be required but may be considered where there is an underlying systemic medical factor

• BOX 3.1.2   Presentation and Management of Necrotising Gingivitis

Predisposing Factors

- Pre-existing gingivitis
- Poor oral hygiene
- Smoking
- Stress

Signs and Symptoms

- Ulceration of the papillae tips or gingival margin
- Formation of a pseudo-membrane
- Pain
- Halitosis

Treatment

- Debridement, though this may be painful
- Mouthwashes can help, particularly chlorhexidine or hydrogen peroxide based
- Antibiotics may be prescribed. Metronidazole is the drug of choice
- When the acute phase has been treated, address the predisposing factors to reduce the chance of recurrence

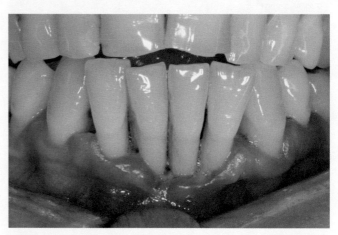

• **Figure 3.1.5** Interproximal cratering following an episode of necrotising gingivitis.

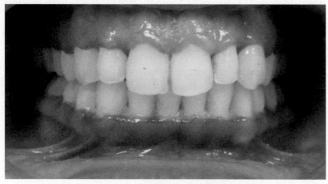

• **Figure 3.1.4** Necrotising gingivitis.

A more aggressive form of necrotising gingivitis can occur that extends to the underlying supporting bone and attachment. So-called necrotising periodontitis may be associated with an underlying immune deficiency, particularly HIV (Robinson 1998) or malnutrition. While the destruction is far more significant, the principles of treatment are the same.

Acute Herpetic Gingivostomatitis

Primary herpetic gingivostomatitis (Box 3.1.3) is an acute local infection by the herpes simplex virus. It presents as multiple small vesicles that can coalesce to produce larger irregular ulcerated lesions surrounded by erythema (Figure 3.1.6). Lesions may be limited to the

• BOX 3.1.3   Presentation and Management of Acute Herpetic Gingivostomatitis

Signs and Symptoms

- Usually pre-school children
- Painful oral ulceration
- Pyrexia
- Increased saliva

Treatment

- Treat symptoms
  - Anti-pyretic medication
  - Maintain fluid intake
- Wait for infection to run its course, usually 1–2 weeks

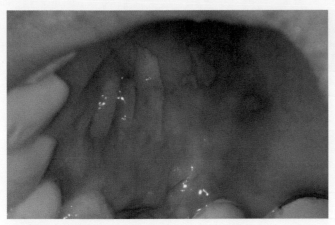

• **Figure 3.1.6** Irregular ulceration and erythema in herpetic gingivostomatitis.

gingiva or include other mucosal areas of the mouth. Historically, in the United Kingdom, the condition was usually seen in young children where it is associated with herpes simplex virus (HSV) 1. However, increasingly, it is seen in young adults where it tends to be associated with HSV-2.

Transmission is by direct contact with the infected lesions or saliva of an individual with an infected lesion.

Treatment Planning for Periodontitis

Outcomes of Periodontal Treatment

Much of dentistry involves planning for treatment where the result can be predicted with some certainty, such as the placement of a restoration in a tooth with a small- or medium-sized carious lesion. Some situations are less predictable both in the short-term response to treatment and the longer-term success of that treatment.

The management of periodontitis often falls into this more unpredictable category, and clinicians therefore schedule reassessment appointments to monitor what has been achieved by treatment to date and to plan the next stage (Box 3.1.4). Ultimately, the aim is to achieve a beneficial outcome for the patient; however, successful treatment of periodontitis can only be judged in the long term by stable attachment levels and the retention of teeth. The difficulty with this approach is that success is being judged retrospectively. When treating patients or trying to assess the clinical success of treatment, surrogate measures, which are associated with periodontal stability, are used. The most commonly reported measure with the greatest predictive ability for tooth loss is probing pocket depth. The British Society of Periodontology and Implant Dentistry has produced guidelines that outline the ideal end points of the treatment of periodontitis (Box 3.1.5). These are helpful for the clinician as they set the aims for any course of periodontal treatment and also set standards against which the patient can be judged during reassessment.

> • **BOX 3.1.4** **Overall Treatment Outcomes in Periodontal Therapy**
>
> • **Definitive** – leading to a definite end point
> • **Provisional** – leading to an intermediate stage in treatment to allow further consideration
> • **Compromise** – leading to a less-than-ideal end point because of unfavourable factors
>   Patients should be aware of the aims of treatment and understand why uncertainty may be an issue.

> • **BOX 3.1.5** **Ideal Treatment Outcomes in Periodontal Therapy**
>
> • All pockets 4 mm or less
> • Bleeding on probing less than 10%
> • Plaque score less than 15%
> • No furcations probeable
>   As defined by the British Society of Periodontology and Implant Dentistry, these are the ideal end points of treatment as they are associated with periodontal stability. These end points may not be achievable in some cases and a compromise may have to be accepted.

> **KEY POINT 5**
>
> Successful treatment of periodontitis can only be judged in the long term by stable attachment levels and the retention of teeth.

For periodontitis, one approach is to divide the phases of treatment into:
• *Cause-related therapy* – generally speaking, non-surgical treatment aimed at managing the cause of the disease and resulting in clinical improvements in the soft tissues
• *Corrective therapy* – surgical procedures such as pocket reduction or elimination that aim to re-establish a normal dento-gingival anatomy, albeit at a different position around the tooth
• *Supportive periodontal therapy* – ongoing regular periodontal therapy aimed at maintaining periodontal health and reducing or preventing further disease progression.

This is not to say that one phase of treatment necessarily progresses to the next, rather that these are staged approaches in managing the disease. With a high level of patient compliance, many periodontal conditions may stabilise with cause-related therapy alone. The best approach for an individual patient, or clinical situation, will depend on the patient's attitude as well as the oral findings. The European Federation of Periodontology (EFP) produced the S3 Clinical Practice Guideline for the Treatment of Stage I-III Periodontitis (Kebschull & Chapple 2020, Sanz et al. 2020). This applied evidence-based clinical recommendations as a *stepwise* approach to treatment (see Chapter 4.3 for further details).

Table 4 Stepwise approach			
Step of therapy	Periodontitis stage I	Periodontitis stage II	Periodontitis stage III (and stage IV in BSP implementation plan)
Step 1: Control of risk factors	Always		
Step 2: Subgingival instrumentation	Only in affected teeth		Only in affected teeth, possibly with adjunctive measures
Step 3: Corrective surgery	N/A		Only in affected teeth after re-evaluation of step 2 procedures; specialists/dentists with specific training; subjects with adequate biofilm control
Supportive periodontal therapy	Always		

• **Figure 3.1.7** The stepwise approach to treating periodontitis. (Reprinted by permission from Springer Nature: Br. Dent. J. Evidence-based, personalised and minimally invasive treatment for periodontitis patients - the new EFP S3-level clinical treatment guidelines, Kebschull, M., Chapple, I., copyright 2020.)

The *Stepwise* Approach to Periodontal Treatment

The stepwise approach (see Appendices 3 and 4) breaks treatment down into a series of stages which follow the classic management strategy for periodontitis and maps them to the new classification system developed in 2017. The extent to which a patient is likely to progress along the stepwise approach can be estimated by their classification (Figure 3.1.7).

The first stage of treatment is considered the pre-requisite to therapy and referred to as step 0 (see Appendix 3). This includes the initial examination and subsequent diagnosis and classification of the periodontal condition. Risk factors should be assessed, and the patients educated on the causes of the disease and relevance of those risk factors. From there, a personal care plan should be developed.

Step 1

Step 1 is aimed at motivating the patient and establishing the behaviour changes required for successful periodontal treatment. Optimal oral hygiene has been shown to be critical to the long-term stability of any post-treatment improvements (Axelsson et al. 2004). Optimal supragingival plaque control is also required to reduce subgingival recolonisation by the periodontal pathogens associated with the disease (Magnusson et al. 1984). For this reason, ideally, an optimal level of oral hygiene should be established before undertaking subgingival instrumentation. As a patient's home care improves, there should be a reduction in inflammation, and this will lead to a reduction in probing depths. Oral hygiene is covered in more detail in Chapters 4.1 and 4.3.

Local risk factors should be addressed, such as the removal of supragingival plaque-retentive factors, as mentioned in the section on the management of gingivitis, along with professional mechanical plaque removal

(PMPR). Consideration should also be given to systemic factors, such as smoking cessation advice or diabetes control.

> ### KEY POINT 6
> Optimal oral hygiene has been shown to be critical to the long-term stability of any post-treatment improvements.

Step 2

This is the cause-related therapy mentioned previously and involves disruption of the biofilm by subgingival instrumentation, possibly including the use of local or systemic adjunctive measures if appropriate (such as local delivery antiseptics or systemic antibiotics).

Subgingival instrumentation is aimed at removing plaque and plaque-retentive factors, such as subgingival calculus, from root surfaces. Significant probing depth reduction can be achieved by non-surgical periodontal treatment, which is almost invariably the first line of treatment. This is technically demanding and requires scheduling sufficient time to allow the treatment to be done thoroughly. There are different ways of approaching the appointment schedules (see Chapters 5.1 and 5.2), depending upon the extent and severity of the disease, the clinician's preferred approach and the patient's acceptance of treatment. There is little evidence to support one approach over another (Eberhard et al. 2008).

Adjunctive use of specific antibiotics may be prescribed for specific cases where the disease is particularly aggressive, such as generalised periodontitis stage III in a young adult. If adjunctive antibiotics are used, then it is essential that all the root-surface instrumentation is completed during the course of antibiotics (see Chapter 5.3).

Step 3

Step 3 follows a periodontal reassessment after a suitable time is allowed for a response to the non-surgical therapy.

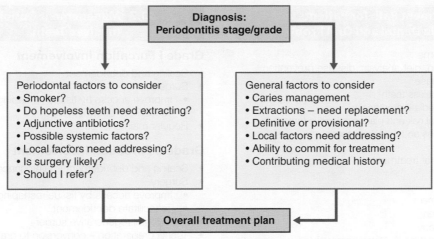

• **Figure 3.1.8** Factors to consider when a diagnosis of periodontitis has been made.

When there are sites where the end points have not been met, then further treatment, as outlined in step 3, is considered. This may involve further non-surgical therapy when further improvements could or should be expected, or surgical intervention where anatomical considerations such as vertical bone loss or furcation involvements limit the likelihood of success by simpler means. Periodontal surgery should not be considered in the absence of adequate level of plaque control by the patient.

Step 4

Step 4 represents supportive periodontal therapy (SPT), which is aimed at maintaining periodontal stability. It can be hoped that the periodontally involved sites have responded to the treatment provided in either step 2 or step 3, and the ideal end points have been achieved. The patient can then be put into an SPT regime appropriate for their needs (Chapter 5.4).

Structuring Periodontal Treatment

The stepwise approach helps structure the management of periodontitis, but this still needs to be tailored to the individual needs of the patient. Figure 3.1.8 gives examples of the factors that could influence the overall treatment plan. As the complexity of a case increases, so does the importance of assessing the prognosis as part of the planning process (Table 3.1.1). The prognosis can relate to individual teeth, based on factors that may be favourable or unfavourable, or to patient factors that will influence the response to treatment. Estimation of prognosis will allow the clinician to make judgements on the likely outcome of treatment both at a tooth level and patient level. Prognosis is covered in detail in Chapter 2.5.

It is also worth considering where periodontal treatment fits into the overall management of a dental patient. Dental education can compartmentalise dentistry into its various specialities and disciplines. There is an obvious benefit to this, particularly when considering that teaching

TABLE 3.1.1	Factors to consider when assessing prognosis	
Assessing prognosis		
Tooth factors	**Patient factors**	
Restorative condition	Susceptibility	
Endodontic condition	Oral hygiene ability	
Periodontal condition	Dexterity	
Attachment level	Motivation	
Bone height	Systemic disease	
Root length	Smoking status	
Root shape/divergence		
Site of defect		
Plaque-retentive factors		
Furcation involvement		

hospitals are divided into departments. However, in dental practice, patients will often present with multiple oral problems, and a decision has to be made about the prioritisation of treatment and how to break down the treatment into a manageable, logical structure. This will ensure that all the oral problems are considered in a systematic way (Box 3.1.6).

Achieving the Ideal End Points of Treatment

The aims of periodontal treatment have been outlined in Box 3.1.5. These treatment outcomes do not eliminate the risk of disease progression but are all associated with maximising the likelihood of stability and a reduced risk of progression. A treatment plan for the management of periodontitis is aimed at achieving these outcomes. The success of each phase of treatment, or after treatment during SPT, is judged on the reassessment which should be scheduled within an appropriate time frame.

Periodontal Reassessment

Clinicians do not cure patients of periodontal diseases; rather they aim to control the disease. As such, there is no actual end to treatment, and the long-term maintenance of periodontal health is an ongoing process (see Chapter 5.4). The purpose of a reassessment appointment is to assess whether the desired clinical end points have been achieved and to decide what the next stage of treatment is for the patient. This may be further active treatment or the prescription of a supportive periodontal maintenance regimen and setting of a recall period, when a formal periodontal review will be performed. The time between active treatment and reassessment should be sufficient for the tissues to respond. Badersten et al. (1984) showed that there may be improvements for up to 9 months following non-surgical treatment. However, most of the change will have occurred and be recordable at 8–12 weeks. Therefore, reassessment appointments are often scheduled 8–12 weeks after active treatment.

The reassessment appointment involves gathering all the relevant periodontal data once again so that these can be compared to previous periodontal examinations. Improvements in clinical parameters, as well as assessment of further disease progression or stability, will all be considered when deciding what the next stage of treatment should be. This might involve further oral hygiene instruction with the aim of improving the long-term stability, further subgingival debridement or periodontal surgery.

Further non-surgical treatment is considered if further improvements can be expected. This may occur when there

is residual inflammation or where there is a thin tissue biotype that can be expected to recede, leading to probing depth reduction, or where tissue shrinkage as a result of the initial therapy has improved access to residual contaminated root surface and calculus deposits. Periodontal surgery still has a place and can be considered when it is appropriate (see Chapter 6.1).

Management of Furcations

Furcation involvements can pose a particular challenge in their management. The positions of the furcation entrances are often in less accessible areas of the mouth, making treatment and access for plaque control more awkward. Furcations are associated with complex tooth shapes within the furcation leading to an unfavourable anatomy for plaque control as well as adversely affecting the healing potential. There is less scope for a reduction in the probing depths after treatment. The classification of furcation involvements is covered in Chapter 2.2. The management options for the treatment of furcations are summarised in Box 3.1.7.

Scaling and Root-Surface Instrumentation (Non-Surgical Treatment)

Scaling and root-surface instrumentation can be particularly challenging in furcation-involved teeth because of the additional difficulties in accessing the root surface. Teeth with narrow furcation entrances and close roots can be very

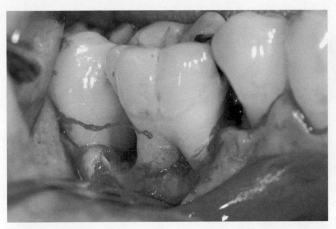

• **Figure 3.1.9** Osteoplasty in the furcation area to improve access for plaque control.

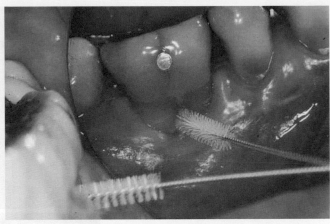

• **Figure 3.1.10** Access between the roots in this class III furcation allows the patient to clean with an interdental brush.

difficult to clean thoroughly, and the tooth surface may have concavities within the furcation that cannot be accessed by even the smallest curette or ultrasonic tip. Furcation entrances may also be interproximal in the case of upper first premolars.

Furcation Surgery

Periodontal surgery to furcation entrances can help overcome the difficulties associated with non-surgical management of furcation entrances. Access to the root surface for debridement is improved by raising a periodontal flap. The local tissues can also be adjusted where possible to improve postoperative maintenance. The furcation entrance itself can be carefully opened by means of judicious use of a water-cooled handpiece. This local osteoplasty (bone removal) and flap modification can improve the postoperative access for maintenance (Figure 3.1.9).

Periodontal regenerative surgery is a technique that aims to stimulate bone growth in intra-bony defects. In theory this could occur between the roots to close the furcation. Whilst regenerative surgery is recognised as a possible treatment option, this has proven to be an unpredictable way of managing furcations.

Tunnel Preparation

The tunnel preparation aims to convert a grade II or grade III furcation into an open grade III furcation that can be maintained by the patient (Figure 3.1.10). It will usually involve raising buccal and lingual flaps and reshaping the tissues to leave the furcation open for interproximal brushing. Occasionally, persistent oral hygiene can convert a grade II or III furcation involvement to one that can be maintained in this way. Hellden et al. (1989) looked at the

survival of teeth that had had tunnel procedures and found the main reason for failure in teeth treated in this way was caries in the furcation.

Root Resection

Root resection is an option for converting an uncleansable furcation defect into one that can be maintained by dividing the tooth and either removing one root (root resection), one half of the tooth (hemisection) or converting a molar unit into two premolar-sized units by dividing the crown and restoring each root as individual premolar-sized units (premolarisation) (Figures 3.1.11 and 3.1.12). These can be complicated treatment options as the tooth needs to be root-treated before the roots can be sectioned and removed, and often the tooth will need to be restored with a full coverage crown afterwards. Lee et al. (2012) recently showed that the average lifespan of a root-resected tooth is around 7 years, so it should still be considered as a possible treatment option to prolong the life of a severely compromised tooth.

Summary

Periodontal treatment, and periodontal treatment planning, should always be considered in the context of the patient's overall treatment needs. Once any acute problems have been resolved, periodontal treatment planning then aims to control the destructive processes that characterise periodontitis. Following a stepwise approach to periodontal treatment planning should ensure a successful and stable periodontal outcome. Central to successful periodontal outcomes is the patient's self-care as well as long-term professional supportive care.

Multiple choice questions on the contents of this chapter are available online at Elsevier eBooks+.

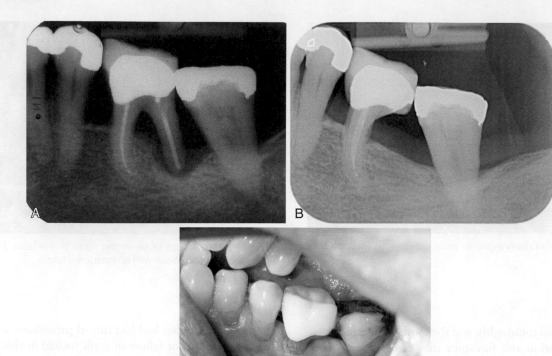

• **Figure 3.1.11** A root-resected lower molar tooth: (A) the tooth on presentation, (B) radiograph and (C) clinical appearance 10 years after surgery.

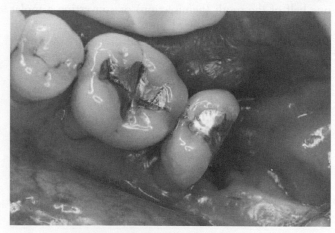

• **Figure 3.1.12** A hemisected lower molar tooth.

References

Axelsson P, Nyström B, Lindhe J. The long-term effect of a plaque control program on tooth mortality, caries and periodontal disease in adults. Results after 30 years of maintenance. *J Clin Periodontol.* 2004;31:749–757.

Badersten A, Nilveus R, Egelberg J. Effect of non-surgical periodontal therapy II. Severely advanced periodontitis. *J Clin Periodontol.* 1984;11:63–76.

Eberhard J, Jervøe-Storm PM, Needleman I, Worthington H, Jepsen S. Full-mouth treatment concepts for chronic periodontitis: a systematic review. *J Clin Periodontol.* 2008;35:591–604.

Hartnett AC, Shiloah J. The treatment of acute necrotizing ulcerative gingivitis. *Quintessence Int (Berl).* 1991;22:95–100.

Hellden LB, Elliot A, Steffennsen B, Steffensen JEM. Prognosis of tunnel preparations in the treatment of class III furcations. A follow-up study. *J Periodontol.* 1989;60:182–187.

Herrera D, Roldan S, Sanz M. The periodontal abscess: a review. *J Clin Periodontol.* 2000;27:377–386.

Kebschull M, Chapple I. Evidence-based, personalised and minimally invasive treatment for periodontitis patients - the new EFP S3-level clinical treatment guidelines. *Br Dent J.* 2020;229(7):443–449.

Lee KL, Corbet EF, Leung WK. Survival of molar teeth after resective periodontal therapy – a retrospective study. *J Clin Periodontol.* 2012;39:850–860.

Löe H, Theilde E, Jenson SB. Experimental gingivitis in man. *J Periodontol.* 1965;36:177–187.

Loesche WJ, Syed SA, Laughon BE, Stoll J. The bacteriology of acute necrotising ulcerative gingivitis. *J Periodontol.* 1982;53:223–230.

Magnusson I, Lindhe J, Yoneyama T, Liljenberg B. Recolonization of a subgingival microbiota following scaling in deep pockets. *J Clin Periodontol.* 1984;11:193–207.

Robinson PG. Which periodontal changes are associated with HIV infection? *J Clin Periodontol.* 1998;25:278–285.

Sanz M, Herrera D, Kebschull M, Chapple I, Jepsen S, Beglundh T, Sculean A, Tonetti M. Treatment of stage I-III periodontitis-The EFP S3 level clinical practice guideline. *J Clin Periodontol.* 2020;47(suppl 22):4–60.

3.2

The Management of Mucogingival Conditions (Gingival Recession)

DAVID GILLAM AND WENDY TURNER

CHAPTER OUTLINE

OVERVIEW OF THE CHAPTER

After providing definitions, this chapter describes the prevalence of gingival recession and dentine hypersensitivity, mechanisms for gingival recession and dentine hypersensitivity, aetiology, classification, predisposing and precipitating factors and management of these conditions.

By the end of the chapter the reader should:

- Understand the causes of gingival recession and dentine hypersensitivity
- Be able to manage these conditions using a non-surgical approach.

The chapter covers the following topics:

- Introduction
- Definitions
- Prevalence of gingival recession and dentine hypersensitivity
- Mechanisms for gingival recession

- Mechanisms of sensory transmission of dentine hypersensitivity
- Aetiology of gingival recession and dentine hypersensitivity
- Classification of gingival recession including the updated guidelines from the World Workshop 2017
- Predisposing factors for gingival recession
- Precipitating factors for gingival recession
- Management – treatment of gingival recession defects and dentine hypersensitivity
- Summary.

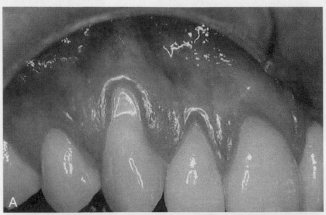

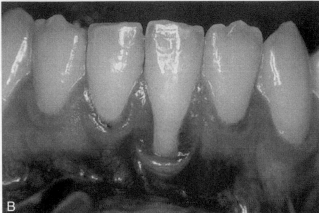

• **Figure 3.2.1** Clinical features of (A) gingival recession defect with so-called toothbrushing trauma and (B) gingival recession associated with localised plaque-induced inflammation lesion. Source: Lindhe J, Lang NP & Karring T, eds: Lindhe's Clinical Periodontology and Implant Dentistry, 2 Volume Set, 7th Edition, 2021.

Introduction

According to the published epidemiological studies, exposure of the root surface may be a consequence of:

1. Overzealous or improper oral hygiene habits in populations and patients with high standards of oral hygiene where gingival recession and dentine hypersensitivity predominantly affects the buccal surfaces of upper canines, premolars and molars (Figure 3.2.1A)
2. Progression/treatment of periodontal diseases in populations and patients with poor plaque control or who have been deprived of professional dental care and education where recession defects may be more widely distributed around all four surfaces of the affected tooth (Figure 3.2.1B).

Patients may also become aware of the problems associated with gingival recession: for example, aesthetics, the appearance of triangular interdental spaces, pain from dentine hypersensitivity and a fear of losing teeth which, in turn, may have an impact on their quality of life.

KEY POINT 1

Exposure of a root surface may be the consequence of overzealous/improper oral hygiene habits and/or progression/treatment of periodontal diseases.

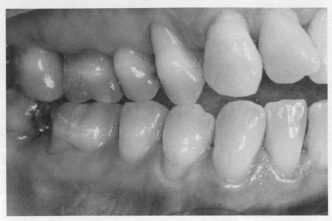

• **Figure 3.2.2** Clinical features of gingival recession with associated dentine hypersensitivity.

Definitions

Gingival Recession

A marginal tissue recession is characterised by the displacement of the location of marginal periodontal tissues apical to the cemento-enamel junction (American Academy of Periodontology 2001). Gingival recession, defined as an apical shift of the gingival margin with respect to the cemento-enamel junction (CEJ), is associated with clinical attachment loss (CAL) and exposure of the root surface to the oral environment (Cortellini & Bissada 2018).

Dentine Hypersensitivity

Pain from dentine hypersensitivity is generally one of the main symptoms of gingival recession together with patients' aesthetic concerns. Dentine hypersensitivity has been defined as "being characterised by short sharp pain arising from exposed dentine in response to stimuli (typically thermal, evaporative, tactile, osmotic or chemical) and which cannot be ascribed to any other form of defect or disease" (Canadian Advisory Board on Dentin Hypersensitivity 2003). From a clinical perspective, the definition of dentine hypersensitivity is essential when treating the condition and is important when considering a differential diagnosis of tooth-related pain (Figure 3.2.2).

Prevalence of Gingival Recession and Dentine Hypersensitivity

There are limited data on studies that specifically look at gingival recession and dentine hypersensitivity. Generally speaking, the two conditions are investigated separately in the published literature and, consequently, there is an overlap of information when discussing aetiology, predisposing factors and clinical features of the two conditions (Kassab & Cohen 2003, Kamal 2005, Gillam & Orchardson 2006). A study by Colak et al. (2012) reported that 7.6% of Turkish patients experienced dentine hypersensitivity upon testing, most of these sensitive teeth had associated buccal gingival recession of up to 3 mm. A study by West et al. (2013) reported an association between clinically elicited dentine hypersensitivity, erosive tooth wear and gingival recession in 18–35-year-old European adults. Secondary analysis on 350 UK participants enrolled in the main European study indicated that while each participant exhibited at least one tooth with gingival recession, many of these teeth did not exhibit dentine hypersensitivity despite prevalent recession and severe erosive tooth wear (Seong et al. 2018).

Mechanisms for Gingival Recession

Baker and Seymour (1976) proposed a hypothesis that would explain gingival recession caused by: (1) good oral hygiene practice (e.g. overzealous toothbrushing) and (2) periodontitis. It is plausible that toothbrushing leads to subclinical inflammation by epithelial permeability, and both the gingival biotype and quality of the underlying bone may influence the degree of localised destruction of the gingival crest. Similarly, the presence of plaque may lead to inflammatory changes within the connective tissue space and subsequent destruction and remodelling of the gingival crest. The resultant clinical appearance of this remodelling will be determined by the periodontal (gingival) biotype; a thin gingival biotype may result in recession whereas, in thick gingival biotypes, the inflammation may be confined to the region of the gingival sulcus and persist as a periodontal pocket.

Mechanisms for Sensory Transmission of Dentine Hypersensitivity Sensitivity

Several mechanisms are described for the transmission of various stimuli across dentine to the pulp, for example: (1) nerves in dentine, (2) the odontoblast as a sensory receptor or transducer and (3) the hydrodynamic theory. Currently, the hydrodynamic theory, as proposed by Brännström (1963), is considered the main mode of stimulus transmission across dentine. Briefly, the hydrodynamic theory describes the process whereby rapid fluid movement (towards the pulp or away from the pulp) in the dentinal tubules responds to either a cold, hot or osmotic stimulus on the exposed dentine surface and subsequently activates the A-δ fibres in the pulp–dentine area by a mechanoreceptor action (Figure 3.2.3).

Evidence from scanning electron microscopy studies has demonstrated the presence of open dentine tubules on the outer surface of sensitive teeth. In addition, the number and width of the open dentinal tubules in sensitive and non-sensitive dentine may have a significant impact on the rate of fluid flow through dentine.

> **KEY POINT 2**
> Dentine hypersensitivity is mediated by a hydrodynamic process.

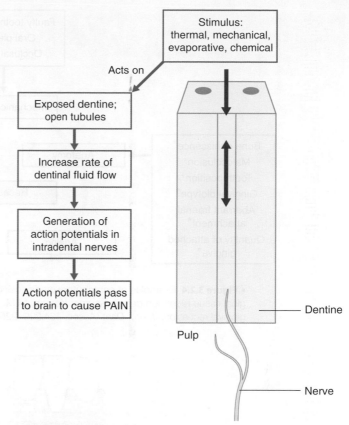

• **Figure 3.2.3** Outline of the hydrodynamic mechanism by which stimuli activate interdental nerves to cause pain. Source: Orchardson, R., Gillam, D.G., 2006. Managing dentine hypersensitivity. *J. Am. Dent. Assoc.* 137,990–998.

Aetiology of Gingival Recession and Dentine Hypersensitivity

Gingival recession should be considered a multifactorial periodontal condition. There are several contributory predisposing and precipitating factors which may interact to cause gingival recession and dentine hypersensitivity (Figure 3.2.4). The aetiological factors associated with dentine hypersensitivity may initiate two specific biological processes, namely, *lesion localisation* and *lesion initiation*. Lesion localisation occurs when the dentine is exposed due to the loss of enamel and/or soft tissue (including the loss of cementum). Once the dentine is exposed, patent dentine tubules will be exposed to the oral environment and lesion initiation may occur. The predominant factor in this process appears to be acid erosion.

The role of gingival recession in dentine hypersensitivity therefore should be considered as a predisposing factor rather than the primary cause. For example, areas of gingival recession may dictate where lesions are initiated; however, dentine hypersensitivity may occur when erosion opens up the exposed dentine tubules.

> **KEY POINT 3**
> Gingival recession is a multifactorial periodontal condition.

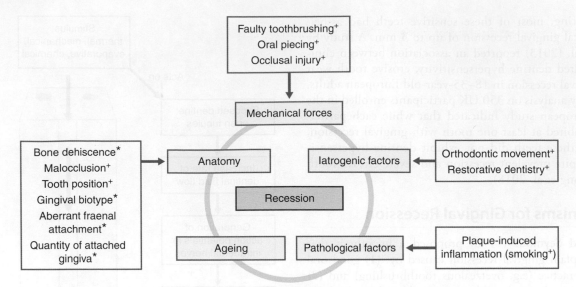

• **Figure 3.2.4** Examples of contributory predisposing* and precipitating+ factors associated with a marginal tissue recession defect. Source: Kassab, M.M., Cohen, R.E., 2003. The etiology and prevalence of gingival recession. *J. Am. Dent. Assoc.* 134,220–225.

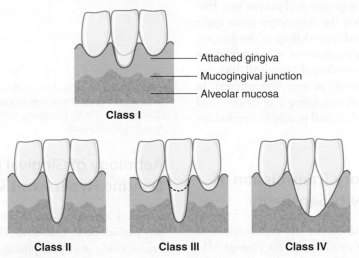

• **Figure 3.2.5** Miller's classification of gingival recession (Miller 1985a).

Classification of Gingival Recession

Several classifications have been previously proposed in the published literature to facilitate both a diagnosis and a template for a therapeutic strategy. Currently, the classification mainly used by clinicians in root-coverage procedures is the Miller classification system (I–IV) (Miller 1985a). One of the advantages of this classification is the ability to correlate treatment prognosis/outcome and anatomical features, whereas previous classification systems used either anatomical features or treatment prognosis only (Figure 3.2.5, Table 3.2.1). However, it should be acknowledged that this classification was proposed when root-coverage techniques were in their infancy and as such the forecast of potential root coverage in the Miller classification (I–IV) no longer matches the treatment outcomes of the most advanced

surgical techniques (Pini-Prato 2010, Cortellini & Bissada 2018). The classification (RT1–RT3) described by Cairo et al. (2011) is a treatment-oriented classification which forecasts the potential for root coverage through the assessment of both the recession depth and the interdental CAL (Table 3.2.2). This classification system for recession has been recommended by the 2017 World Workshop (Cortellini & Bissada 2018).

In the Cairo RT1 classification (Miller class I & II) 100% root coverage can be predicted. In the Cairo RT2 classification (overlapping Miller class III) several randomised clinical trials indicate the limit of interdental CAL within which 100% coverage is predictable when applying different root coverage procedures. In the Cairo RT3 classification (overlapping Miller class IV) full root coverage is not achievable (Cortelinni & Bissada 2018).

TABLE 3.2.1 Miller's classification of marginal tissue recession defects

Classification	Distinguishing feature	Description
Miller (1985a)	Takes into consideration factors that may influence both treatment and anticipated therapeutic outcomes	Class I Marginal tissue recession that does not extend to the mucogingival junction with no interproximal tissue loss Class II Marginal tissue recession that extends to or beyond the mucogingival junction, with no periodontal attachment loss in the interdental area Class III Marginal tissue recession that extends to or beyond the mucogingival junction, with periodontal attachment loss in the interdental area or malpositioning of teeth Class IV Marginal tissue recession that extends to or beyond the mucogingival junction, with severe bone or soft tissue loss in the interdental area, to a level apically to the buccal/labial soft tissue margin and/or severe malpositioning of teeth (see Figure 3.2.5)

(Miller 1985a)

TABLE 3.2.2 The recession classification system (Cairo et al. 2011) as recommended by the World Workshop 2017

Recession type (RT)	Clinical features
RT1	Gingival recession with no loss of interproximal attachment. Interproximal CEJ is clinically not detectable at both mesial and distal aspects of tooth.
RT2	Gingival recession associated with loss of interproximal attachment. The amount of interproximal attachment loss is less than or equal to the buccal attachment loss.
RT3	Gingival recession associated with loss of interproximal attachment. The amount of interproximal attachment loss is higher than the buccal attachment loss.

Source: Reprinted from *Journal of Clinical Periodontology* 45:(Supplement 20):S190–198, Pierpaolo Cortellini, Nabil F. Bissada (2018), with permission from John Wiley & Sons.

Predisposing Factors for Gingival Recession

Anatomical Recession (Tooth Position)

Several anatomical factors are associated with gingival recession:

- Tooth position in the dental arch (e.g. a prominent buccally positioned upper canine)
- Overcrowding with tooth displacement out of the arch (with bone dehiscence)
- Bulbous root structure
- Enamel pearls.

Quantity of Attached Gingiva

Historically, it has been suggested that the absence of an adequate width of attached gingiva may reduce resistance to plaque accumulation and lead to both recession and pocket formation. There is no published evidence, however, to suggest that a lack of an "adequate" zone of attached gingiva results in an increased incidence of soft tissue recession in patients maintaining a proper level of plaque control (Cortellinni & Bissada 2018).

A recent consensus concluded that a minimum amount of keratinised tissue is not needed to prevent attachment loss when adequate plaque control is being maintained. However, attached gingiva is important to maintain gingival health in patients with suboptimal plaque control (Cortellinni & Bissada 2018).

Periodontal (Gingival) Biotype

Soft tissue biotype can affect the outcome of periodontal treatment and root-coverage procedures. Several investigators have defined a thin tissue biotype as a thickness of <1.5 mm and a thick tissue biotype as a tissue thickness >2 mm (Claffey & Shanley 1986). Clinicians traditionally have used a probe to discriminate thin from thick gingiva based on the transparency of the probe through the gingival tissues, although this method may have inherent flaws (Fu et al. 2010). Recent studies examining tissue biotype and its relation to the underlying bone morphology would appear to suggest that periodontal (gingival) biotype is significantly related to labial plate thickness, alveolar crest position, keratinised tissue width, gingival architecture (thickness), tooth dimension and probe visibility but is unrelated to gingival recession (Cook et al. 2011, Cortellini & Bissada 2018). Examples of normal, thin and thick gingival tissues can be seen in Figure 3.2.6. Table 3.2.3 shows management options for thick and thin periodontal (gingival) biotypes in the absence and presence of gingival recession.

> **KEY POINT 4**
>
> The new classification system for gingival recession recognises the importance of the periodontal (gingival) biotype, interproximal attachment loss and the characteristics of the root surface

Bone Morphology

The alveolar bone crest is usually approximately 1–2 mm apically to the CEJ, but tooth position in the arch can affect the bone morphology around a tooth. Clinically, gingival recession is often accompanied by an alveolar bone dehiscence, although it is not clear whether the underlying bone dehiscence develops before, or in parallel with, gingival recession.

Malocclusion

Angle's class II division II malocclusion has been associated with direct trauma on the labial gingival margins of lower incisors and on the palatal margins of upper incisors. This particular incisor relationship may therefore generate recession defects at these areas, often resulting in indentations in the gingiva (Tugnait & Clerehugh 2001). A deep overbite in the absence of adequate overjet may also lead to the stripping of the gingival margins. Severe class III malocclusions combined with a deep bite and occlusal trauma caused by upper teeth to lower anterior teeth may also result in damage to the gingival margin.

High Attachment of Frenum

Several investigators have previously suggested that a high fraenal attachment may predispose a site to gingival recession, for example, when the attachment close to the gingival margin compromises the plaque removal from the area by the patient (Marini et al. 2004, Ustun et al. 2008). According to Chapple & Hamburger (2006), contrary to popular belief, there is no evidence in the published literature for a direct effect from so-called frenal pull in the initiation of gingival recession, as the frenum rarely has any muscle fibres.

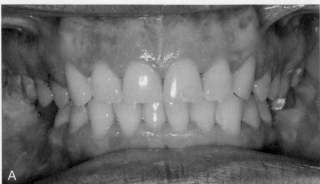
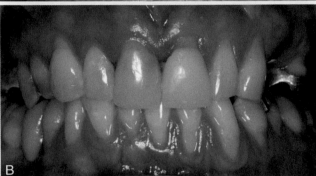
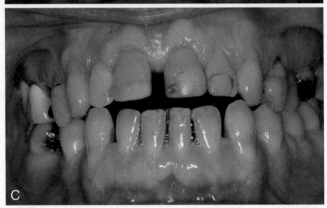

• **Figure 3.2.6** Clinical pictures of (A) normal, (B) thin and (C) thick gingival biotypes.

TABLE 3.2.3	Management options for different periodontal (gingival) biotypes	
Presence/absence of gingival recession	Periodontal (gingival) phenotype	Management options
Absence of gingival recession	Thick gingival biotype	Prevention through good oral hygiene and monitoring.
	Thin gingival biotype	Attention and careful monitoring by the clinician. With respect to cases with severe thin gingival biotype, mucogingival surgery should be considered to prevent future mucogingival damage. This applies especially in cases in which additional orthodontics, restorative dentistry or implant therapy are planned.
Presence of gingival recession	Thick biotypes	Conservative clinical approach– charting and monitoring periodontal and root surface lesions.
	Thin biotypes and when motivated by patient concern	Mucogingival surgery for root coverage and CEJ reconstruction when needed. This applies especially in cases in which additional orthodontics, restorative dentistry or implant therapy are planned.

Precipitating Factors for Gingival Recession

According to Marini et al. (2004) there are several factors that may contribute to the onset of gingival recession (see Figure 3.2.4).

Plaque, Calculus and Periodontal Diseases

Published studies would appear to correlate the prevalence of generalised recession with high levels of bacterial deposits around teeth and the presence of active or past periodontitis. Attachment loss may therefore manifest either as recession of the gingival margin, pocket formation or their combination. A localised plaque-induced inflammatory lesion may also induce development of a recession defect as observed in Figure 3.2.1B.

Toothbrush Trauma

Gingival recession has been reported to be relatively common in populations with high standards of oral hygiene, where it is usually located at buccal surfaces of canines, premolars and molars (see Figure 3.2.1A) and associated with wedge-shaped hard tissue defects. Results from these studies would suggest that potentially overzealous or improper toothbrushing habits may be associated with gingival recession. However, there is no evidence of a cause-and-effect relationship between toothbrushing and gingival recession.

Tooth Movement

Labial tooth movement may result either from occlusal trauma accompanied by periodontal diseases or from orthodontic movement (Tugnait & Clerehugh 2001) (Figure 3.2.7). According to Wennström (1996), provided the tooth is moved within the envelope of alveolar bone, gingival recession will not occur irrespective of the quality (volume) and quantity (width) of attached gingiva. However, if labial tooth movement results in the development of alveolar bone dehiscence, there is a greater risk of gingival recession. The use of computerised tomography to visualise the morphology of the buccal or lingual bone plates in the planning phase of orthodontic therapy may help prevent gingival recession during orthodontic therapy, as the thickness of the bone around individual teeth and any bony dehiscences/ fenestrations can be identified before treatment is initiated.

Smoking

Smoking is a significant risk factor for the development of periodontal diseases. Increased prevalence and severity of recession has also been reported in populations who either smoke or use smokeless tobacco (Robertson et al. 1990, Banihashemrad et al. 2008). Several mechanisms have been proposed for the effect of smoking on gingival recession, for example, (1) systemically compromising the innate and

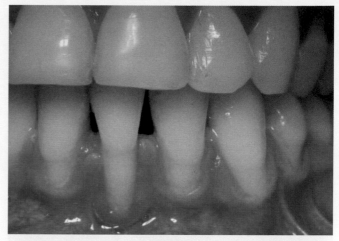

• **Figure 3.2.7** Gingival recession following orthodontic treatment (Courtesy of Prof. Georgios N. Belibasakis).

adaptive immune response and (2) topically reduced tissue vascularity influencing any subsequent wound healing of the affected tissues.

Healing after Periodontal Treatment

Pocket reduction following non-surgical periodontal treatment is achieved by the control of inflammation which may result in gingival recession. Surgical treatment of periodontal defects may also result in more recession postoperatively (Lindhe & Nyman 1980). Patients should therefore be warned about the possibility of post-treatment recession in all forms of periodontal therapy.

Restorative Dentistry

Subgingival and overhanging restoration margins can be considered a local risk factor in the development of periodontal diseases. Any subgingival placement of restorations (fillings, crowns, etc.) may therefore produce an inflammatory lesion in response to plaque accumulation which can impinge on the supracrestal tissue attachment (biological width) of the connective tissue, possibly resulting in loss of attachment or enlargement of the gingival tissues (Figure 3.2.8).

Removable Partial Dentures

Several investigators have suggested that removable partial dentures may compromise every aspect of the periodontal health of abutment teeth, including the incidence of gingival recession. For example, poorly designed removable partial dentures may traumatise the periodontal tissues either physically or as a result of plaque accumulation (Tugnait & Clerehugh 2001, Ercoli & Caton 2018). According to Wright and Hellyer (1995), however, the accumulation of plaque may be considered the main causative factor associated with gingival recession rather than any aspect of denture design per se.

per.

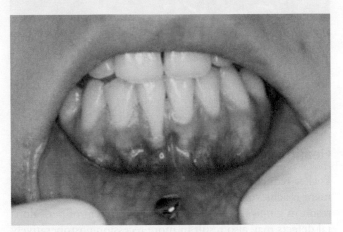

• **Figure 3.2.8** Inflammatory response of the gingivae following the subgingival placement of restoration margins.

• **Figure 3.2.9** Gingival recession due to trauma caused by a lower lip stud. Source: Reprinted by permission from Springer Nature: *Br. Dent. J.* Gingival recession due to trauma caused by a lower lip stud, JJ O'Dower et al., Copyright 2002.

Self-Inflicted Trauma/Chemical Trauma

Case reports detailing the effects of patient behaviour, such as fingernail picking at the gingival margin, or lip and tongue piercings, have shown localised gingival recession (Figure 3.2.9) (O'Dwyer & Holmes 2002). Similarly, topical cocaine application can also promote rapid gingival recession and dental erosion (Kapila & Kashani 1997).

Clinical Outcomes of Gingival Recession

Common clinical outcomes reported to be associated with gingival recession include:
- Dentine hypersensitivity
- Aesthetic concerns
- Plaque retention and inflammation
- Tooth abrasion
- Root caries and non-carious cervical lesions (NCCL).

Dentine Hypersensitivity

Dentine hypersensitivity is usually one of the main symptoms of gingival recession that may encourage patients to seek advice from a dental professional. Generally, this pain is transient in nature, and simple monitoring and reassurance

may be sufficient when dealing with different forms of postoperative sensitivity. Identification of the exact cause of dentine hypersensitivity is paramount if successful treatment is to be achieved. This process will involve taking a thorough history of the complaint together with a clinical examination to eliminate any other possible dental cause, such as defective restoration margins or dental caries (differential diagnosis). The use of a cold air syringe and an explorer probe may help in the detection of sensitive areas of the tooth.

> **KEY POINT 5**
> Dentine hypersensitivity is, by definition, a diagnosis of exclusion.

Aesthetics

A high smile line is usually a predisposing factor that contributes to the patient's concerns regarding the appearance of gingival recession. Elongation of the clinical crowns of teeth contrasts with the darker root dentine and, additionally, the presence of "black triangles" as a consequence of generalised recession is often seen in patients with periodontitis and often compromises the aesthetics (Figure 3.2.10). These elements may generate psychological issues which are further aggravated by the established association of recession with ageing. Concern about the aesthetic effects of recession is often one of the main reasons for patients attending the dental clinic.

> **KEY POINT 6**
> Aesthetics and pain arising from dentine hypersensitivity are key motivators for a patient to see a dentist.

Plaque Retention and Gingival Inflammation

Receding gingival margins are often exposed to plaque accumulation due to patients' inability to perform oral hygiene effectively at those sites. This may be due to either discomfort associated with dentine hypersensitivity or difficulties in cleaning the gingival margin of the recession defect.

Tooth Abrasion

It has been suggested that aggressive toothbrushing may cause exposure of the root surface which could continue if the brushing technique is not corrected. Other toothbrushing characteristics have also been reported to increase the risk of abrasion, for example, filament finishing and stiffness, in contrast to other studies that suggest abrasives in toothpastes are more likely to lead to loss of tooth or gingival tissue than toothbrushing per se.

Root Caries and Non-Carious Cervical Lesions

According to Banting (2001), the location of root caries has been positively associated with age and gingival recession, and this is consistent with the concept that root caries occur in a location adjacent to the crest of the gingiva where dental

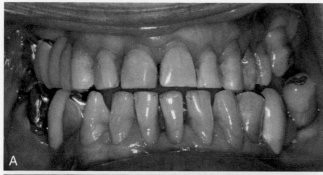

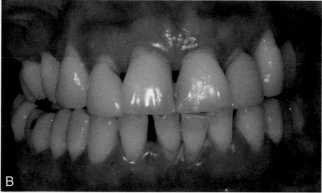

• **Figure 3.2.10** (A) Contrast of darker root dentine and enamel and (B) interdental soft tissue loss leading to the appearance of "black triangles".

plaque accumulates. High counts of *Streptococcus mutans* and high plaque scores at the gingival margin have been associated with the initiation of root caries lesions. Non-carious cervical lesions (NCCL) have also been associated with gingival recession and can be classified according to their appearance (wedge-shaped, disc-shaped, flattened and irregular areas). Several studies have indicated that the prevalence and severity of NCCL increases with age, and the presence of these dental lesions with subsequent concavities on the root surface may obliterate the CEJ (Cortellini & Bissada 2018).

Management and Treatment of Gingival Recession Defects and Dentine Hypersensitivity

The management and treatment of gingival recession defects and associated dentine hypersensitivity may be based on non-surgical and surgical treatment strategies (Table 3.2.4).

Non-Surgical Management of Gingival Recession and Dentine Hypersensitivity

Management may comprise:
1. Preventive care
2. Non-surgical correction of the defects.

1. Preventive Care

Once a diagnosis of gingival recession has been confirmed, the degree of recession may be measured clinically using a periodontal probe. The use of study casts and clinical photographs may also be helpful in monitoring any progression of gingival recession over time.

Non-surgical periodontal therapy and oral hygiene advice are the two cornerstones of periodontal therapy. Gingival recession may be the result of plaque accumulation due to incorrect oral hygiene habits, and subsequent correction would therefore contribute to the stability of the gingival margin.

Additionally, patients should receive advice and/or treatment to alleviate symptoms arising from gingival recession outcomes, mainly dentine hypersensitivity. Dietary advice on the consumption of acidic drinks commonly associated with erosion and on high-sugar-concentration products that provide the nutritional environment for root caries lesions may also be provided. Instructing the patient to use an atraumatic brushing oral hygiene technique or changing from a manual to a powered toothbrush may also be beneficial. Smoking cessation advice may also be appropriate for some patients. Dentine hypersensitivity arising from periodontal therapy may be initially alleviated by the application of desensitising polishing pastes prior to the provision of a desensitising toothpaste for home use. Application of desensitising products, such as toothpastes and bonding agents to occlude or seal the dentine tubules, have also been proposed for the treatment of dentine hypersensitivity. High fluoride concentration varnishes and dentifrices may be used in treating both dentine hypersensitivity and root caries (see Table 3.2.3). Following the initial management of gingival recession, orthodontic therapy may also be indicated to correct malpositioned teeth or replacement of fixed or removable prosthesis to allow the patient to maintain a healthy oral environment.

2. Non-Surgical Correction of Recession Defects

When recession defects cannot be treated by surgical root coverage procedures, for example, when the recession defect is due to periodontitis, restorative techniques may be used. The presence of "black triangles" can be masked by using a flexible silicone gingival veneer. The use of a tooth-coloured composite as a minimally invasive adhesive restoration may also be recommended to resolve associated carious lesions and alleviate pain symptoms from dentine hypersensitivity. Restoration of cervical defects with glass ionomer cements may also have the added advantage of fluoride release over a prolonged period of time. Aesthetic concerns raised by the presence of recession defects may thus be resolved by either non-surgical or surgical correction.

Surgical Treatment of Gingival Recession Defects

The main techniques that have been described in the published literature for the treatment of gingival recession by root coverage include pedicle soft tissue grafts, free soft tissue grafts and guided tissue regeneration.

TABLE 3.2.4	Non-surgical and surgical interventions for patients with gingival recession and dentine hypersensitivity	
Non-surgical treatment		**Surgical treatment**
In-surgery procedures		Periodontal flap surgery/periodontal plastic techniques
Clinical measurement of the gingival recession defect and taking study casts and clinical photographs to monitor condition over time Identification and correction of predisposing or precipitating factors Dietary and oral hygiene advice Manufacture of silicone gingival veneers Orthodontic treatment Restorative correction of recession defect and subgingival margins of fillings and crowns Desensitising polishing pastes Desensitising gels for bleaching procedures Polymers: Sealants/varnishes/resins/dentine bonding agents Laser obturation of dentinal tubules Bleaching gels + desensitising agent Pulpal extirpation (root canal treatment)		Guided tissue regeneration Coronally advanced flap +/− enamel matrix derivatives Coronally advanced flap + connective tissue graft Free gingival graft (acellular dermal matrix allograft)
Over-the-counter (toothpastes and mouth rinses)		
Strontium chloride/strontium acetate Potassium nitrate/chloride/citrate/oxalate Calcium compounds: Calcium carbonate and arginine and casein phosphopeptide + amorphous calcium phosphate Bioactive glass Hydroxyapatite Fluoride in higher concentration Amine/stannous fluoride		

Pedicle Soft Tissue Grafts

The two main procedures in this category are the laterally positioned pedicle graft and the coronally advanced flap which is often used with enamel matrix derivatives, connective tissue graft or acellular dermal matrix allograft material, depending on the amount of remaining keratinised tissue.

Free Soft Tissue Grafts

Free soft tissue grafts are used for root coverage procedures either as epithelial (free gingival grafts) or subepithelial connective tissue grafts.

Guided Tissue Regeneration

Guided tissue regeneration procedures using resorbable or non-resorbable membranes with or without enamel matrix derivatives.

According to Miller (1985b) complete root coverage can be anticipated in Miller class I and II recession defects, whereas only partial root coverage can be expected when part of the interproximal tissue is lost (Miller class III). Root coverage is not predictable in Miller class IV.

From the published literature, the optimal result of a root coverage procedure would be the complete resolution of the marginal tissue recession defect as measured on the denuded/covered root surface, with minimal probing depths in conjunction with an acceptable chromatic and texture harmony of the treated with the adjacent sites (Cortellini & Prato

2012). According to Cortellini & Bissada (2018) there is currently insufficient evidence to conclude that root coverage procedures predictably reduce dentine hypersensitivity.

KEY POINT 7
Treatment of a patient with gingival recession is usually non-surgical.

Summary

The management of gingival recession and any associated sequelae, such as dentine hypersensitivity, caries, NCCL or aesthetics, may be based on either a non-surgical or surgical approach depending on the extent and severity of the problem. The implementation of a preventive treatment approach that incorporates the identification and subsequent treatment or management of both the aetiological and predisposing factors is essential irrespective of whether a non-surgical or surgical approach is proposed. Monitoring the condition over time to maintain the status quo and prevent any further deterioration of the problem is an essential component of the management strategy.

Dentine hypersensitivity is essentially a diagnosis of exclusion, and as such a differential diagnosis should be initiated to determine the exact cause of the patient's pain. Identification of the exact cause is imperative if subsequent treatment is to be effective.

Multiple choice questions on the contents of this chapter are available online at Elsevier eBooks+.

References

American Academy of Periodontology. *Glossary of Periodontal Terms.* Chicago: American Academy of Periodontology; 2001.

Baker DL, Seymour GJ. The possible pathogenesis of gingival recession. A histological study of induced recession in the rat. *J Clin Periodontol.* 1976;3:208–219.

Banihashemrad SA, Fatemi K, Najafi MH. Effect of smoking on gingival recession. *J Dent Res.* 2008;5(1):1–4.

Banting D. *The diagnosis of root caries A presentation to the NIH Consensus Development Conference on Diagnosis and Management of Dental Caries Throughout Life.* Washington, DC; 2001.

Brännström M. A hydrodynamic mechanism in the transmission of pain producing stimuli through the dentin. In: Anderson DJ, ed. *Sensory Mechanisms in Dentine.* London: Pergamon Press, Oxford; 1963:73–79.

Cairo F, Nieri M, Cincinelli S, Mervelt J, Pagliaro U. The interproximal clinical attachment level to classify gingival recessions and predict root coverage outcomes: an explorative and reliability study. *J Clin Periodontol.* 2011;38:661–666.

Canadian Advisory Board on Dentin Hypersensitivity. Consensus-based recommendations for the diagnosis and management of dentine hypersensitivity. *J Can Dent Assoc (Tor).* 2003;69:221–228.

Chapple IL, Hamburger J. Periodontal medicine: a window on the body. Quintessential of Dental Practice. *Periodontology.* 2006;5:164–165.

Claffey N, Shanley D. Relationship of gingival thickness and bleeding to loss of attachment in shallow sites following nonsurgical periodontal therapy. *J Clin Periodontol.* 1986;13:654–657.

Colak H, Demirer S, Hamidi M, Uzgur R. Prevalence of dentine hyper-sensitivity among adult patients attending a dental hospital clinic in Turkey. *West Indian Med J.* 2012;61(2):174–179.

Cook DR, Mealey BL, Verrett RG, Mills MP, Noujeim ME, Lasho DJ, et al. Relationship between clinical periodontal biotype and labial plate thickness: an in vivo study. *Int J Periodontics Restorative Dent.* 2011;31:345–354.

Cortellini P, Bissada NF. Mucogingival conditions in the natural dentition: Narrative review, case definitions, and diagnostic considerations. *J Clin Periodontol.* 2018;45(Supplement 20):S190–S198.

Cortellini P, Prato PG. Coronally advanced flap and combination therapy for root coverage. Clinical strategies based on scientific evidence and clinical experience. *Periodontol 2000.* 2012;59:158–184.

Ercoli C, Caton JG. Dental Prostheses and tooth-related factors. *J Periodontol.* 2018;89 Supp 1:S223–S236.

Fu J-H, Yeh C-Y, Chan H-L, Tatarakis N, et al. Tissue biotype and its relation to the underlying bone morphology. *J Periodontol.* 2010;81:569–574.

Gillam DG, Orchardson R. Advances in the treatment of root dentin sensitivity: mechanisms and treatment principles. *Endod Top.* 2006;13:13–33.

Kamal H. *Prevalence of dentine hypersensitivity in gingival recession-African and Middle-East IADR Federation Conference.* September 27–29th Abstract presentation); 2005.

Kapila YL, Kashani H. Cocaine-associated rapid gingival recession and dental erosion. A case report. *J Periodontol.* 1997;68:485–488.

Kassab MM, Cohen RE. The etiology and prevalence of gingival recession. *J Am Dent Assoc.* 2003;134:220–225.

Lindhe J, Nyman S. Alterations of the position of the marginal soft tissue following periodontal surgery. *J Clin Periodontol.* 1980;7:525–530.

Marini MG, Greghi SLA, Passanezi E, Sant'ana ACP. Gingival recession: prevalence, extension and severity in adults. *J Appl Oral Sci.* 2004;12:250–255.

Miller PD. A classification of marginal tissue recession. *Int J Periodontics Restorative Dent.* 1985a;5:8–13.

Miller PD. Root coverage using a free soft tissue autograft following citric acid application. III. A successful and predictable procedure in areas of deep-wide recession. *Int J Periodontics Restorative Dent.* 1985b;5:15–37.

O'Dwyer JJ, Holmes A. Gingival recession due to trauma caused by a lower lip stud. *Br Dent J.* 2002;192:615–616.

Orchardson R, Gillam DG. Managing dentine hypersensitivity. *J Am Dent Assoc.* 2006;137:990–998.

Pini-Prato G, Franceschi D, Cairo F, Nieri M, Rotundo R. Classification of dental surface defects in areas of gingival recession. *J Periodontol.* 2010;81:885–890.

Robertson PB, Walsh M, Greene J. Periodontal effects associated with the use of smokeless tobacco. *J Periodontol.* 1990;61:438–443.

Salvi GE, Lindhe J, Lang NP. Treatment planning of patients with periodontal diseases. In: Lindhe J, Lang NP, Karring T, eds. *Clinical Periodontology and Implantology.* Vol. 2. 5th ed. Oxford: Blackwell Munksgaard; 2008:655–674 (Ch 31).

Seong J, Bartlett D, Newcombe RG, Claydon NCA, Hellin N, West NX. Prevalence of gingival recession and study of associated related factors in young UK adults. *J Dent.* 2018;76:58–67.

Tugnait A, Clerehugh V. Gingival recession – its significance and management. *J Dent.* 2001;29:381–394.

Ustun K, Sari Z, Orucoglu H, Duran I, Hakki SS. Severe gingival recession caused by traumatic occlusion and mucogingival stress: a case report. *Eur J Dent.* 2008;2:127–133.

Wennström JL. Mucogingival therapy. *Ann Periodontol.* 1996;1:671–701.

West NX, Sanz M, Lussi A, Bartlett D, Bouchard P, Bourgeois D. Prevalence of dentine hypersensitivity and study of associated factors: a European population-based cross-sectional study. *J Dent.* 2013;41(10):841–851.

Wright PS, Hellyer PH. Gingival recession related to removable partial dentures in older patients. *J Prosthet Dent.* 1995;74:602–607.

3.3

TREATMENT PLANNING: PERIODONTAL PROBLEMS IN CHILDREN AND ADOLESCENTS

VALERIE CLEREHUGH AND ARADHNA TUGNAIT

CHAPTER OUTLINE

OVERVIEW OF THE CHAPTER

This chapter outlines the different periodontal diseases that can affect children and adolescents and outlines the principles for periodontal screening and management of children and adolescents under 18 years of age.

By the end of the chapter the reader should be able to:

- Outline the various key periodontal diseases that can affect children and adolescents
- Understand the role of periodontal screening using the simplified basic periodontal examination (sBPE) in patients under 18 years old
- Explain the different steps of periodontal therapy based on the European Federation of Periodontology (EFP) S3-level clinical practice guidelines and the British Society of Periodontology and Implant Dentistry (BSP) implementation of them

- Understand the factors that may influence the decision to treat young patients in a general dental practice or refer to a specialist.

The chapter covers the following topics:

- Introduction
- Periodontal diseases that can affect children and adolescents
- Periodontal history, examination and simplified basic periodontal examination (sBPE)
- Treatment planning and periodontal therapy for the younger age groups
- The decision to treat in general dental practice or refer to a specialist.

Introduction

A wide range of periodontal diseases can affect children and adolescents, just as in adults (Clerehugh & Tugnait 2001, Clerehugh et al. 2004, Clerehugh 2008), but the 2017 World Workshop on the Classification of Periodontal and Peri-implant Diseases and Conditions (Caton et al. 2018) reflects that our understanding of them has changed since the previous 1999 International Workshop classification (Armitage 1999) (see Box 3.3.1). Furthermore, a new method for staging and grading periodontitis was agreed upon that influences the management of patients, whether they are children, adolescents or adults (Tonetti et al. 2018). The BSP has published an implementation plan for periodontal diagnosis in the context of the 2017 classification for clinical practice in the United Kingdom (Dietrich et al. 2019), along with guidance on implementation of the EFP S3-level evidence-based guidelines for stage I–III periodontitis in UK clinical practice (West et al. 2021).

> ### KEY POINT 1
>
> Many different periodontal diseases can affect children and adolescents (see Box 3.3.1) but the 2017 World Workshop Classification on Periodontal and Peri-implant Diseases and Conditions reflects that our understanding of them has changed since the previous 1999 classification.

This chapter will focus on:

- Gingivitis
- Periodontitis
- Necrotising periodontal diseases
- Recession
- Gingival overgrowth.

Early diagnosis and treatment planning are essential to ensure successful management in the younger age groups, and periodontal screening is a key aspect of this. In 2012, BSP and the British Society of Paediatric Dentistry (BSPD) jointly produced guidelines for periodontal screening and management of children and adolescents under 18 years of age, and these were updated in 2021 (Clerehugh & Kindelan 2021, www.bsperio.org.uk) using a simplified version of the basic periodontal examination used in adults (sBPE). The principles of periodontal management need to be applied to the younger age groups when treating the conditions in Box 3.3.1, and the decision needs to be taken whether to treat in the primary dental care setting or to refer to a specialist.

Periodontal Diseases that can Affect Children and Adolescents

Periodontal Health

In children and adolescents with a healthy periodontium, the gingival sulcus is typically 0.5–3 mm deep on a fully erupted tooth, and the alveolar crest has been shown to be between 0.4 and 1.9 mm apical to the cement–enamel junction (CEJ) in teenagers (Hausmann et al. 1991).

> ### • BOX 3.3.1   Classification of Periodontal Diseases/Conditions in Children/Adolescents based on 2017 World Workshop Classification of Periodontal and Peri-Implant Diseases and Conditions (Caton et al. 2018)
>
> **Periodontal health, gingival diseases/conditions**
>
> Periodontal health and gingival health
> Gingivitis, dental plaque biofilm induced
> Gingival diseases, non-dental plaque biofilm induced
>
> **Periodontitis**
>
> Necrotising periodontal diseases
> Periodontitis
> Periodontitis as a manifestation of systemic disease
>
> **Other conditions affecting the periodontium**
>
> Systemic diseases or conditions affecting the periodontal
>   supporting tissues
> Periodontal abscesses and endodontic–periodontal lesions
> Mucogingival deformities and conditions
> Traumatic occlusal forces
> Tooth and prosthesis-related factors
>
> Reprinted from *Journal of Clinical Periodontology*, 30(10):15, Caton, J.G., Armitage, G., Berglundh, T. et al. (2018), with permission from John Wiley & Sons.

Periodontal health was classified for the first time in the 2017 World Workshop Classification on Periodontal and Peri-implant Diseases and Conditions (Caton et al. 2018) that replaced the previous 1999 international classification (Armitage et al. 1999). According to the 2017 World Workshop Classification, a case of periodontal health on an intact periodontium is defined by the absence of inflammation (i.e. bleeding on probing [BOP] at less than 10% sites) and the absence of attachment loss and bone loss from previous periodontitis, with probing depths ≤3 mm); there is also a category which acknowledges periodontally healthy tissues on a reduced and stable periodontium arising from historical successfully treated periodontitis (Chapple et al. 2018).

Gingivitis

Plaque-Induced Gingivitis

If supragingival plaque accumulates, an inflammatory cell infiltrate develops in the gingival connective tissue and the weak junctional epithelial attachment is disrupted, leading to an increase in gingival sulcus depth and formation of a false gingival pocket, in which subgingival plaque can collect; supragingival calculus and subgingival calculus may form on the clinical crown. This is entirely reversible with effective plaque biofilm and calculus removal supragingivally and subgingivally. At this stage, the most apical extent of the junctional epithelium (JE) is still at the CEJ, and there is no periodontal loss of attachment or bone loss.

Epidemiological studies report a low prevalence of plaque-induced gingivitis in preschool children, reaching a peak in prevalence around puberty. Puberty gingivitis is the increased inflammatory gingival response to dental plaque mediated by the hormonal changes associated with puberty, perhaps also in association with changes in the bacterial composition of the dental plaque (Bimstein & Eidelman 1988, Bimstein & Matsson 1999). The 2013 Child Dental Health Survey in England, Wales and Northern Ireland found that out of a representative sample of 13,628 children aged 5, 8, 12 and 15 years, only 22% of 5-year-olds had visible gingival inflammation, compared with 46% of 8-year-olds, 60% of 12-year-olds and 52% of 15-year-olds (Pitts et al. 2015).

According to the 2017 World Workshop Classification, a case of gingivitis on an intact periodontium and on a reduced periodontium without a history of periodontitis is defined as >10% bleeding sites with probing depths <3 mm (Chapple et al. 2018). Localised gingivitis is defined as 10–30% bleeding sites; generalised gingivitis is defined as >30% bleeding sites. Importantly from an epidemiological perspective, a periodontitis case cannot simultaneously be defined as a gingivitis case. This means that a patient with a history of periodontitis with gingival inflammation is still classed as a periodontitis case. From a clinical perspective, successfully treated periodontitis patients may achieve a reduced, stable periodontium where probing depths are ≤4 mm and there is an absence of clinical inflammation (BOP). However, BOP may occur at certain sites, and where probing depths are ≤3 mm, this would be classified as gingival inflammation in a stable periodontitis patient; close monitoring is required due to the potential for relapse and high risk of recurrence of periodontitis.

Necrotising Gingivitis

Necrotising gingivitis (NG) has a fusiform-spirochaetal microbial aetiology and is more generally found in patients in developing countries who typically exhibit various risk factors, including smoking, immunosuppression – in particular HIV-positive status – stress, malnourishment or poor diet (Herrera et al. 2018). Extreme living conditions and severe (viral) infections such as measles, herpes viruses, chicken pox, malaria or febrile illnesses may be predisposing conditions in children (Papapanou et al. 2018). Key diagnostic features include:

- Pain
- Necrosis and ulceration of the interdental papillae which have a "punched out" appearance
- Bleeding, which may be spontaneous
- Secondary fetor oris
- Pseudo-membrane may be present
- May manifest in children and teenagers
- May progress to necrotising periodontitis (NP).

NG is the only form of gingivitis for which systemic antibiotics may normally be indicated as part of the treatment.

Non-Plaque-Induced Gingival Lesions

Children may also present with non-plaque-induced gingival lesions. For such lesions, a specialist referral may be indicated (Clerehugh et al. 2004, Clerehugh & Kindelan 2021).

• BOX 3.3.2 Local and Systemic Periodontal Risk Factors

Local
- Anatomical factors
- Overhanging/poorly contoured restorations
- Removable partial dentures
- Orthodontic appliances
- Root fractures and cervical root resorption
- Calculus
- Local trauma
- Fraenal attachments
- Mouth breathing and lack of lip seal

Systemic
- Smoking
- Poorly controlled type 1 and type 2 diabetes mellitus
- Ethnic origins
- Genetics
- Male gender
- Polymorphonuclear leucocyte function
- Socio-economic status (low educational level)
- Acquired systemic infection (e.g. HIV)
- Severe malnutrition

Periodontitis

The key features of periodontitis are:

- Loss of attachment of the periodontal connective tissues
- Apical migration of the JE beyond the CEJ and transformation of the JE to pocket epithelium (often thin and ulcerated)
- Alveolar bone loss.

Local and systemic periodontal risk factors can influence the rate, severity and extent of progression of periodontitis (Box 3.3.2). The system of staging and grading periodontitis was introduced for the first time in the 2017 World Workshop on Classification (Tonetti et al. 2018), see Chapter 2.1 and Appendices 1 and 2. Risk factors have not previously been included in the classification of periodontitis, but the 2017 World Workshop scheme allows for the presence of recognised periodontal risk factors (especially smoking and diabetes; see Box 3.3.2) to be able to modify the assigned grade of periodontitis (Tonetti et al. 2018). It is also important to incorporate current disease status into the periodontitis diagnosis (stable, unstable or in remission) by considering the presence of true probing pocket depths (PPD) of 4 mm or more and BOP, which reflect the inflammatory status and drive treatment planning (Chapple et al. 2018, Dietrich et al. 2019). Details can be found in Chapter 2.1 and Appendix 2.

Although current evidence, as documented in the 2017 World Workshop (Caton et al. 2018), does not support the distinction between the conditions previously classified as chronic and aggressive periodontitis in the 1999 International Classification (Lang et al. 1999), it is important for the dental practitioner to be able to identify those adolescents at an incipient (early) stage of periodontitis who are amenable to treatment in general dental practice (typically stage I, grade A) and those minority of cases who would previously have been classified as aggressive periodontitis with a more severe, rapidly progressing, destructive form of periodontitis who would now be categorised typically as stage II, III or IV, grade C and who would benefit from referral to a specialist (Wadia et al. 2019, Walter et al. 2019a, b, Clerehugh & Kindelan 2021).

Radiographic bone loss has been observed around the primary dentition in some children, and this reinforces the notion that periodontitis can develop at an early age (Matsson et al. 1995, 1997).

In the mixed dentition, it is important to be aware of the potential problem of false pocketing occurring around partially erupted teeth.

Incipient Periodontitis

In the permanent dentition, the transition from gingivitis to the early stages of periodontitis, namely incipient periodontitis, can occur in the early teenage years, affecting a substantial number of teenagers. It is characterised by 1–2 mm loss of clinical attachment interproximally, periodontal pockets 4–5 mm deep and crestal alveolar bone loss of about 0.5 mm which is usually horizontal (Figure 3.3.1).

A 5-year longitudinal study of 167 adolescents (Clerehugh et al. 1990) showed that 3% had attachment loss of 1 mm or more on at least one of the molar, premolar or incisor teeth when examined at age 14 years, increasing

to a prevalence of 37% at 16 years and 77% at 19 years. Periodontal pathogens typical of those found in the subgingival microflora of adults with periodontitis have also been found in the subgingival plaque of adolescents with incipient periodontitis, including *Porphyromonas gingivalis, Prevotella intermedia, Aggregatibacter actinomycetemcomitans* and *Tannerella forsythia* (Clerehugh et al. 1997, Hamlet et al. 2004).

Stage II, III or IV Grade C Periodontitis in Younger Age Groups

The condition that would previously have been diagnosed as localised aggressive periodontitis, although not deemed in the 2017 World Workshop on Classification to have a sufficiently well-defined aetiology or pathophysiology to have its own classification, has in fact been acknowledged to have a well-recognised clinical presentation: typically with an onset around puberty and localised first molar/incisor presentation with interproximal clinical attachment loss which is much more severe and more rapidly destructive than expected and inconsistent with the levels of plaque biofilm deposits present. Historically it has typically been found in adolescents from Africa/Middle East with Aggregatibacter actinomycetemcomitans as the implicated infecting agent (Fine et al. 2018, Papapanou et al. 2018). A. actinomycetemcomitans is very adept at evading the host defences and can be difficult to eradicate (Figure 3.3.2). Hence the management may well involve adjunctive systemic antimicrobials at the

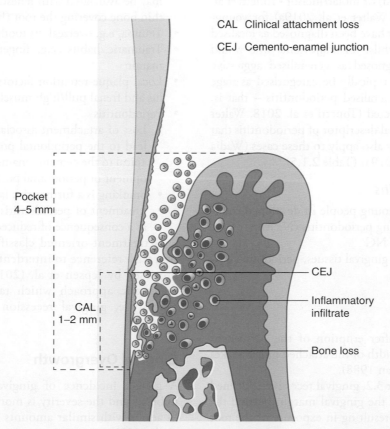

CAL   Clinical attachment loss

CEJ   Cemento-enamel junction

Pocket 4–5 mm

CAL 1–2 mm

CEJ

Inflammatory infiltrate

Bone loss

• **Figure 3.3.1** Incipient periodontitis.

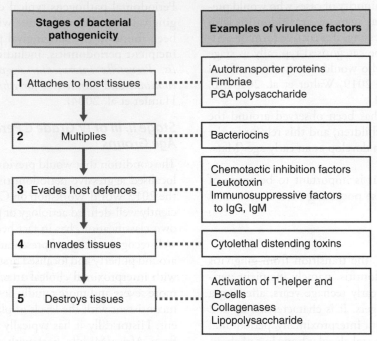

Aggregatibacter actinomycetemcomitans

Stages of bacterial pathogenicity	Examples of virulence factors
1 Attaches to host tissues	Autotransporter proteins Fimbriae PGA polysaccharide
2 Multiplies	Bacteriocins
3 Evades host defences	Chemotactic inhibition factors Leukotoxin Immunosuppressive factors to IgG, IgM
4 Invades tissues	Cytolethal distending toxins
5 Destroys tissues	Activation of T-helper and B-cells Collagenases Lipopolysaccharide

• **Figure 3.3.2** *Aggregatibacter actinomycetemcomitans.*

cause-related corrective phase of therapy, but careful consideration would be required on a case-by-case basis.

Within the staging system there is a category for describing the extent and distribution of periodontitis as localised (up to 30% of teeth affected) or molar/incisor (Tonetti et al. 2018, Wadia et al. 2019, Walter et al. 2019a) for youngsters who would previously have been diagnosed as localised aggressive periodontitis, whilst for adolescents who would previously have been diagnosed as generalised aggressive periodontitis, they would typically be categorised as stage II, III or IV, grade C, generalised periodontitis – that is, 30% or more of teeth affected (Tonetti et al. 2018, Walter et al. 2019a). The additional descriptor of periodontitis that is "currently unstable" may also apply to these cases (Wadia et al. 2019, Walter et al. 2019a) (Table 2.1.5).

Necrotising Periodontitis

Although uncommon in young people in developed countries like the UK, necrotising periodontitis (NP):

• May be an extension of NG
• Features necrosis of the gingival tissues, periodontal ligament and alveolar bone.

Recession

During the early years, after eruption of the permanent tooth, an increase in the width of the attached gingiva takes place (Bimstein & Eidelman 1988).

As explained in Chapter 3.2, gingival recession is defined as the apical migration of the gingival margin beyond the cement–enamel junction, resulting in exposure of the root surface.

Factors associated with recession, especially if the gingiva is thin, are:

• Anatomy
• Tooth position, or orthodontic tooth movement, which may be associated with fenestration or dehiscence in the thin bone covering the root (Figure 3.3.3)
• Trauma, e.g. overzealous toothbrushing
• Traumatic habits, e.g. finger picking of the gingival margin
• Local plaque-retention factors, e.g. supragingival calculus and frenal pull/high muscle attachments
• Periodontitis
  • Loss of attachment associated with periodontitis can lead to the periodontal pocket margin being located apical to the cement–enamel junction, with the development of periodontal pockets and alveolar bone loss
  • Smoking is a further risk factor for recession
  • Treatment of periodontitis can also lead to recession as a consequence of reduced marginal inflammation.

A treatment-oriented classification of gingival recession with reference to interdental loss of attachment was proposed by Jepsen et al. (2018), along with a clinical diagnostic approach which takes account of gingival phenotype, gingival recession and associated cervical lesions.

Gingival Overgrowth

A greater incidence of gingival overgrowth is seen in puberty, and the severity is more intense in children than in adults with similar amounts of dental plaque (Tiainen et al. 1992).

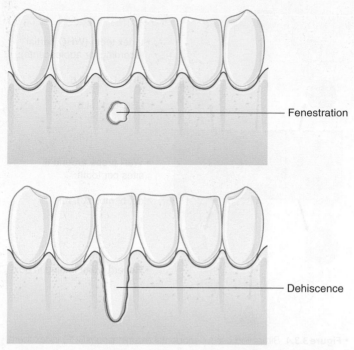

• **Figure 3.3.3** Fenestration and dehiscence may be associated with gingival recession, especially where overlying gingiva is thin and subjected to trauma, e.g. from overzealous toothbrushing.

There are a number of contributing factors to gingival overgrowth:

- Usually associated with plaque-induced inflammation
- Drugs: phenytoin for management of epilepsy; ciclosporin (immunosuppressant); calcium channel blockers
- Hormonal (pregnancy; contraceptive pill)
- Hereditary gingival fibromatosis
- Neoplasia, including leukaemia
- Scurvy, vitamin C deficiency
- Mouth breathing, which can exacerbate existing plaque-induced gingivitis.

The enlarged gingival tissue may be difficult to clean, thereby acting as a plaque-retention factor, and aesthetics may be a concern.

Periodontal History, Examination and Simplified Basic Periodontal Examination

Periodontal History and Examination

> #### KEY POINT 2
> A thorough history and examination are necessary for periodontal diagnosis and subsequent treatment planning and will identify systemic and local periodontal risk factors (Box 3.3.2).

The routine dental examination of children and adolescents should include an extra-oral and intra-oral assessment. Variables to note are gingival colour, contour, swelling, the presence and location of inflammation, recession or suppuration. Oral hygiene and the presence of supragingival

calculus deposits should be noted. Local periodontal risk factors – e.g. plaque-retention factors, location of high fraenal attachments, malocclusion, the presence of mouth breathing and incompetent lip seal – should be identified. Mouth breathing, increased lip separation and decreased upper lip coverage have all been associated with higher levels of plaque and gingival inflammation. The influence of mouth breathing tends to be restricted to palatal sites, whereas decreased lip coverage influences gingival inflammation at both palatal and labial sites (Wagaiyu & Ashley 1991). Radiographs and sensitivity tests may be necessary.

Just as for adults, periodontal screening is recommended in children and adolescents, but a simplified version of the basic periodontal examination (BPE) has been developed for the under 18-year-old group (sBPE), and guidelines on its use have been updated by Clerehugh and Kindelan in association with the BSP and the BSPD in 2021 (Clerehugh & Kindelan 2021) (Figure 3.3.4).

Simplified Basic Periodontal Examination (sBPE)

Periodontal screening using the simplified BPE (sBPE) is appropriate for children and adolescents under 18 years of age seen in general dental practice and community and hospital settings.

> #### KEY POINT 3
> A simplified version of the BPE (sBPE) is a quick, acceptable method for periodontal screening in the under 18-year-old age group in general dental practice and community and hospital settings.

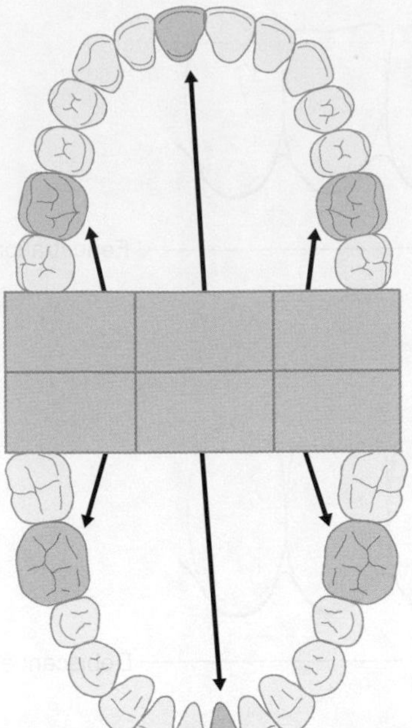

- Index teeth (WHO partial recording for adolescents):

  UR6, UR1, UL6

  LR6, LL1, LL6

- Walk probe around 6 sites per tooth:

  db, b, mb, dl, l, ml

- Record worst finding in box

• **Figure 3.3.4** Simplified basic periodontal examination (sBPE) index teeth.

sBPE Codes

0 Healthy (no bleeding on probing, no calculus/overhangs or pocketing ≥3.5 mm detected). Black band entirely visible.

1 Bleeding on probing (no calculus/overhangs or pocketing ≥3.5 mm detected). Black band entirely visible.

2 Calculus (supragingival and/or subgingival) or plaque-retention factor (no pocketing ≥3.5 mm detected). Black band entirely visible.

3 Shallow pocket (4 mm or 5 mm), i.e. probing depth ≥3.5 mm but ≤5.5 mm. Black band partially visible.

4 Deep pocket (6 mm or more), i.e. probing depth >6 mm. Black band disappears.

* Furcation

KEY POINT 4

sBPE is performed on six index teeth (UR6, UR1, UL6, LL6, LL1 and LR6) using a WHO 621 probe with a 0.5 mm spherical ball on the tip and a black band at 3.5–5.5 mm to delineate healthy sulcus (probing depth 3 mm or less) from pockets (probing depth 4 mm or more), employing a light probing force of 20–25 g.

The sBPE is performed on the following six index teeth: UR6, UR1, UL6, LL6, LL1 and LR6 using the WHO 621 probe with a light probing force of 20–25 g. This has a 0.5 mm spherical ball on the tip and a black band at 3.5–5.5 mm to delineate healthy sulcus depth (<3.5 mm) and periodontal pockets of 4 mm or more (see Figure 3.3.5).

There are, however, certain points that need to be considered when adapting this for use in children and adolescents (Clerehugh 2008, Clerehugh & Kindelan 2021, www.bsperio.org.uk):

1. At 7–11 years of age, in the mixed dentition phase, the index teeth should only be examined for bleeding of the gingiva, calculus and/or overhangs of fillings, i.e. sBPE codes 1 and 2 only, to avoid the problem of false pockets on the erupting/recently erupted first permanent molar and incisor teeth

2. At 12–17 years of age, the full range of sBPE codes can be used on the six index teeth. It would be unusual to find periodontal breakdown at other teeth without the index teeth being affected

3. An sBPE should be undertaken in all new child or adolescent patients and prior to commencing orthodontic treatment in the under 18s

4. Whether in the mixed or permanent dentition stage, the examination of these index teeth is quick, easy and well tolerated and is sufficient to identify children who would benefit from a more detailed examination.

Although a brief periodontal examination similar to the sBPE has been reported to be acceptable for children as young as 3 years of age (Rapp et al. 2001), it would not normally need to be undertaken in the primary dentition.

As a guide for when to do sBPE:

- If sBPE = 0, screen again at routine recall visit or within 1 year, whichever is sooner
- If sBPE = 1 or 2, treat and screen again at routine recall or after 6 months, whichever is sooner
- If sBPE = 3, undertake initial periodontal therapy, including any other affected teeth in the involved sextant(s). After 3 months, do a full periodontal assessment, including 6-point probing pocket depths on the index tooth and other teeth in the involved sextant(s).
- If sBPE = 4 or * on any index tooth, do a full periodontal assessment, including 6-point probing pocket depths, throughout the entire dentition. Consider referral to a specialist. Undertake initial periodontal therapy as for code 3 in the meantime (Figure 3.3.5).

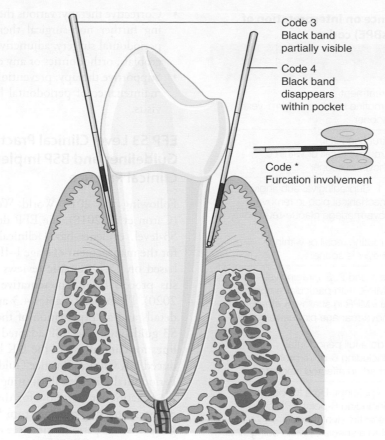

Code 3
Black band
partially visible

Code 4
Black band
disappears
within pocket

Code *
Furcation involvement

• **Figure 3.3.5** Section through tooth - diagram of sBPE codes 3, 4, *.

Please see Table 3.3.1 for guidance on the interpretation of sBPE codes for clinical practice.

Use of Radiographs

In health, the alveolar bone crest is 0.4–1.9 mm from the CEJ around permanent teeth but may be greater than 2 mm in primary teeth. This distance may increase with facial growth and if an adjacent primary tooth is lost or a neighbouring permanent tooth erupts. Horizontal bite-wing radiographs for the detection of caries can be useful in assessing a young patient's periodontal condition on posterior teeth (Faculty of General Dental Practitioners 2018). Selected periapical radiographs may be indicated for the anterior and/or posterior teeth. Panoramic films are commonly used for orthodontic purposes to assess the state of the developing dentition. The chance to assess bone levels on intra-oral or panoramic films should always be seized, even if the film was not originally taken to assess the periodontal condition.

For sBPE codes of 3, 4 or *, consideration should normally be given to a radiographic examination when it is justified and has the potential to change the management or prognosis, taking account of best available radiological practice. Assessment of bone loss is a key aspect of staging and grading periodontitis and reaching a periodontal diagnosis (see Chapter 2.1 and Appendices 1 and 2).

A radiographic report should be included in the patient's case notes. In addition to caries and other pathology, findings of periodontal significance to record include:

- Bone levels/loss
- Type of bone loss (horizontal or vertical)
- Calculus
- Furcations
- Apical pathology
- Endodontic-periodontal lesion
- Root caries
- Deficient or overhanging restoration margins
- Poorly contoured restorations
- Widened periodontal ligament space.

KEY POINT 5

For sBPE codes of 3, 4 or *, consideration should normally be given to a radiographic examination when it is justified and has the potential to change the management or prognosis, in line with best radiological practice. Assessment of bone loss is a core component of staging and grading of periodontitis.

Periodontal Diagnosis

The diagnosis of any periodontal conditions present in a child or adolescent will follow the history, examination and any special tests; a treatment plan can then be drawn up. Guidance on periodontal diagnosis in the context of

TABLE 3.3.1 Summary guidance on interpretation of simplified BPE (sBPE) codes

sBPE code	Summary
0	No periodontal treatment Screen again at routine recall or within 1 year, whichever is sooner
I	Oral hygiene instruction (OHI) Screen again at routine recall or within 6 months, whichever is sooner
2	OHI as for code 1. Supragingival/subgingival professional mechanical plaque removal (PMPR). Remove/manage plaque-retention factors Screen again at routine recall or within 6 months, whichever is sooner
3	OHI as for codes 1 and 2. Supragingival/subgingival PMPR, with particular emphasis on subgingival PMPR in shallow 4 mm–5 mm pockets. Remove/manage plaque-retention factors After 3 months, do a full periodontal assessment, including 6-point probing pocket depth (PPD) chart, in affected sextants
4 or *	Unusual in young patients. Do a full periodontal assessment, including 6-point PPD chart, throughout the entire dentition Consider referral to a specialist while doing initial therapy, as code 3

Table reproduced from Clerehugh & Kindelan (2021) by courtesy of the authors and with permission from the British Society of Periodontology and Implant Dentistry (www.bsperio.org.uk/publications).

the 2017 World Workshop Classification of periodontal diseases and conditions and its implementation in clinical practice has been produced by the BSP (Dietrich et al. 2019). Appendix 2 shows how to reach a diagnosis in conjunction with use of the periodontal screening systems used in the UK (appropriate for both BPE for adults and sBPE for children under 18), and then shows the use of staging and grading for periodontitis cases, assessment of current periodontitis status, risk factor assessment and finally reaching a diagnosis statement in clinical practice.

Treatment Planning and Periodontal Therapy

Periodontal therapy has traditionally been undertaken in three phases: initial, corrective and supportive, each with a number of associated stages:

- Initial therapy: cause related; targeted at controlling the plaque biofilm, managing any modifiable periodontal risk factors and completing the initial phase of non-surgical periodontal therapy in order to control the infection and inflammation and halt the progress of disease.

- Corrective therapy: various therapeutic measures, including further non-surgical therapy or, in selected cases, periodontal surgery, adjunctive local or systemic antimicrobials, orthodontics or any definitive restorative work.
- Supportive therapy: prevention of disease recurrence and maintenance of periodontal health, with tailored recall visits.

EFP S3 Level Clinical Practice Treatment Guidelines and BSP Implementation for UK Clinical Practice

Following the 2017 World Workshop on Classification (Caton et al. 2018), the EFP developed a set of stringent S3-level, evidence-based clinical recommendations (CRs) for the management of stage I–III periodontitis. These were based on 15 systematic reviews and a moderated consensus process from representative stakeholders (Sanz et al. 2020). Please see Chapter 4.3 and Appendix 3 for further details and an explanation of the development of the EFP S3 guidelines. The BSP adapted these EFP S3-level guidelines for clinical use in the UK healthcare system and produced UK Clinical Practice Guidelines for the Treatment of Periodontal Diseases, illustrating the four-step sequence for the practitioner to follow for the treatment of periodontal diseases, covering the spectrum from periodontal health to gingivitis and periodontitis (see Appendix 4).

Preventive advice, health education and oral hygiene instruction are key to successful management of plaque-induced gingivitis and prerequisites to the successful management of periodontitis in the younger age groups. The young patients and their families/caregivers should have a diagnosis and discussion of the causes of the child/young person's periodontal condition, treatments options, risk-benefits and a care plan. The following steps 1–4 can then provide a stepwise approach for successful treatment outcomes of their periodontal diseases/periodontitis (Appendices 3 and 4).

Step 1 Building Foundations for Optimal Treatment Outcomes

Step 1 aims to lead to behaviour change/motivation to successfully control the plaque biofilm (OHI); uses possible adjunctive therapies for gingival inflammation; uses professional mechanical plaque removal (PMPR) to remove supragingival plaque and calculus and also any subgingival plaque and calculus on the crown of the tooth; employs risk factor control.

Step 2 Subgingival Biofilm & Calculus Control/Removal

Step 2 aims to control (reduce/eliminate) the subgingival plaque biofilm and subgingival PMPR to remove subgingival plaque biofilm and subgingival calculus from the root surface; may also involve the use of: adjunctive physical or chemical agents; adjunctive local or systemic host-modulating agents; adjunctive subgingival locally delivered antimicrobials; adjunctive systemic antimicrobials.

Step 3 Management of Non-Responding Sites (≥4 mm with BOP or ≥6 mm)

Step 3 aims at treating non-responding sites (probing depth >4 mm with BOP or >6 mm); aims to gain access to further subgingival instrumentation or to achieve regeneration or resection in lesions (infrabony or furcation) that increase complexity in managing periodontitis.

Step 4 Maintenance/Supportive Periodontal Therapy

Step 4 aims to maintain periodontal stability through supportive periodontal care in all treated periodontitis patients; combines preventive/therapeutic interventions from steps 1 and 2; requires regular recall intervals, tailored to patient's individual needs; should be managed as a recurrent disease with updated diagnosis and treatment plan; requires compliance with OHI regimens and healthy lifestyle, which are integral.

KEY POINT 6

Preventive advice, health education and oral hygiene instruction are key to successful management of plaque-induced gingivitis and are also prerequisites to the successful management of periodontitis in the younger age groups. The BSP UK Clinical Practice Guidelines for the Treatment of Periodontal Diseases provides a stepwise approach for successful treatment outcomes of periodontal diseases/ periodontitis in the under 18 age group.

KEY POINT 7

All phases of periodontal therapy require ongoing guidance on oral hygiene practices to control gingival inflammation.

Plaque Control

According to the Children's Dental Health Survey of 2013 (Tsakos et al. 2015), twice daily toothbrushing was reported in 79% of 12-year-olds (compared with 76% in 2003) and in 84% of 15-year-olds (versus 80% in 2003); between 37%–49% of children in all age groups reported using an electric toothbrush. The use of dental floss, although small, was evident, with 21% of 15-year-olds reporting its use. Mouthwash use was reported in all age groups, rising from 22% of 5-year-olds up to 67% of 15-year-olds. Oral health messages for the child population should incorporate relevant information about the use of these common oral hygiene adjuncts. Smoking prevalence was very low (2%) in 12-year-olds, but because 11% of 15-year-olds reported being a current smoker and 29% reported having ever smoked cigarettes, smoking cessation advice is of paramount importance in these teenage years.

Under optimal conditions, the careful and regular removal of dental plaque biofilm can prevent the occurrence and progression of early periodontal diseases (Badersten et al. 1975, Agerbaek et al. 1977, Axelsson & Lindhe 1977, Hamp et al. 1978, Ashley & Sainsbury 1981). It is however recognised that attainment and maintenance of optimal oral hygiene requires reinforcement by dentists or professionals complementary to dentistry (Siam et al. 1980). There is strong reinforcement of this message in the Public Health England/Department of Health's Delivering Better Oral Health (DBOH) evidence-based toolkit for prevention, now in its third edition (2017); a fourth edition is currently being compiled (Public Health England 2020).

Toothbrushing and Motivation

Plaque biofilm-induced gingivitis in children and adolescents can be managed by thorough mechanical plaque removal and good oral hygiene (Oh et al. 2002, Needleman et al. 2005), which has additional benefits in terms of reduced risk of caries. Public Health England/Department of Health Guidelines on Delivering Better Oral Health should be followed (2017); they recommend commencing toothbrushing as soon as the first primary tooth erupts. Children under 3 years of age should use a toothpaste containing no less than 1000 ppm fluoride, whilst a family toothpaste (1350–1500 ppm fluoride) is indicated for maximum caries control in children above 3 years of age, ensuring adequate parental supervision for use of small amounts. As manual dexterity to carry out good plaque control for themselves varies from child to child, guidance from the DBOH toolkit (Public Health England 2017) is that parents/caregivers should brush/supervise toothbrushing at ages 0–3 years and supervise children 3–6 years of age. No particular technique of toothbrushing has been shown to be better than any other, rather the need to systematically clean all tooth surfaces should be emphasised by the clinician. The patient's existing toothbrushing technique may need to be modified to achieve this. It is recognised that disclosing tablets can help to indicate areas that are being missed. It is recommended that toothbrushing is carried out twice a day with a fluoridated toothpaste.

An appropriately sized toothbrush should be recommended for children and adolescents; the DBOH toolkit (Public Health England 2017) has recommended a small-headed toothbrush with medium texture bristles. The 2013 Child Dental Health Survey has shown that around 40% of children overall used an electric toothbrush (39% of 5-year-olds, 49% of 8-year-olds, 37% of 12-year-olds, 41% of 15-year-olds). Although there is evidence that some powered toothbrushes, with a rotation-oscillation action, may be more effective for plaque control than manual toothbrushes (Robinson et al. 2003, 2005, Deacon et al. 2010, Yaacob et al. 2014), it is probably more important that the toothbrush, whether manual or powered, is used effectively twice daily. The practitioner can thus recommend good, effective brushing with a manual or powered toothbrush twice daily using a fluoridated toothpaste. The choice of toothbrush may be influenced by patient preference.

Professional support to patients and parents in the form of preventive or educational programmes has been shown to improve patient motivation, leading to improved levels of oral health (Hochstetter et al. 2007). A recent systematic review with meta-analysis involving adolescents and mothers of young children, as well as adults, showed that mobile applications and text messages compared with conventional oral hygiene instructions were a useful adjunct in improving oral hygiene and oral health knowledge and reducing gingival inflammation (Toniazzo et al. 2019). The reader is directed to Chapter 4.3 on patient adherence to healthcare advice and some of the difficulties to be overcome when motivating patients to clean their teeth to a higher standard.

Flossing

Although evidence relating to the effectiveness of flossing in children for the improvement in gingival and periodontal health is sparse, it may be beneficial to recommend supervised flossing of children's teeth for those at high risk of caries. The Public Health England DBOH toolkit (2017) recommends for children aged 12–17 years to clean daily between the teeth to below the gum line before toothbrushing, using dental floss or tape for small spaces between the teeth, or, for larger spaces, using interdental brushes.

The BSP have produced an infographic for children called, "Let's keep children smiling," portraying the message that they should be efficient at flossing or using interdental brushes at around the age of 10 years (available at www.bsperio.org.uk).

Non-Surgical Periodontal Therapy
Management of Gingivitis and Periodontitis

Step 1 of the stepwise approach contains the key elements for the management of plaque-biofilm-induced gingivitis in the child or adolescent (see Chapter 4.3 and Appendices 3 and 4). It is directed at the removal of supragingival and subgingival plaque and calculus deposits on the clinical crown of the tooth via PMPR, in conjunction with risk factor control and patient education and engagement in tailored home plaque control measures; adjunctive therapeutic agents to help control inflammation may also be indicated (Sanz et al. 2020, West et al. 2021). Management of any modifiable risk factors needs to be incorporated into treatment planning, including smoking cessation advice if applicable to children and teenagers.

For periodontitis cases, step 1 needs to be successfully completed before progressing on to step 2. This involves reinforcement of oral hygiene measures, risk factor control and behaviour change before proceeding with subgingival PMPR. Incipient periodontitis (stage I, grade A) in teenagers can often be managed in dental practice. The more challenging cases (stages II, III, IV, Grade C) in the younger age groups and consideration for adjunctive use of systemic antimicrobials may best be undertaken by a specialist to whom referral may be appropriate (Clerehugh & Kindelan 2021). Re-evaluation of the outcome of step 2 drives the decision to move to step 3 (managing non-responding sites) or to step 4 (supportive periodontal therapy [SPT]) (see Chapter 5.4 for further information on this topic).

Younger patients are able to comply with this treatment, but more attention may need to be paid to behavioural aspects (see Chapter 4.3) to acclimatise them to treatment.

Although the effects of plaque on the gingival and periodontal tissues may be transient for the duration of the orthodontic therapy (Ristic et al. 2007), high plaque accumulation can develop in patients undergoing fixed orthodontic treatment (Atack et al. 1996, Turkkahraman et al. 2005) which can result in demineralisation of the adjacent enamel and gingival inflammation (Lovrov et al. 2007). Patients accepted for orthodontic treatment, particularly fixed appliance therapy, should demonstrate an adequate level of oral hygiene. Toothbrushing using the Bass technique with use of approximal brushes and interspace brushes (Goh 2007) is recommended by orthodontic specialists. Reminder therapy has been shown to be a valuable strategy in contributing to the reduction of plaque and gingival indices and white spot lesions in patients undergoing orthodontic treatment according to a systematic review and meta-analysis of high-quality evidence (Lima et al. 2018). A systematic review showed some limited evidence that use of mobile phones can be effective in improving adherence to oral hygiene advice in orthodontic patients (Sharif et al. 2019). The daily use of a 0.05% sodium fluoride mouthwash (225 ppm) should be advised at a different time from toothbrushing for patients undergoing fixed appliance therapy (Benson et al. 2004, Public Health England 2017).

Role of Systemic Antimicrobials

Systemic antimicrobials are not indicated for the management of plaque-induced gingivitis or the cases of incipient periodontitis (typically stage I, grade A) that may be found in adolescents who would normally be treated in the primary dental care setting in general dental practice. There are some specific exceptions:

1. Severe, rapidly destructive disease
Stage II, III, IV, grade C periodontitis in young individuals who would previously have been diagnosed as aggressive periodontitis in the old classification (Armitage et al. 1999) may be considered for adjunctive systemic antibiotic therapy, but such cases are often best managed by specialists (Clerehugh & Kindelan 2021), including:
- molar-incisor pattern of periodontitis affecting first molars/incisors that may occur in adolescents around puberty, which would previously have been classified as localised aggressive periodontitis.
- localised pattern of periodontitis in young people, which would previously have been classified as localised aggressive periodontitis.
- generalised periodontitis, grade C in young adults, which would previously have been diagnosed as generalised aggressive periodontitis.

In these situations, systemic antimicrobials would only be administered as adjuncts to disruption of the biofilm achieved through subgingival PMPR (Teughels et al. 2020, West et al. 2021) (Figure 3.3.6). According to a recent systematic review and meta-analysis (Teughels et al. 2020), the best treatment outcomes have been observed using a

Evidence-based recommendation (2.16)

A. Due to concerns about patient's health and the impact of systemic antibiotic use to public health, its routine use as adjunct to sub-gingival instrumentation in patients with periodontitis is **not recommended.**

B. The adjunctive use of specific systemic antibiotics **may be considered** for specific patient categories (e.g. generalised periodontitis grade C in young adults).

Supporting literature Teughels et al. [45]

Quality of evidence RCTs (n=28) with a double-blind, placebo-controlled, parallel design. Risk of bias was low for 20 of the studies, while 7 studies had a high risk. PPD reduction at 6 months; MET+AMOX: n=8, 867 patients. PPD reduction at 12 months; MET+AMOX: n= 7, 764 patients, MET: n=2, 259 patients.

A. Grade of recommendation grade A - ↓↓

B. Grade of recommendation grade 0 - ↔

A. Strength of consensus consensus (0% of the group abstained due to potential CoI)

B. Strength of consensus consensus (0% of the group abstained due to potential CoI)

BSP implementation

*This evidence-based recommendation (A) is **adopted.***

A. We do not recommend the routine use of systemic antimicrobials as an adjunct to sub-gingival instrumentation in patients with periodontitis, due to concerns with overuse of systemic antimicrobials on individual patient health and on the wider aspects of public health.

*This evidence-based recommendation (B) is **adopted.***

B. *The adjunctive use of specific systemic antibiotics may be considered for specific patient categories (e.g. periodontitis grade C^2 in younger adults where a high rate of progression is documented)*

Updated evidence: No new applicable evidence was identified

Strength of consensus: ***Unanimous consensus*** (0% abstentions due to potential CoI)

• **Figure 3.3.6** Do adjunctive systemic antibiotics improve the clinical outcome of subgingival instrumentation? (Reprinted from West N et al. BSP implementation of European S3 - level evidence-based treatment guidelines for stage I-III periodontitis in UK clinical practice. *Journal of Dentistry* 2021;106:1–72:103562.)

combination of adjunctive systemic amoxicillin (adult dose, 250 mg or 500 mg three times per day) plus metronidazole (adult dose, 200 mg or 400 mg three times per day), although no conclusive consistent evidence emerged for optimum duration which ranged from 3–14 days in the studies cited; to a lesser extent metronidazole alone or azithromycin alone also showed significant clinical benefits in terms of probing pocket depths, clinical attachment level, bleeding on probing, frequency of pocket closure and residual pockets. The debate as to whether to use in the initial phase of treatment or after 3 months subgingival PMPR is ongoing, and the need for cautious and judicious use of systemic antimicrobials is paramount because of antibiotic resistance and potential side effects from their use (Teughels et al. 2020).

2. Necrotising gingivitis

Treatment includes an adult dose of metronidazole 400 mg three times per day for 3 days, in association with debridement, to target the fusiform-spirochaetes in the subgingival plaque, as in British National Formulary guidance by National Institute for Health and Care Excellence (NICE) (https://bnf

.niced.org.uk/treatment-summary/oropharyngeal-infections-antibacterial-therapy.html); doses should be scaled pro rata for children/adolescents according to age as per the BNF.

3. Periodontal abscess with systemic involvement

When local measures are not sufficient, treatment should include the administration of phenoxymethylpenicillin 500 mg four times daily, or alternatively amoxicillin 500 mg three times daily (or, if penicillin allergy, clarithromycin 500 mg twice daily) for up to 5 days, review at 3 days, plus metronidazole 400 mg three times per day if signs of spreading infection, e.g. lymph node involvement. Doses pro rata according to age in younger age groups.

KEY POINT 8

Systemic antimicrobials are not indicated for the management of plaque-induced gingivitis or for most cases of periodontitis in young people, with a few specific exceptions: uncommon but severe and rapidly destructive forms of periodontitis in young patients (typically staged and graded as stage II, III or IV, grade C); necrotising gingivitis; periodontal abscess with systemic involvement.

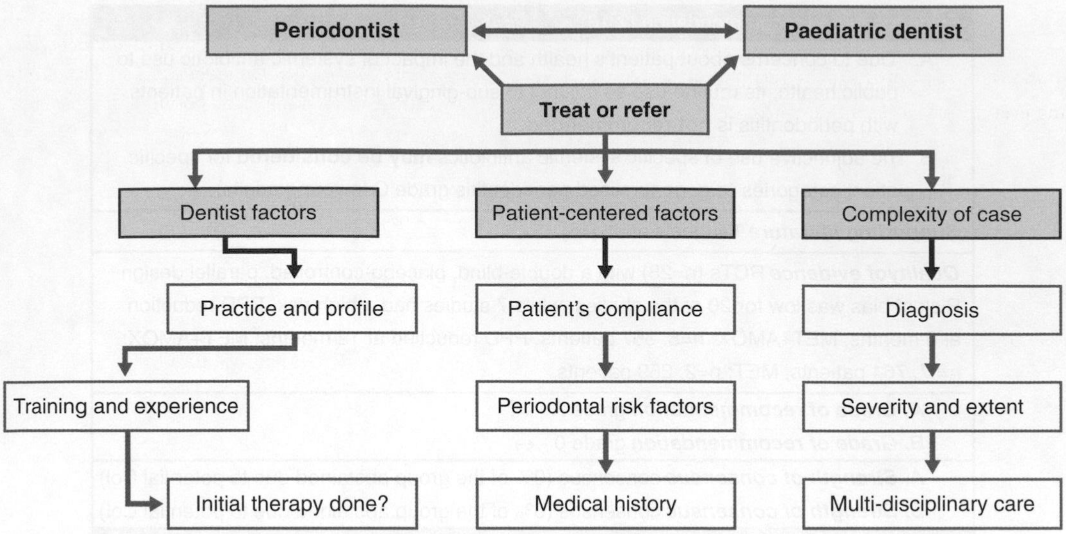

• **Figure 3.3.7** The decision to treat or refer young cases in practice depends on a number of factors.

Management of Recession

The recession should be monitored and management should use a two-tiered approach:

1. Aimed at halting the recession by taking account of the aetiological factors
2. Managing the consequences of recession.

When considering the aetiological factors, the patient needs:

- An atraumatic brushing technique
- Advice on habits associated with gingival trauma (e.g. finger-picking habits), replacement of poorly designed partial dentures
- Orthodontic treatment planning – avoidance of movement which might lead to thinning of the buccal or lingual plate, especially where the gingiva is thin
- Treatment of periodontitis and oral health education on prevention of further destruction
- Smoking cessation advice.

When managing the consequences of recession, the clinician needs to treat:

- Dentine hypersensitivity
  - Anti-sensitive teeth dentifrices; dietary advice; topical fluorides; restoration(s)
- Root caries
  - Topical fluorides; dietary advice; restoration(s)
- Restoration of aesthetics
  - Findings from the literature suggest that mucogingival surgery is not needed before the patient reaches adulthood (Bosnak et al. 2002). Referral to a specialist in paediatric dentistry or periodontology should be considered by the primary care clinician.

Management of Gingival Overgrowth

Treatment for gingival overgrowth should begin with rigorous home care for optimal plaque biofilm control and frequent appointments for PMPR as in steps 1 and 2 of the S3-level treatment approach. Although this often leads to improvement, resective (gingivectomy) surgery (step 3) may be necessary to correct the gingival contour where function and aesthetics are a concern, especially with respect to drug-induced gingival overgrowth. The management of such patients may require referral to dental paediatric or periodontal specialists who will liaise with appropriate medical colleagues.

Treat or Refer

The decision to treat young patients in a primary dental care setting or refer to a specialist is dependent on a number of factors (Figure 3.3.7).

As per the updated BSP Guidelines for Periodontal Screening and Management for Children and Adolescents under 18 years of age (Clerehugh & Kindelan 2021), the periodontal conditions and cases that may be considered for referral include:

- Stage II, III periodontitis not responding to treatment
- Grade C or stage IV periodontitis
- Medical history that significantly affects periodontal treatment or requires multi-disciplinary care
- Periodontitis as a direct manifestation of systemic disease
- Systemic/genetic diseases that can affect periodontal supporting tissues
- Root morphology/furcation defects adversely affecting prognosis on key teeth
- Non-plaque-induced conditions requiring complex or specialist care
- Cases requiring diagnosis/management of rare/complex clinical pathology
- Drug-induced gingival overgrowth needing surgery
- Cases requiring evaluation for periodontal surgery

Multiple choice questions on the contents of this chapter are available online at Elsevier eBooks+.

A series of videos demonstrating how to assess the periodontium are also available online.

References

Agerbaek N, Paulsen S, Nelson B, Glavind L. Effect of professional tooth-cleaning every third week on gingivitis and dental caries in children. *Community Dent Oral Epidemiol*. 1977;6:40–41.

Armitage GC. Development of a classification system for periodontal diseases and conditions. *Ann Periodontol*. 1999;4:1–6.

Ashley FP, Sainsbury RH. The effect of a school based plaque control programme on caries and gingivitis – a three-year study in 11–14 year old girls. *Br Dent J*. 1981;150:41–45.

Atack NE, Sandy JR, Addy M. Periodontal and microbiological changes associated with the placement of orthodontic appliances: a review. *J Periodontol*. 1996;67:78–85.

Axelsson P, Lindhe J. The effect of a plaque control programme on gingivitis and dental caries in school children. *J Dent Res Special issue*. 1977:C142–C148.

Badersten A, Egelberg J, Koch G. Effect of monthly prophylaxis on caries and gingivitis in school children. *Community Dent Oral Epidemiol*. 1975;3:1–4.

Benson PE, Parkin N, Millet DT, Dyer FE, Vine S, Shah A. Fluorides for the prevention of white spots on teeth during fixed brace treatment. *Cochrane Database Syst Rev*. 2004;(3). https://doi.org/10.1002/14651855.CD003809.pub2.

Bimstein E, Eidelman E. Morphological changes in the attached and keratinized gingival and gingival sulcus in the mixed dentition period. A 5-year longitudinal study. *J Clin Periodontol*. 1988;15:175–179.

Bimstein E, Matsson L. Growth and development considerations in the diagnosis of gingivitis and periodontitis in children. *Pediatr Dent*. 1999;21:186–191.

Bosnak A, Jorgić-Srdjak K, Marcević T, Plancak D. The width of the clinically-defined keratinized gingival in the mixed dentition. *ASDC J Dent Child*. 2002;69:266–270.

Caton JG, Armitage G, Berglundh T, Chapple ILC, Jepsen S, Kornman KS, Mealey BL, Papapanou PN, Sanz M, Tonetti MS. A new classification scheme for periodontal and peri-implant diseases and conditions – Introduction and key changes from the 1999 classification. *J Clin Periodontol*. 2018;45(Suppl 20):S1–S8.

Chapple ILC, Mealey BL, et al. Periodontal health and gingival diseases and conditions on an intact and a reduced periodontium: Consensus report of workgroup 1 of the 2017 World Workshop on the Classification of Periodontal and Peri-Implant Diseases and Conditions. *J Clin Periodontol*. 2018;45(Suppl 20):S68–S77. https://doi.org/10.1111/jcpe.12940.

Clerehugh V. Periodontal diseases in children and adolescents. *Br. Dent. J*. 2008;204:469–471.

Clerehugh V, Kindelan S. British Society of Periodontology. Guidelines for periodontal screening and management of children and adolescents under 18 years of age. 2012. Available at www.bsperio.org.uk/publications. (accessed 20 January 2021).

Clerehugh V, Kindelan S. *British Society of Periodontology. Guidelines for periodontal screening and management of children and adolescents under 18 years of age*; 2021. Updated July 2021. Available at www.bsperio.org.uk/publications (accessed 05/05/22) and www.bspd.co.uk/Professionals/Resources/Clinical-Guidelines-and-Evidence-Reviews (accessed 05.05.22).

Clerehugh V, Tugnait A. Diagnosis and management of periodontal diseases in children and adolescents. *Periodontol 2000*. 2001;26: 46–168.

Clerehugh V, Lennon MA, Worthington HV. Five-year results of a longitudinal study of early periodontitis in 14 to 19-year-old adolescents. *J Clin Periodontol*. 1990;17:702–708.

Clerehugh V, Seymour GJ, Bird PS, Cullinan M, Drucker DB, Worthington HV. The detection of *Actinobacillus actinomycetemcomitans*, *Porphyromonas gingivalis* and *Prevotella intermedia* using an ELISA in an adolescent population with early periodontitis. *J Clin Periodontol*. 1997;24:57–64.

Clerehugh V, Tugnait A, Chapple ILC. *Periodontal Management Of Children, Adolescents And Young Adults*. London: Quintessence Publishing Co. Ltd; 2004.

Clerehugh V. Periodontal diseases in children and adolescents. *Br Dent J*. 2008;204:469–471.

Deacon SA, Glenny AM, Deery C, Robinson PG, Heanue M, Walmsley AD, Shaw WC. Different powered toothbrushes for plaque control and gingival health. Cochrane Database of Systematic Reviews. 2010.

Department of Health. *Delivering Better Oral Health. An Evidence Based Toolkit for Prevention*. 2nd ed. Department of Health; 2009. Gateway Reference 8504.

Dietrich T, Ower P, Tank M, West NX, Walter C, Needleman I, Hughes FJ, Wadia R, Milward MR, Hodge PJ, Chapple ILC. Periodontal diagnosis in the context of the 2017 classification system of periodontal diseases and conditions – implementation in clinical practice. *Br Dent J*. 2019;226:16–22.

Faculty of General Dental Practitioners (UK). Selection criteria for dental radiography. London: FGDP, eds Horner, K., Eaton, K.A., third edition, updated 2015 and 2018. Also available online at https://www.fgdp.org.uk/selection-criteria-dental-radiography/5-radiographs-periodontal-assessment (accessed 05 March 2021).

Fine DH, Patil AG, Loos BG. Classification and diagnosis of aggressive periodontitis. *J Clin Periodontol*. 2018;45(Suppl 20):S95–S111. https://doi.org/10.1111/jcpe.12942.

Goh HH. Interspace/interdental brushes for oral hygiene in orthodontic patients with fixed appliances. *Cochrane Database Syst Rev*. 2007;18(3):CD005410. https://doi.org/10.1002/14651858.CD005410.pub2.

Hamlet S, Ellwood R, Cullinan M, Worthington H, Palmer J, Bird P, et al. Persistent colonisation with Tannerella forsythensis and loss of attachment in adolescents. *J Dent Res*. 2004;83:232–235.

Hamp SE, Lindhe J, Farrell J, Johansson LA, Karlsson R. Effect of a field programme based on systematic plaque control on caries and gingivitis in school children after three years. *Community Dent Oral Epidemiol*. 1978;6:17–23.

Hausmann E, Allen K, Clerehugh V. What alveolar crest level on a bitewing radiograph represents bone loss? *J Periodontol*. 1991;62:570–572.

Herrera D, Retamal-Valdes B, Alonso B, Feres M. Acute periodontal lesions (periodontal abscesses and necrotizing periodontal diseases) and endo-periodontal lesions. *J Clin Periodontol*. 2018;45(Suppl 20):S78–S94. https://doi.org/10.1111/jcpe.12941.

Hochstetter AS, Lombardo MJ, D'eramo L, Piovano S, Bordoni N. Effectiveness of a preventive programme on the oral health of preschool children. *Promot Educ*. 2007;14(3):155–158.

Jepsen S, Caton JG, et al. Periodontal manifestations of systemic diseases and developmental and acquired conditions: Consensus report of workgroup 3 of the 2017 World Workshop on the Classification of Periodontal and Peri-Implant Diseases and Conditions. *J Clin Periodontol*. 2018;45(Suppl 20):S219–S229. https://doi.org/10.1111/jcpe.12951.

Lang N, Bartold PM, Cullinan M, Jeffcoat M, Mombelli A, Murakami S, et al. Consensus report: aggressive periodontitis. *Ann Periodontol*. 1999;4:53.

Lima IFP, de Andrade Vieira W, de Macedo Bernardino Í, Costa PA, Lima APB, Pithon MM, Paranhos LR. Influence of reminder therapy for controlling bacterial plaque in patients undergoing orthodontic treatment: a systematic review and meta-analysis. *Angle Orthod.* 2018;88(4):483–493.

Lovrov S, Hertrich K, Hirschfelder U. Enamel demineralization during fixed orthodontic treatment – Incidence and correlation to various oral hygiene parameters. *J Orofac Orthop.* 2007;68:353–363.

Matsson L, Hjersing K, Sjödin B. Periodontal conditions in Vietnamese immigrant children in Sweden. *Swed Dent J.* 1995;19:73–81.

Matsson L, Sjödin B, Käson Blomquist H. Periodontal health in adopted children of Asian origin living in Sweden. *Swed Dent J.* 1997;21:177–184.

Needleman I, Suvan J, Moles DR, Pimlott J. A systematic review of professional mechanical plaque removal for prevention of periodontal diseases. *J Clin Periodontol.* 2005;32:229–282.

Oh T, Ebar R, Wang H. Periodontal diseases in the child and adolescent. *J Clin Periodontol.* 2002;29:400–410.

Papapanou PN, Sanz M, et al. Periodontitis: Consensus report of Workgroup 2 of the 2017 World Workshop on the Classification of Periodontal and Peri-implant Diseases and Conditions. *J Clin Periodontol.* 2018;45(Suppl 20):S162–S170. https://doi.org/10.1111/jcpe.12946.

Pitts, N., Chadwick, B., Anderson, T. Children's Dental Health Survey 2013. Report 2: Dental Disease and Damage in Children, England, Wales and Northern Ireland. Health and Social Care Information Centre; National Statistics publication, published 19th March 2015. Available at www.hscic.gov.uk (accessed 21/03/2021).

Public Health England. *Delivering Better Oral Health: An Evidence-Based Toolkit for Prevention.* 3rd ed. 2017. PHE gateway number: 2016224. Available from: www.gov.uk/government/publications/delivering-better-oral-health-an-evidence-based-toolkit-for-prevention (accessed on 03/04/21).

Public Health England. *Developing Better Oral Health: Guideline Development Manual*; 2020. London, PHE gateway number: GW-965.

Rapp GE, Garcia RV, Motta AC, Andrade IT, Bião MA, Carvalho PB. Prevalence assessment of periodontal disease in 3–6-year-old children through PSR – a pilot study. *J Int Acad Periodontol.* 2001;3:75–80.

Ristic M, Vlahovic Svabic M, Sasic M, Zelic O. Clinical and microbiological effects of fixed orthodontic appliances on periodontal tissues in adolescents. *Orthod Craniofac Res.* 2007;10:187–195.

Robinson PG, Deacon SA, Deery C, Heanue M, Walmsley AD, Worthington HV, Glenny AM, Shaw WC. Manual versus powered toothbrushing for oral health. *Cochrane Database Syst Rev.* 2003;1. https://doi.org/10.1002/14651858.CD002281.pub2.

Robinson P, Deacon SA, Deery C, Heanue M, Walmsley AD, Worthington HV, et al. Manual versus powered toothbrushing for oral health. *Cochrane Database Syst Rev.* 2005;2. https://doi.org/10.1002/14651858.CD002281.pub2.

Sanz M, Herrera D, Kebschull M, Chapple I, Jepsen S, Beglundh T, Sculean A, Tonetti MS; On behalf of the EFP Workshop Participants and Methodological Consultants. Treatment of stage I–III periodontitis—The EFP S3 level clinical practice guideline. *J Clin Periodontol.* 2020;47:4–60. https://doi.org/10.1111/jcpe.13290.

Sharif MO, Newton T, Cunningham SJ. A systematic review to assess interventions delivered by mobile phones in improving adherence to oral hygiene advice for children and adolescents. *Br Dent J.* 2019;227(5):375–382.

Siam JD, Peterson JK, Matthews BL, Voglesong RH, Lyman BA. Effects of supervised daily plaque removal by children after 3 years. *Community Dent Oral Epidemiol.* 1980;8:171–176.

Teughels W, Feres M, Oud V, Martín C, Matesanz P, Herrera D. Adjunctive effect of systemic antimicrobials in periodontitis therapy: A systematic review and meta-analysis. *J Clin Periodontol.* 2020;47:212–281. https://doi.org/10.1111/jcpe.13264.

Tiainen L, Asikainen S, Saxen L. Puberty-associated gingivitis. Community Dent. *Oral Epidemiol.* 1992;20:87–89.

Tonetti MS, Greenwell H, Kornman KS. Staging and grading of periodontitis: Framework and proposal of a new classification and case definition. *J Clin Periodontol.* 2018;45(Suppl 20):S149–S161. https://doi.org/10.1111/jcpe.12945.

Toniazzo MP, Nodari D, Muniz FWMG, Weidlich P. Effect of Health in improving oral hygiene: a systematic review with meta-analysis. *J Clin Periodontol.* 2019;46(3):297–309.

Tsakos G, Chadwick B, Anderson T. *Children's Dental Health Survey 2013. Report 1. Attitudes, Behaviours and Children's Dental Health. Health and Social Care Information Centre.* National Statistics publication; 2015. published 19th March 2015, Available at https://digital.nhs.uk/data-and-information/publications/statistical/children-s-dental-health-survey/child-dental-health-survey-2013-england-wales-and-northern-ireland#related-links (accessed 21/03/2021).

Turkkahraman H, Sayin MO, Bozkurt FY, Yetkin Z, Kaya S, Onal S. Archwire ligation techniques, microbial colonization, and periodontal status in orthodontically treated patients. *Angle Orthod.* 2005;75:231–236.

Wadia R, Walter C, Chapple ILC, Ower P, Tank M, West NX, Needleman I, Hughes FJ, Milward MR, Hodge PJ, Dietrich T. Periodontal diagnosis in the context of the 2017 classification system of periodontal diseases and conditions: presentation of a patient with periodontitis localized to the molar teeth. *Br Dent J.* 2019;226:180–182.

Wagaiyu EG, Ashley FP. Mouthbreathing, lip seal and upper lip coverage and their relationship with gingival inflammation in 11–14-year-old schoolchildren. *J Clin Periodontol.* 1991;18:698–702.

Walter C, Chapple ILC, Ower P, Tank M, West NX, Needleman I, Hughes FJ, Wadia R, Milward MR, Hodge PJ, Dietrich T. Periodontal diagnosis in the context of the 2017 classification system of periodontal diseases and conditions: presentation of a pair of young siblings with periodontitis. *Br Dent J.* 2019 a;226:23–26.

Walter C, Ower P, Tank M, West NX, Needleman I, Hughes FJ, Wadia R, Milward MR, Hodge PJ, Dietrich T. Periodontal diagnosis in the context of the 2017 classification system of periodontal diseases and conditions: presentation of a middle-aged patient with localized periodontitis. *Br Dent J.* 2019 b;226:98–100.

West N, Chapple I, Claydon N, D'Aiuto F, Donos N, Ide M, Needleman I, Kebschull M. BSP implementation of European S3 - level evidence-based treatment guidelines for stage I-III periodontitis in UK clinical practice. *J Dent.* 2021;106:1–72:103562. https://doi.org/10.1016/j.jdent.2020.103562.

Yaacob M, Worthington HV, Deacon SA, Deery C, Walmsley AD, Robinson PG, Glenny AM. Powered versus manual toothbrushing for oral health. *Cochrane Database Syst Rev.* 2014:6. https://doi.org/10.1002/14651858.CD002281.pub3.

3.4

REFERRAL TO A PERIODONTAL SPECIALIST

ALAN WOODMAN

CHAPTER OUTLINE

OVERVIEW OF THE CHAPTER

This chapter explains the who, what, why, when, where and how of periodontal referrals.

It incorporates the British Society of Periodontology and Implant Dentistry (BSP) guidance on referral and associated dento-legal issues.

By the end of the chapter, and after having completed the online questions and exercises, the reader should:

- Understand the indications for the referral of periodontal patients
- Appreciate the mechanisms of effective referral
- Be confident in explaining to patients the benefits and possible outcomes of referral
- Be able to construct a satisfactory referral letter
- Understand the long-term relationship between the referrer, referee and the patient.

The chapter covers the following topics:

- Introduction
- Why refer?
- Who to refer to
- What to refer – radiographic criteria, restorative criteria, implants
- When to refer
- Where to refer
- What to expect from a referral
- After the referral
- Dento-legal issues.

Introduction

For most patients, the early recognition and treatment of periodontal diseases allows clinicians to achieve a predictable outcome and a stable periodontium. This can be maintained for life with continued supportive care and allows for the successful provision of other dental treatment. *The important role of the hygienist in achieving*

this long-term outcome cannot be overstated. However, a small proportion of patients may either initially present to the clinician with a more advanced condition, because of previous non-attendance or lack of appropriate treatment, or display a high level of susceptibility or show a greater disease complexity due to health, behavioural, anatomical or dental complications. Such patients may seem to the receiving clinician to demand, or deserve, particular skills which they themselves feel unable to offer, and thus referral to a specialist in periodontics is deemed desirable.

This chapter aims to advise the clinician on the rationale for periodontal referral and the practical aspects of achieving a successful result for the patient. The referral should be seen as a shared, continuing and cyclical partnership among the several participants (Figure 3.4.1).

KEY POINT 1

Early recognition of periodontal diseases will minimise the need for late referral.

Why Refer?

A decision to refer to a colleague will be based upon:
- The clinician's experience, confidence and perceived ability to manage the patient's condition
  - If the situation is carefully explained to the patient and a choice clearly given, most patients only see referral as a positive benefit, not as a "failure" in their clinician, but it is important to be able to answer their initial queries about the referral
  - In the medical environment, patients do not expect their general practitioner (GP) to handle all their problems and referral is common
- The age and general health status of the patient
  - Periodontitis presenting in a younger patient is generally regarded as a greater concern – *aggressive disease* at any age justifies referral, but referral is *essential* for the adolescent patient
  - Concurrent health problems may influence the onset of periodontal diseases and their treatment outcomes, particularly:
    Unstable diabetes
    Drug-induced gingival enlargement (DIGE), which is increasingly prevalent as more patients receive calcium channel blockers as part of anti-hypertensive therapy
    A history of head and neck radiotherapy
    A known significant bleeding dyscrasia/disorder
    A significant immunocompromised or suppressed state
- The complexity of the treatment likely to be required. For example:
  - Multiple deep infra-bony lesions, where surgical care is likely to be recommended
  - The presence of suspected posterior perio-endo lesions, where complex endodontic treatment, or possible root resection, is required
  - Extensive pocketing associated with tooth mobility, where splinting may be indicated
  - Isolated pockets affecting important abutment teeth
  - The presence of concurrent muco-gingival disease
  - The presence of peri-implant disease or the close proximity of implants to the disease site(s)
  - A requirement for intramuscular (IM) or intravenous (IV) medication as a component of clinical management

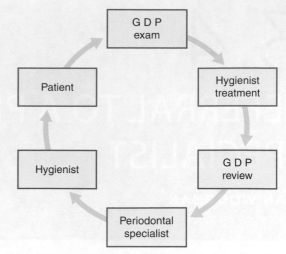

• **Figure 3.4.1** The participants in periodontal care and treatment.

- The patient's preference or request to see a specialist
  - Patients have become increasingly aware of treatment alternatives via the internet and other media and may demand another approach if, in their view, existing treatments seem unsuccessful
  - Such a request should not be assumed to be a criticism, but it must carefully be discussed to determine the reasons for the patient's decision and to maintain a professional relationship post-referral
  - The specialist will always be discreet and tactful when replying to the patient's inevitable query, "Why has this not been done before, by my dentist/hygienist . . . ?"

KEY POINT 2

The dental hygienist or therapist may be the backbone of successful periodontal care but will always provide more effective support with good general dental practitioner (GDP) input and interest.

KEY POINT 3

It is very important that the specialist maintains proper professional respect when dealing with such patient queries to ensure that the long-term relationship between the referrer, patient and specialist remains mutually supportive.

Who to Refer

Three broad groups of patients may be regarded as suitable for referral:
- Patients with concurrent complicating medical conditions, discussed previously, but most commonly:
  - Unstable diabetes
  - Those presenting with DIGE, especially those taking calcium channel blockers (e.g. nifedipine) for hypertension
- Compliant but non-responding patients:
  - Non-smokers – who have made good efforts with their oral hygiene but failed to achieve the outcome expected after initial hygienic phase treatment
  - Smokers – who show a poor response to initial treatment, but they must be advised that:

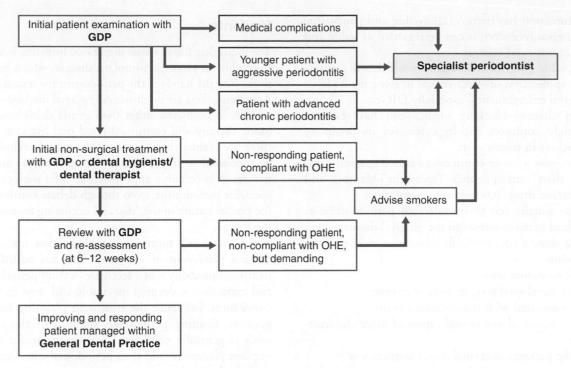

• Figure 3.4.2 Protocol for referral.

the outcome of treatment will be less predictable, whoever undertakes it,

progress will be slower to achieve, and

surgical treatment may not be a practical option if they continue to smoke

advising a patient to seek smoking cessation advice prior to referral makes a very valuable contribution to their care, both in the short and long term.

- Non-compliant but demanding patients:
  - These patients have not adequately complied with oral hygiene advice during initial or maintenance therapies, and thus show little or no improvement, yet demand further treatment but will not accept extractions
  - Referral of such patients is not ideal, but some may respond to a different approach or different clinician. If they still do not respond after specialist care, an alternative strategy must be adopted, usually involving the extraction of teeth
  - It may be that simply giving a second (specialist) opinion will suffice and convince the patient to accept the original GDP proposals
  - Providing a comprehensive history of the treatment attempted is particularly important for these patients, to assist the specialist in making a reasoned judgement about any possible treatment options.

A protocol for referring periodontal patients is shown in Figure 3.4.2.

What to Refer

Clinical Criteria

Certain features of periodontal diseases are logical prerequisites for referral (but not all have to be present at the same time). Patients suited to referral will usually show some of the following features:

- Non-resolving sites, either as multiple pockets or isolated deep lesions
- Pocket depth ≥5 mm
- Significant anatomical difficulty such as:
  - the close proximity of roots, either due to closely approximated teeth, or
  - narrow furcation spaces
  - "extra" roots, such as third roots in upper premolars, or lower molars, fourth roots in upper molars or, less commonly, bifid roots in canines or incisors
  - thick crestal bone
  - thick, obstructive, gingival tissues
- Mobility of grade 1 or 2
- If mobility exceeds this, i.e. grade 3, extraction is the most likely outcome and referral is rarely justified unless splinting is proposed
- Persistent bleeding on probing from pockets – in spite of good oral hygiene
- Persistent desquamative gingival surfaces
- History of periodontal abscess(es)
- Suspected perio-endo/endo-perio lesion
- Unstable furcation involvement – i.e. a furcation to which access is denied by either the gingival tissues or an unfavourable root anatomy
  - Furcations which show roots divergent by >30 degrees may be maintained in the long term and are suitable for referral
  - A convergence or divergence of <30 degrees is unpredictable
  - If further complicated by mobility or occlusal stresses such convergent teeth should *not* be the subject of referral

- If a furcation has become cleansable and patent due to gingival recession, it can be regarded as stable and should not need referral
- Unacceptable gingival architecture – which will complicate the application of effective oral hygiene methods
  - Gingival enlargement – especially DIGE
  Calcium channel–blocking medications have become increasingly common anti-hypertensives in favour of beta-blockers in recent years
  They are now a more common cause of gingival overgrowth than anti-epileptics (epanutin/Dilantin) and anti-rejection drugs (cyclosporin, tacrolimus)
  Their use usually has to be tolerated periodontally, as the medical benefits outweigh the gingival disadvantages and GPs show understandable reluctance to change the prescription
- Gingival recession, which
  May have developed progressively over time
  May be associated with fraenal attachments
  May have occurred as a complication of successful treatment
  Leaves the patient concerned about aesthetics or
  Permits persistent cervical sensitivity, resistant to topical therapies
- Elective "crown-lengthening" surgery to improve the restorability of teeth.

Radiographic Criteria

It is expected that patients referred to a specialist would exhibit at least one of these features:
- >30% loss of bony support
  - which can *only* be judged if the radiograph shows the *whole tooth*, thus
  - peri-apical or orthopantomogram (OPT) views *are essential* for confirmation of diagnosis
- Irregular (vertical) bone loss
- Infra-bony lesions
- Perio-endo/endo-perio lesion(s)
- Concurrent but unrelated endodontic lesion(s) on periodontally affected teeth.

Restorative Criteria

Prior to referral, it is important to consider the restorability of periodontally affected teeth. There is no point in carrying out complicated periodontal treatment to retain a tooth which cannot then be restored.

However, the presence of periodontal lesions in certain circumstances assumes priority for complex care, where the alternative, tooth loss, would have serious consequences for the existing restoration or prostheses:
- Abutment teeth for existing bridges/dentures
- Last functional molar in any quadrant
- Teeth complicated by suspected occlusal co-factors
- Potential loss of posterior support if tooth/teeth lost.

Implants

The increasing use of osseo-integrated implants has resulted, inevitably, in more peri-implant disease, which has tended to fall into the hands of the periodontist for remedial action. At present, there are no universally agreed methods of coping with these problems, other than gentle debridement, antibiotic therapy and continued good oral hygiene, although there are claims that regenerative surgical techniques can be successful in improving the bone contours around the fixtures. It is certainly appropriate to refer such cases to the specialist periodontist, even though debate continues about the precise nature of the "disease" occurring around the failing fixture.

An increasing number of periodontists undertake the surgical placement of implants. This has added a useful treatment modality when teeth are beyond periodontal care and extraction is deemed inevitable and may, in some circumstances, influence the treatment planning for referred patients. Gaining periodontal stability of the remaining teeth is generally considered a prerequisite for successful implant placement and thus periodontal care usually must precede the implant phase.

> ### KEY POINT 4
> You may not wish to undertake periodontal treatment yourself, but remember that your dental hygienist/therapist is specifically trained to undertake non-surgical periodontal therapy.
> In all but the most severe cases, let the hygienist/therapist carry out some initial treatment rather than assuming the worst outcome!

> ### KEY POINT 5
> Clear, concise and comprehensive records on paper or computer are absolutely essential in periodontal therapy and facilitate any referrals.
> Such records also offer medico-legal protection to the clinician.
> Make a record of *all* discussions, communications and advice given to patients about their problems and treatment.

When to Refer

As with any medical condition, early referral is the ideal. However, the timing of the presentation of the case is not always within the clinician's control and most cases are referred later than the specialist would prefer.

Unless the patient presents with an established aggressive periodontitis, it is usually appropriate for the GDP or dental hygienist to carry out some initial hygienic phase therapy, which is the accepted start of all periodontal treatment.
- Referral should be considered if, following review of such initial hygienic phase therapy after 3 months, extensive pocketing remains with bleeding from the pockets
- If pockets reappear after a period of stability

- If, on presentation, prior to initial treatment, a new patient shows basic periodontal examination (BPE) code 4 in several sextants, especially in the younger or medically challenged patient
- If the patient has advanced chronic periodontitis
- If the restorative co-factors are challenging in addition to the poor periodontal condition.

The BPE may be regarded as a guide to referral, but clinicians are strongly recommended to undertake a full periodontal assessment and comprehensive periodontal examination (CPE) to justify referral and to enhance their own records of the patient's condition at referral for dentolegal prudence, particularly if the patient is a poor complier with oral hygiene advice and appointments.

It is likely that patients considered suitable for referral will have demonstrated a BPE code of 4 in one or more sextants; however, a widespread distribution of code 3 may also initiate referral, especially as this may be associated with DIGE.

The relationship between the complexity of treatment and the BPE is explained in the British Society of Periodontology and Implant Dentistry (BSP) document "Referral Policy and Parameters of Care", which attempts to outline complexity in terms of the types of patient, condition, complications and potential treatments to assist in making a decision to refer.

Ultimately, the timing of the referral will be the referring clinician's decision and will be made after discussion with the patient.

Where to Refer

In the UK, the options available to the GDP and patient, which are limited by location and professional demography, are as follows:

- University dental school periodontal or restorative consultant
  - This is inconvenient for those living outside the main cities
  - The cases required for undergraduate training are usually only moderately severe
  - The dental school need for complex cases will be proportionate to the number of postgraduates undertaking treatment
  - However, if available, treatment will be free.
- NHS general hospital restorative consultant
  - Unfortunately, such departments rarely have funding for prolonged treatments and hygienist support, but advice and treatment planning may be, at best, available but will be free
- Community dental service periodontal specialist
  - Such posts are few and far between but will usually be free
- Dentist with special interest in periodontics (DWSIs)
  - A small number of GDPs have followed this route in practice and may be able to provide an enhanced periodontal service locally. This is most likely to be under private terms
- Private specialist in periodontics

- Since the creation of a specialists list by the General Dental Council (GDC), such periodontal specialists have become available but, as they are exclusively practising under private contract, this may prove expensive for many potential patients.
- It is essential that referring clinicians discuss the possibility and extent of fees which could be incurred for initial consultation when recommending referral and that they ensure patients understand their liabilities. Most specialists will provide a guide to their fees.
- Subsequent fees will be discussed between the specialist and the patient following the consultation. Referring clinicians should avoid discussion with the patient about specialists' fees for treatment.
- If there is certainty about the availability of specialists in a particular area, the British Society of Periodontology and Implant Dentistry website (www.bsperio.org.uk) offers a suitable search capability. The GDC Specialists List, contained in the dentists register, also has similar information (https://www.gdc-uk.org/registration/your-registration/specialist-lists).

> ### KEY POINT 6
> There is no fast track to periodontal health.
> Paying privately for periodontal treatment does not necessarily equate to better treatment, but usually means that more time is spent with the clinician.
> Remember the time spent on periodontal health education is as rewarding clinically as the active treatment.

> ### KEY POINT 7
> In the UK (and other countries with state-funded care), there are strict budgetary restraints on all expenditure within the National Health Service.
> This may limit some surgical procedures involving expensive regenerative materials, even within the dental schools, unless research funding is available.

> ### KEY POINT 8
> Never assume the financial status or commitment of your patients.
> Always give the patient the full choice of options for referral.
> Many patients will choose to prioritise their personal spending on dental care so that they may keep their teeth for longer.

How to Refer

Essential information required in any communication, either online, by email or by letter should contain:
- Referring clinician's details and contact information
- Patient's details, date of birth and address
- Patient's contact information and availability
- Medical alert/status of the patient
- Patient's original complaint/wishes
- Brief description of periodontal and general dental condition
- Specific concerns, especially related restorative complications or plans
- Outline of treatment provided and response, if any

- Copies of charts, radiographs (new and old) and study casts if available
- Purpose of referral – is this for:
  - Second opinion
  - Treatment planning, or
  - Treatment.

Examples of suitable formats for referral and referral exercises are included in the online section of this chapter.

KEY POINT 9

Always state:
- Why they are coming
- What you have tried
- What the patient wants
- Where any specific sites are to be found
- What medical issues might be a compromise to treatment.

KEY POINT 10

Always try to send:
- Previous CPE chart(s)
- Relevant radiographs or copies (old radiographs are particularly useful to provide a historical record of disease progression)
- Photographs of acute sites
- Models – if occlusal or recession problems are the subject of the referral.

KEY POINT 11

Always provide:
- Clear details of:
  Your address & contact
  Patient's address
  Patient's contact
  Patient's availability
- Give the patient details of:
  Who they are seeing
  Any possible cost
  Why you want them to go

What to expect from a Referral

What to Expect as a Referring Clinician

- Probably more initial non-surgical "re-treatment"
- A period of review and reassessment usually 6 weeks to 3 months post-treatment
- Possibly endodontic co-treatment may be recommended (undertaken by the referrer or another specialist)
- Possibly occlusal co-treatment (by the specialist or, less likely, by the referrer)
- Possibly a recommendation for surgical treatment
- The need for continued long-term hygienist support, either initially or permanently within the referral practice.

How to Prepare your Patient

- Always try to explain the origins of their disease, the reasons for your concern and the need for referral

• BOX 3.4.1A	Results of a 6-Year Audit of Activity of a Specialist in Periodontics
New patient consultations	2036
Initial non-surgical treatment by the periodontist	997
Initial non-surgical treatment by dental hygienist	959
Patients receiving occlusal analysis	993
Patients subsequently provided with an acrylic occlusal splint	91
Patients proceeding to surgical care after review of initial treatment	523
Supportive care reviews with the periodontist*	4710
Supportive care reviews with the dental hygienist	12256
Patients receiving acrylic labial gingival veneers for aesthetics	178
Periodontal splints applied (webbing/composite)	334
Periodontal splint repairs subsequently undertaken	639
Metal (Rochette/Maryland) splints applied	61

*Joint appointments with the dental hygienist.

- Always ensure that the alternatives to further periodontal treatment are explained
- Do not assume that a surgical approach will be undertaken
- Do not second-guess what the specialist will say – let the specialist outline the treatment needs in due course
- If appropriate, warn the patient of the likelihood of a poor response to treatment in the presence of modifiable risk factors, such as smoking and poor oral hygiene.

Many specialists in periodontics undertake a broad spectrum of periodontal and closely allied treatments, such as implant dentistry, occlusal therapies and apical surgery. Others restrict their practice to "pure" periodontics.

The choice of specialist will depend upon the referring clinician's undergraduate teaching, interests and beliefs, the perceived needs of your patient and the availability of a specialist in the local area.

The clinical audits (Box 3.4.1A and B) illustrate the activities typical of a specialist in periodontics, showing the varied tasks undertaken within a "broad spectrum" specialist periodontal practice over a 6-year period (2004–2010).

KEY POINT 12

The patient should receive:
- A clear statement of the problem
- The objectives of treatment
- A clear plan of proposed treatment
  Including:
- The number of appointments planned
- Who will be treating the patient
- An estimate of costs
- The anticipated treatment time.

• BOX 3.4.1B	Specialist in Periodontics: Surgical Activities Over a 6-Year Period

Surgical treatments	523
Including tissue regeneration with:	
Emdogain (nil teeth lost)	20
Ceramic (5% teeth lost)	34
BioOss/Gide (3% teeth lost)	187
Also:	
Frenectomies	31
Connective tissue grafts	7
And:	
Apicectomies	48
Vital root resections	63
Number requiring subsequent:	
Endodontic treatment	14
Extraction	6

After Referral

The Specialist's Report

Following consultation, the specialist will provide the referring clinician (and the patient) with a report on the condition of the patient, the findings, diagnosis and proposed treatment.

This may be a copy of a report prepared for the patient or a separate report. Many specialists will copy all correspondence to the patient and referring dentist to each party, thus enabling complete transparency regarding any fees involved and the treatment offered.

If paying for treatment, the patient will receive an estimate of the likely fees involved for any proposed treatment within the specialist practice.

Patients may seek to discuss these reports (and the estimate of likely fees) with the referring clinician for guidance and/or reassurance before committing to treatment. This is quite reasonable, although most patients will agree to treatment at or shortly after their consultation.

In essence the specialist report should outline:
- The current dental status of the patient
- The current periodontal status of the patient
- The particular periodontal sites of concern
- Any concurrent restorative concerns
- Any concurrent endodontic concerns
- Any observed soft tissue concerns
- Any observed occlusal concerns
- Any medical contraindications or co-factors
- A proposed treatment plan, which must also be clear to the patient.

Any perceived concurrent treatment requirements will be discussed, for example:
- Endodontic
- Restorative – new or replacement prostheses/restorations

- Occlusal or orthodontic treatment in complex cases.

Such treatments may be undertaken either by the referring clinician or managed by the specialist or another specialist colleague, depending upon the complexity and wishes of the patient and the referring clinician.

The report may also indicate where the necessary supportive periodontal treatment (SPT) should be undertaken after initial treatment – within the specialist practice or the referring clinician's practice. However, most specialist periodontists prefer to keep the patient under their close supervision for a recovery period of at least 1 year.

SPT, the longer-term outcome of all periodontal treatment, is usually undertaken by the dental hygienist under the supervision of the referring clinician. Many periodontists, however, prefer to keep SPT under their control. There is reliable research evidence that such long-term care in specialist practice is more successful in reducing subsequent tooth and attachment loss than that carried out in general dental practice.

If the patient remains under the care of the specialist for a long period of time, it is customary to provide the referring clinician with a periodic review of the patient's status, especially if a change in the treatment plan is proposed, for example, progress to surgical therapy or the need for extractions.

Examples of such reports and estimates can be found in the online section which complements the printed part of this book.

Legal and Ethical Issues

Guidance on these issues can be found in the GDC document: Standards for the Dental Team (http://www.gdc-uk.org/Dentalprofessionals/Standards/Documents/Standards for the Dental Team.pdf).

As dentistry has entered increasingly litigious times, the frequency of complaints against practitioners for failing to diagnose and/or treat periodontal diseases has risen considerably, and the various defence organisations regularly remind their clients of the need for comprehensive record keeping, early recognition of disease and good communication with their patients to minimise risk.

From an ethical standpoint, the patient has a right to expect referral for any condition if their primary care clinician feels unable to provide treatment to a satisfactory standard. Thus, ignoring or delaying necessary periodontal treatment cannot be excused when the option of referral to a colleague is available.

Similarly, a failure to take adequate steps to diagnose and thus subsequently fail to treat periodontal diseases will be deemed unacceptable by regulating authorities.
- Responsibility for recognising the need for referral lies with the diagnosing clinician

- Responsibility for providing the appropriate care after referral lies with the specialist
- The specialist will work under different conditions from the generalist:
  - They are expected to undertake more complex tasks
  - They are assumed, by definition, to be more experienced and competent in their field
  - Thus, any failure of treatment will be judged a more serious breach of their "duty of care".
- Patients' expectations will be higher when receiving specialist treatment; thus to avoid disappointment:
  - Setting realistic and clearly understood goals is essential at the outset of specialist care
  - Gaining informed consent must be achieved
  - Having ensured that all options for treatment have been fully explained.

The referring clinician has often known the patient for a considerable time and has been able to establish a good rapport. It is worth remembering that the specialist is meeting and treating a stranger and such rapport will take time to build. The interpersonal skills of the specialist are as important as their clinical skills in ensuring a harmonious relationship between them, their patient and their referring clinicians.

On Conclusion of Specialist Care

- It is essential that the specialist informs the referring clinician of the outcome of treatment, the likely future care required and the prognosis for the patient's periodontal and general dental condition as a result of the treatment provided.
- After surgical procedures there may be a recommended interval for radiographic reviews.
- A clear statement of the oral hygiene advice given and continuing techniques expected will be beneficial for future dental hygiene support.

The specialist must always remain available for advice or remedial treatment, even though they may have returned the patient to the referring clinician.

Problems can occur when care is shared between the specialist and, for example, the dental hygienist in the original referring practice, often during the supportive phase of care. Should the patient's condition deteriorate, an awkward situation can arise. It is advisable to follow the specialist's

recommendations for SPT closely and ensure that the treatment provided is adequate.

Managing the Patient Who Declines Referral

Not all patients will accept the need for referral. This may be for many reasons:
- anxiety
- lack of understanding
- lack of interest in keeping teeth
- financial concerns
- other health issues
- lack of time
- loss of time from work, etc.

In such cases, it is *imperative* that the patient's records are fully annotated with the referral offered, the reasons why referral was recommended and the reasons for this being declined.

Keeping a statement of these facts signed by the clinician and the patient is a prudent action and may limit possible future dento-legal difficulties.

> **KEY POINT 13**
> If a patient declines referral *always* make a full record of this and their reasons for saying no!

Multiple choice questions on the contents of this chapter are available online at Elsevier eBooks+.

A series of case studies and referral letters are also available online.

References and Further Reading

Baker P, Needleman I. Risk management in clinical practice. Part 10. Periodontology. *Br Dent J.* 2010;209:557–565.

Dental Protection Society. *Riskwise.* 2012;43.

Gaunt F, Devine M, Pennington M, Varnazza C, Gwynnett E, Steen N, Heasman P, et al. The cost-effectiveness of supportive periodontal care for patients with chronic periodontitis. *J Clin Periodontol.* 2010;35(8 Suppl):67–82.

General Dental Council, 2005. Standards for dental professionals. Accessed from: www.gdc.org-uk (on 22 October 2012) and http://www.gdc-uk.org/Newsandpublications/Publications/Publications/StandardsforDentalProfessionals[1].pdf (on 24 October 2010).

The Role of Self-Care and Oral Hygiene Methods

SECTION 4

The Role of Self-Care and Oral
Hygiene Methods

4.1

PATIENT EDUCATION AND SELF-PERFORMED BIOFILM CONTROL

ELAINE TILLING

CHAPTER OUTLINE

Introduction

Patients' Health Beliefs

Motivating Patients to Clean Optimally

Tailoring Oral Health Advice

Techniques for Oral Hygiene

    Self-Assessment of Home Plaque Control

Delivery of Oral Hygiene Advice

Toothbrushing

    Manual

    Brushing Technique

    Powered Brushes

Interdental Cleaning

    Elastomeric Toothpicks

    Floss

    Flossing Techniques

    Interdental Brushes

    Oral Irrigators

    Subgingival Cleaning

Adjunctive Antiseptic Agents

    Dentifrices (Toothpastes)

    Mouth Rinses

    Chlorhexidine

Conclusions

OVERVIEW OF THE CHAPTER

This chapter explains the role of self-care in periodontal therapy, oral hygiene methods, the pivotal role of the patient in the long-term success of periodontal management and the complexity of behavioural change in health.

By the end of the chapter the reader should:

- Understand the impact of factors affecting compliance and motivation in self-performed biofilm control
- Describe the practical application of the key principles of the Health Belief Model in relation to self-performed biofilm control
- Be able to demonstrate the various techniques for the mechanical disruption of biofilm using a range of oral hygiene tools
- Recognise the pivotal role of the patient in the outcome of periodontal treatment
- Describe the role of some of the active ingredients in commercially available dentifrices and mouthwashes.

The chapter covers the following topics:

- Introduction
- Patients' health beliefs
- Motivating patients to clean optimally
- Tailoring oral healthcare advice
- Techniques for oral hygiene
- Delivery of oral hygiene advice
- Toothbrushing
- Interdental cleaning
- Dentifrices
- Mouthwashes
- Conclusions.

Introduction

The strategic focus of many health education interventions has been on clearly defined diseases and targeted at changing the behaviours of high-risk individuals. The concept of health as a collective responsibility is not new, but the growing emphasis on the critical role of the individual in their general health and well-being is increasingly recognised. The health educational model for the promotion of oral health emphasises lifestyle and behavioural change through educational awareness. Health professionals tend to dominate in this top-down, disease-led focus. It has been popular within the dental profession as it fits with the clinical approach in the care and treatment of individual patients. However, this model has its limitations, as it underestimates the dynamic complexity of motivation for behavioural change. Establishing and maintaining effective biofilm (plaque) control is not just about having the manual dexterity to clean effectively but about the many factors that strongly influence compliance and motivation. These factors include attitude, understanding, beliefs and lifestyle, all of which need to be taken into consideration when trying to effect permanent change in a patient's habits. There is some debate regarding the impact of self-performed biofilm control for chronic periodontitis. A systematic review (Hujoel et al. 2005) highlighted the lack of consistent epidemiological evidence on the role of plaque/biofilm in the aetiology of periodontitis. With many medical conditions, including periodontal diseases, the behaviour of the individual in terms of modifying risk factors associated with disease is increasingly becoming part of care pathways. In patients diagnosed with periodontal diseases, the pivotal role of the individual in oral biofilm control is recognised in the clinical recommendations (CR) detailed in Figure 4.3.3 in Chapter 4.3. The *stepwise* approach mapped to the new classification system for periodontal and peri-implant diseases by the World Workshop in 2017 (see Chapter 2.1 for full details) is described in Chapter 4.3 and illustrated in Figure 4.3.2. From this it is clear that the responsibility for daily plaque removal is placed firmly on the patient, and supportive periodontal care provided by the clinician is dependent upon the individual's adherence to effective daily home care. The efficacy of the plethora of oral hygiene aids and methods of use are subject to constant change of clinical opinion. However, in the absence of further evidence and professional consensus, the pragmatic and reasonable stance, based upon the weight of evidence for the association between oral biofilm and gingival inflammation, is that the regular and thorough removal of the biofilm using a range of oral hygiene aids remains the mantra for all.

KEY POINT 1

Adequate daily plaque control is key to the prevention and/or stabilisation of periodontal diseases, and this is the responsibility of the patient.

Patients' Health Beliefs

The Health Belief Model (HBM), developed in the 1950s by a group of American Public Health Service psychologists, focuses on compliance and the relationship between patients' beliefs and their behaviour. The HBM, modified later by Rogers (1998), also considers social and economic factors. However, like all models, it has its shortfalls, as human behaviour is not always rational!

The practical use of this model can take different formats and utilise some or all of the principles of: perceived susceptibility, perceived severity, motivation to change, perceived barriers and perceived benefits, which are summarised in Table 4.1.1.

Motivating Patients to Clean Optimally

A biofilm of dental plaque will build on a clean tooth surface within 24 hours and causes gingivitis in 48 hours (Löe et al. 1965). Some of the early clinical signs of gingival inflammation (redness of the gingival margin, swelling and spontaneous bleeding) rarely manifest in chronic gingivitis, leading to underestimation of disease levels by both patients and practitioners (Lang et al. 2009). The lack of pain and associated bleeding serve to relegate the importance of

TABLE 4.1.1   Principles of the Health Belief Model

Perceived susceptibility	In practice, advising the patient that they have a largely incurable chronic disease (in a sensitive manner) gains their attention. Then, by informing them of the prevalence of periodontal disease within the population, they can begin to see that they are different to the majority
Perceived severity	Using the radiographs, periodontal charting and bleeding indices can show the patient the extent of the disease affecting them
Motivation to change	Encouraging the patient to respond positively to their oral health needs can be tackled by directly relating their own disease levels to the likely outcomes using a variety of risk assessment tools
Perceived barriers	Establishing that the exceptionally high level of plaque control required is far more than for the "average patient" helps the patient understand the level of commitment required by them
Perceived benefits	Reduction in discomfort, tooth mobility and tooth loss as well as the potential benefits to overall health are all realistic outcomes of successful treatment

oral hygiene in our day-to-day lives despite the generally accepted understanding that twice daily toothbrushing with fluoridated toothpaste is the best way to reduce the risk of both caries and periodontal diseases. The words of MacKintosh still have relevance today: "Everybody says that prevention is better than cure and hardly anyone acts as if they believed it" (MacKintosh 1953).

Given the prevalence and nature of periodontal diseases, instruction in self-performed, mechanical plaque removal has been the bedrock of oral disease prevention for the past century; maintaining a good level of oral hygiene is the key to sound oral health and prevention of periodontal diseases for the majority of patients. Ensuring patient adherence with oral hygiene advice, to reduce the risk of oral disease and maintain oral health, is a difficult and demanding goal for the dental profession. Indeed, one of the most debated issues in public health is that of the effectiveness of health education. Although there is evidence that oral health education/promotion can be effective in bringing about change in patients' knowledge and in improving patients' oral health, there is good evidence that bespoke or tailored oral hygiene advice appears to be the most effective means of delivery of oral hygiene advice, particularly for long-term adherence and patients with chronic periodontitis (Schou 1998).

Research indicates a number of factors that influence adherence with oral hygiene advice. They include:

- Patients who present with good levels of oral hygiene are more likely to comply with advice than patients who present with poor oral hygiene at the start of treatment (Borkowska et al. 1998)
- Socio-economic status is consistently related to oral hygiene levels and other health-related behaviours (Schou 1998)
- Patients who believe that they have some personal control over their health which may influence outcome are the most likely to comply with advice (Kyak et al. 1998)
- Non-life-threatening chronic conditions tend to inspire less compliance with health advice than life-threatening illness (Wilson 1987).

Tailoring Oral Health Advice

Oral hygiene advice should:
- Take into account the individual's personal needs and background factors
- Involve the patient in the instructional process, for example with the use of digital or printed self-instruction materials
- Be followed up by a bespoke maintenance programme.

Studies indicate that individually tailored oral health educational advice can be extremely effective in improving long-term adherence to oral hygiene in periodontal treatment. One such study (Jonsson et al. 2009), which was a randomised evaluator-blinded, controlled trial, used two different active treatments with 113 adult subjects allocated to an experimental or a control group. The individually tailored oral health educational programme was based on cognitive behavioural principles and the adaptation for each of the participants was based on their thoughts, medium- and long-term goals and oral health status. The effect of the programme on gingival index (GI), plaque indices (PlI), self-reporting, and the participants' own global rating of treatment was evaluated 3 and 12 months after oral health education and non-surgical treatment. Between baseline and the 12-month follow up, those in the experimental group improved both GI and PlI more than in the control group, reported higher frequency of daily interdental cleaning and were more certain that they could maintain the attained level of behavioural change. The largest difference was seen at interproximal surfaces (Jonsson et al. 2009).

Techniques for Oral Hygiene

Self-Assessment of Home Plaque Control

Ensuring that a patient can assess the effectiveness of their own home care is critical in helping the patient to understand that they are able to take responsibility for their long-term oral hygiene. The use of disclosing agents to check brushing techniques and identify problem areas or by monitoring visible gingival inflammation can be effective tools for empowerment. Explanation of the role of inflammation and bleeding as disease indicators can aid compliance by challenging the patient to reduce or eliminate them. The choice of "empowerment tool" or aid to understanding is a matter of individual choice and tailored to the patient's level of understanding and often the stage in their treatment. Disclosing the biofilm is a simple and effective way of establishing "missed areas" at the start of treatment – linking the presence of bleeding to the role of inflammation in the disease process may have more impact and acceptance during the maintenance phase of treatment. Patients often believe that they are getting bleeding from "brushing too hard", which often results in patients brushing less. Taking the time and effort to explain the disease process and what to do about it on a one-to-one basis is essential whichever empowerment tool is used. Educational literature can be a useful endorsement of the advice given but should not take the place of a detailed verbal explanation (see Figure 4.3.6).

Delivery of Oral Hygiene Advice

Effective delivery of healthcare messages requires two core competencies: technical and specialist skills, as well as knowledge and the ability to communicate and educate. The use of commercially available tools and visual aids, such as anatomical models and diagrams, can aid patient understanding of the complex concepts such as demonstrating cleaning techniques for furcation sites. Just as simple and effective is the use of your hands and the patient's sleeve to explain the more difficult concepts of subgingival cleaning for example (Figure 4.1.1). Educational psychologists from the Michigan State University and the University of Iowa who studied the use of

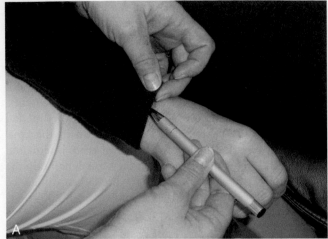

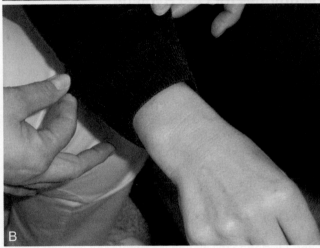

• **Figure 4.1.1** (A) Using the patient's sleeve to demonstrate a periodontal pocket; (B) using the same model to demonstrate gingival recession.

gesturing in teaching complex mathematical theory concluded that gestures clarify or provide conceptual information that is not readily apparent in the accompanying speech (Cook et al. 2013). The use of readily available props such as your hands also has the benefit of being completely free (Figure 4.1.1).

Establishing a mutual cooperation and responsibility between the patient and the clinician for the management of periodontal diseases is critical to a successful clinical outcome. The patience and time required to establish this for both parties should not be underestimated.

The "when", "with what" and "how" part of the advice is more effectively received if tailored to the individual patient. No single method, cleaning tool or cleaning programme for biofilm control suits all.

KEY POINT 2

"When": Oral hygiene measures can be undertaken at any time of the day and should fit in with the patient's daily routine. It is the time spent cleaning and thoroughness rather than frequency of technique that is the most important factor (Honkala et al. 1986).

KEY POINT 3

"With what": While evidence for efficacy of specific oral hygiene aids must be considered, often what the patient prefers to use and is therefore more likely to use is the more effective option. Adaptation of tools and cleaning techniques can be achieved with time and effort.

KEY POINT 4

"How": The actual techniques used to accomplish biofilm control will vary according to the specific needs of the patient and can depend upon, for example: manual dexterity, gingival architecture, physical access to the oral cavity, depth of pockets, size of the tongue, frenal attachments.

The timing of the clinical intervention should be tailored to the individual and clinical need; patients are more likely to appreciate the importance of their own home care if they see the positive results of reduction in inflammation, discomfort and pocket depths without any initial clinical intervention.

KEY POINT 5

Patient-focused interventions that encourage self-management of the patient's own oral health are key to positive clinical outcomes.

Toothbrushing

This may be manual or powered and should take into account the patients' abilities, preference and needs.

Manual

The plethora of manual toothbrushes now available can serve to confound selection by their very number and diversity in terms of design, size, shape and filament type, length and density. Studies have failed to establish clinical superiority for almost every characteristic examined (Frandsen 1985).

Most modern manual toothbrushes use a nylon filament type. Nylon, as a polymer with good chemical resistance, hard wearing and has antistatic properties (more hygienic), is the filament type that predominates the toothbrush market in the developed world. The filaments of a toothbrush are usually arranged in roughly 40 tufts in three or four rows.

The filament texture of choice should be soft, as the filament diameter should be able to penetrate the gingival sulcus unlike the larger filament diameters of the hard filament brushes. The harder filaments can traumatise the soft tissues and can contribute to tooth surface loss by abrasion. Soft filaments should be recommended to all patients because they minimise soft tissue trauma and toothbrush abrasion while maximising biofilm removal, particularly around the gingival margins and in the gingival crevice. A toothbrush with a small-to-medium head with soft, round-ended nylon filaments is recommended.

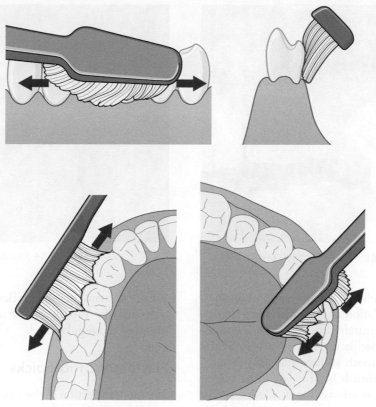

• **Figure 4.1.2** Modified Bass technique.

Features of a recommended toothbrush:
- Small head: small enough to be used effectively everywhere in the mouth to ensure full quadrant coverage
- Ergonomic handle: providing a comfortable stable grip for manoeuvring
- Nylon round-ended soft-to-medium filament.

Brushing Technique

Many brushing techniques have been advised over the years, but the basic requirements of an effective toothbrushing technique are few:

The technique should:
- Clean all accessible surfaces
- Be atraumatic to both hard and soft tissues
- Be simple and easy to learn and perform
- Be methodical in its application to ensure full mouth cleaning.

One of the most frequently recommended methods is the modified Bass (mini-scrub) (Figure 4.1.2). This technique aims to clean the gingival crevice, and so the brush head is held at 45 degrees to the axes of the teeth, with the end of the filaments pointing into the gingival crevice. Gentle pressure is applied towards the gingiva and then the brush is moved in small backwards and forwards movements, so the filaments are forced gently into the crevice and embrasure sites.

Working with the patient to determine the actual pattern of cleaning in terms of covering all the quadrants and all the accessible surfaces is key to this and any other technique employed. Time spent on establishing an effective brushing technique with the patient will have a positive impact on clinical outcome and should be established before any treatment intervention. Empowering the patient to reduce inflammation with an effective oral hygiene regimen can have a lasting impact on their motivation to improve their oral health. Moreover, the resolution of gingival inflammation as a result of effective home care will reduce the discomfort of any future clinical intervention – a motivator in itself.

Powered Brushes

Now well accepted as part of home care, electronic toothbrushes have become a mainstay in oral hygiene support programmes. Systematic reviews of studies of powered toothbrushing using oscillating-rotating heads, compared with manual toothbrushing in patients undergoing the initial phase of periodontal therapy, have found that subjects using a power toothbrush during initial treatment had reduced supragingival plaque to lower levels and showed statistically less bleeding on probing than subjects using a manual toothbrush (Robinson et al. 2003). Timing mechanisms alerting the user to the recommended 2-minute brushing duration are also a feature of some powered brushes and serve to reinforce the 2-minute brushing time that studies have indicated is required for optimal biofilm control.

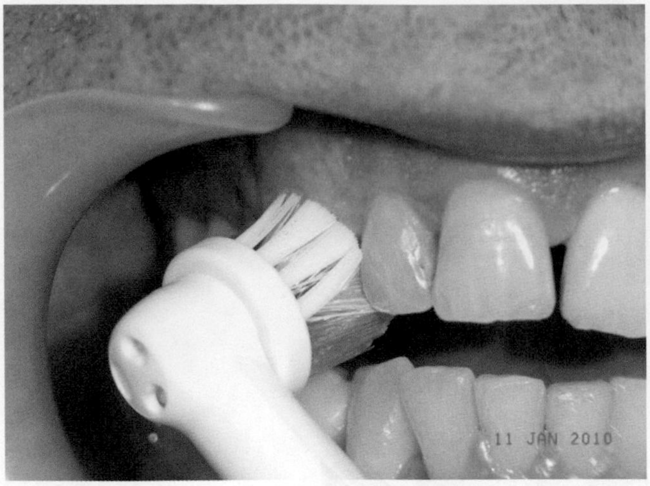

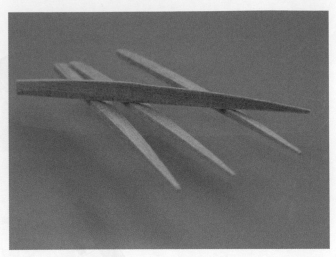

• **Figure 4.1.3** Use of a powered (counter-rotational) brush.

• **Figure 4.1.4** Interdental woodsticks.

Patients need to be taught to use power toothbrushes, as the placement and angulation of the brush head is critical to effectiveness and is entirely different from a manual brushing technique – the oscillating filaments provide the biofilm disruption on the tooth surface and into the gingival crevice, but the toothbrush head needs to be angled and positioned correctly to maximise the oscillating action (Figure 4.1.3).

Interdental Cleaning

Although toothbrushing is regarded as the most important oral hygiene measure, the regular use of interdental cleaning aids is important for all adult patients but particularly for patients with periodontitis. For effective and atraumatic interdental cleaning to be achieved, time and care should be devoted to helping patients select the best product to fit the interdental site and the correct technique for its use (Slot et al. 2020). Because the interdental area is the site of greatest plaque retention, gingival inflammation usually starts in the interdental papilla and spreads around the gingival margin. Interdental cleaning is therefore an essential part of home-care regimens for all, but especially for patients with periodontitis. Research has shown that periodontal pathogens can re-establish within 4 to 8 weeks in the numbers observed before professional debridement (Sbordone et al. 1990), and therefore maintenance of regular self-performed biofilm disruption is crucial to a successful clinical outcome.

Given that periodontitis and gingivitis lesions are predominantly interdental and that the interdental sites are most frequently coated in plaque (Hugoson et al. 1986), regular, thorough interdental cleaning is essential for prevention of disease.

Of the products specially designed for interdental cleaning, toothpicks have been available for the longest time (Kashani 1998). A wide range of toothpick products, both wooden and plastic, are currently available on the market (Figure 4.1.4). Toothpicks can only be used where there is

sufficient interdental space. Bergenholtz et al. (1974) demonstrated the superiority of triangular wood points over round or rectangular ones.

Elastomeric Toothpicks

The modern version of the wooden toothpick is made from a plastic core and often covered with a silicon or rubber cleaning surface. Usually conical in shape, these devices are available in a size range of small, medium and large; they do not require specific sizing for individual patients or sites. They offer an effective option for supragingival plaque control for patients that are new to interdental cleaning.

Floss

In the UK, dental floss was first recommended for interdental cleaning at the end of the 1960s (Drum 1968). For patients with gingivitis, flossing is recognised as an effective method for removing approximal plaque, with studies reporting daily use of floss resulting in reduction of plaque scores and gingivitis (Cronin & Dembling 1996). Flossing is not supported as an effective method for interdental cleaning for patients with diagnosed periodontal diseases undergoing supportive care (Slot et al. 2020).

Dental floss can be waxed or unwaxed, thread-like or tape, and impregnated with flavouring or antibacterial and/ or anti-caries products. Little evidence supports the superior efficacy of any specific type of floss (Lamberts et al. 1982) – most of the evidence for the effectiveness of floss lies with the benefits of supragingival biofilm disruption in patients that have not been diagnosed with periodontal diseases.

Implant floss is a specific type of floss that has a stiff threading end and includes a thicker/often spongey textured section to clean under prostheses. This is often the only option that allows patients to clean around implant abutments.

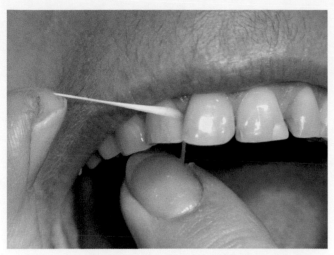

• **Figure 4.1.5** Flossing technique.

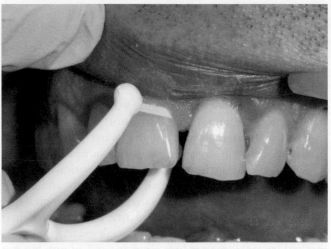

• **Figure 4.1.7** Use of a floss holder.

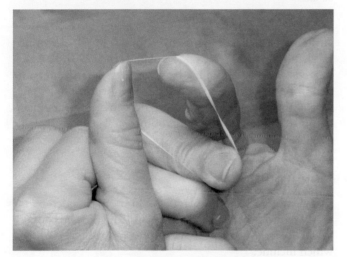

• **Figure 4.1.6** Use of a floss loop.

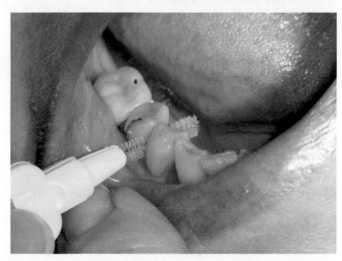

• **Figure 4.1.8** An interdental brush.

Flossing Techniques

To be effective, the floss needs to be adapted to the tooth surface by gently wrapping the floss around the tooth once past the contact site.

The anchorage method of wrapping the floss around the fingers to prevent slipping is useful for some (Figure 4.1.5), but the method of tying the floss in a circle and using the floss between thumb and forefinger on a continuous loop is a little easier (Figure 4.1.6). That said, flossing does not suit all patients as the dexterity required is sometimes beyond the capability or certainly the patience of many.

Devices to make flossing a little easier do exist and vary in design and complexity, some of which allow the floss to be used in the recommended way (Figure 4.1.7). Well-designed floss holders can make flossing easier and therefore more likely to be carried out regularly.

KEY POINT 6

It is important to emphasise to patients that all interdental aids, such as interdental brushes, floss and single-tufted brushes, can be highly effective but are best used following professional advice.

Interdental Brushes

The growth in the popularity of interdental brushes is largely attributed to ease of use and effectiveness (Figure 4.1.8). If a patient can use a pen, then they can usually manage to use an interdental brush effectively. Biofilm disruption in the interdental area can be simply achieved using an interdental brush, with studies reporting the superiority of biofilm removal over that of floss and interdental sticks (Waerhaug 1976, Christou et al. 1998, Worthington et al. 2019).

Available in an ever-increasing number of ISO standard sizes 0–8, it is important for the clinician to ensure that the correct size of brush for the site is used. The maximum biofilm disruption is achieved if the filaments of the brush fit the interdental space fully. Studies have shown that the regular use of interdental brushes can keep the proximal surfaces and some subgingival surfaces free from biofilm to a depth of 2.5 mm below the gum margin (Waerhaug 1976). Adapting the wire core of the brushes by bending allows the brushes to be used comfortably without catching the soft tissue on the opposing side of the interdental space. Interdental cleaning should be carried out once a day before toothbrushing. For patients undergoing supportive periodontal care interdental brushes are recommended alongside toothbrushing wherever anatomically possible.

Oral Irrigators

Oral irrigators or water flossers use water under pressure to flush the interdental sites. Oral irrigators were first designed to be used supragingivally, applying water pressure to displace and remove plaque, relying on pressure to irrigate subgingival regions (Goyal 2012). Since then, various tips have been designed that may be used subgingivally and several manufacturers provide products that enable subgingival use. Whilst these have gained in popularity, consensus for their clinical efficacy is sparce, with only weak evidence suggesting oral irrigators may reduce gingivitis at 1 month but not at 3 or 6 months (Worthington et al. 2019).

Subgingival Cleaning

In deeper periodontal lesions, improved plaque control alone can have very little effect on the gingival condition, pocket depth or the subgingival flora (Corbett & Davies 1993), and so for these patients, tailored oral hygiene education and methods are often delivered in conjunction with professional subgingival debridement.

In addition to interdental cleaning, the introduction of single-tufted brushes to clean subgingivally can significantly enhance clinical outcome (Kinane 1998) (Figure 4.1.9).

> ### KEY POINT 7
> Periodontitis is predominantly an interdental lesion.
> Toothbrushing alone cannot adequately disrupt the biofilm in the interdental spaces, making the use of an interdental aid an essential part of home care.

Adjunctive Antiseptic Agents

Toothpastes and mouth rinses are widely accepted by patients as part of their daily oral hygiene routine. There are also several other chemical plaque control formulations that have been marketed in recent years, although none have been shown to offer any significant benefit over the established toothpastes and mouth rinses.

Dentifrices (Toothpastes)

Dentifrice was originally used to promote better oral hygiene by chemical cleaning of the teeth. With advances in product formulation, it has become a valuable vehicle for delivering a variety of both health and cosmetic benefits. The widespread use of dentifrice has played a significant role in the practice of good oral hygiene and promotion of good oral health (Balg & He 2005). Dentifrices have evolved to provide a vehicle for delivering potential cosmetic, hygienic and therapeutic effects to the teeth and oral mucosa (Stamm 2007). These therapeutic agents, with anti-plaque and

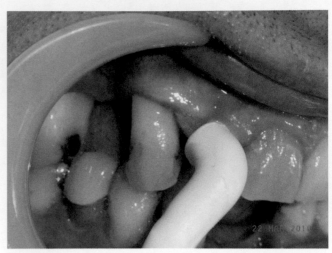

• **Figure 4.1.9** A single-tufted brush being used for subgingival plaque control.

anti-gingivitis effects, are useful adjuncts to self-performed mechanical plaque removal (Stephen et al. 1990). Research suggests that the combined use of a triclosan/copolymer dentifrice may be effective in reducing or controlling gingivitis in those areas demonstrating the most gingival inflammation. Typical ingredients of toothpastes are listed in Table 4.1.2.

Mouth Rinses

The chemical control of plaque biofilm can be aided by the use of mouth rinses. Mouth rinses were first mass-produced in the late 1800s and are used for a number of purposes, which include:

- To clear the mouth of food debris
- As a carrier of antibacterial agents
- As a carrier of anti-caries agents
- To reduce the activity of odour-producing organisms.

The simplest and possibly the most frequently used mouth rinse is a warm, dilute saline solution recommended for postsurgical care. However, the commercial availability of a plethora of mouth rinses attests to public demand for a perceived easy option for home care. Excluding professionally recommended mouthwashes, clinicians need to make it clear that mouthwashes should only be used as an adjunct to mechanical removal of the biofilm. Many combinations of formulations exist to achieve the objectives and are listed in Table 4.1.3.

Chlorhexidine

Of the agents listed in Table 4.1.3, chlorhexidine gluconate is by far the most effective agent against the oral biofilm. It is a bis-biguanide which has an immediate bactericidal action and a prolonged bacteriostatic action due to adsorbtion. Adsorbtion occurs because the chlorhexidine molecule is strongly positively charged (cationic) and binds to negatively charged (anionic) surfaces such as bacterial cell

TABLE 4.1.2   Typical ingredients in toothpastes and their actions

Excipient	Use	Note
Sodium fluoride Stannous fluoride Xylitol	Anti-caries	
Triclosan Zinc chloride Sodium hexametaphosphate	Anti-plaque	
Tetrapotassium pyrophosphate Sodium hexametaphosphate	Anti-calculus	
Hydrogen peroxide Sodium hexametaphosphate	Whitening agent	
Lichen Silica Carbonates & phosphates	Anti-adhesive/abrasive	
Carrageenan, xanthan gum	Thickening agents	
Strontium chloride Arginine Potassium nitrate/citrate Novamin	Dentine hypersensitivity	All work on the hydrodynamic theory of dentine hypersensitivity and seek to occlude, calcify or place a protective seal over the dentinal tubules
Sodium lauryl sulphate	Surfactant/frothing agent	Should be avoided by patients with recurrent aphthous ulceration as this surfactant can irritate the mucosa
Sodium benzoate, methyl paraben, and ethyl paraben	Preservative	All have been linked with mucosal irritation

walls, the oral mucosa and tooth surface. Chlorhexidine can disrupt bacterial cell walls within 20 seconds and then enter the cell itself to attack the cytoplasmic membrane and cause cell death. When chlorhexidine adsorbs to teeth and the periodontal tissues, it prevents microorganisms from attaching and inhibits the development of biofilm. It remains active on oral surfaces for 12 hours or more (Briner et al. 1986) and has been shown to be highly effective in reducing biofilm accumulation and gingivitis (Jenkins et al. 1993).

Chlorhexidine gluconate is produced in a variety of forms. It is most effective as a mouth rinse containing 0.20% or 0.12% chlorhexidine. One of the advantages of the mouth rinse is that it reaches areas of the mouth (interdental sites and gingival crevices) which are more likely to be missed when toothbrushing. Table 4.1.3 sets out further uses of chlorhexidine gluconate and its disadvantages. It can also be used in a gel and as chlorhexidine-impregnated chips, which are small enough to be placed in periodontal pockets where the chlorhexidine leaches out (see Chapter 5.3).

In the UK, the Medicines and Healthcare Products Regulatory Agency (MHRA) has issued a patient safety alert on the risk of anaphylactic reactions from the use of medical devices and medicinal products containing chlorhexidine. Such an occurrence is extremely rare but, nevertheless, care should be taken before prescribing chlorhexidine to ensure that the patient's medical history is reviewed and an enquiry made about possible sensitivity to chlorhexidine.

KEY POINT 8

Chemical agents can be a useful adjunct to, but are not a replacement for, mechanical biofilm control.

Conclusions

Successful treatment of periodontal diseases requires the active involvement of the patient at the outset of treatment. A collaborative approach to treatment planning and long-term supportive care fosters ownership and empowerment in the patient. The "when", "what with" and "how" aspects of self-performed biofilm control should be patient-led and professionally supported. The individual patient's oral hygiene regimen should be monitored, modified and developed by both patient and dental professional in what has to be a mutually responsible partnership if successful clinical outcomes are to be achieved.

Multiple choice questions on the contents of this chapter are available online at Elsevier eBooks+.

TABLE 4.1.3 Common mouthwash ingredients

Excipient	Mode of action	Indications for use	Notes/disadvantages
0.12 or 0.2% Chlorhexidine gluconate	Antibacterial Cationic	Plaque inhibition; gingivitis; maintenance of oral hygiene; post-periodontal surgery or treatment; aphthous ulceration; oral Candida	Superficial discoloration of tongue, teeth and tooth-coloured restorations, usually reversible; transient taste disturbances and burning sensation of tongue on initial use Less common: oral desquamation; parotid swelling; skin reactions Extremely rare: generalised allergic reactions, hypersensitivity and anaphylaxis
Triclosan	Antibacterial Non-ionic	Plaque inhibition; gingivitis; maintenance of oral hygiene	Has had some negative reports regarding its carcinogenic potential in the presence of chlorine and heat. Although there is some evidence of hormone regulation in animals and potential damage to the immune system, the benefits for the inclusion in oral hygiene products may well outweigh the potential risk
Cetylpyridinium chloride (CPC)	Antibacterial Cationic quaternary ammonium	Plaque inhibition; gingivitis	Can cause superficial staining
Phenolic compounds	Antibacterial	Gingivitis when used in conjunction with toothbrushing	
Hydrogen peroxide	Antibacterial Oxygenating agent	Gingivitis; aphthous ulceration; pericoronitis	
Zinc gluconates	Antibacterial Inhibits volatile sulphur compound production	Halitosis	
Fluorides	Anti-caries	High caries risk used in conjunction with toothbrushing	Not suitable for under age 7 – ingestion risk for children not able to spit out
Alcohol	Enhance antibacterial activity, stabiliser for active ingredients, e.g. essential oils		Suggested links with mouth cancer due to drying/chelating effects of mucosa has led to an increased number of alcohol-free products
Humectants	Prevent drying out		
Surfactant	To keep ingredients in solution		
Flavourings	Enhance taste		
Colouring agents	Point of difference for sales		
Water	Vehicle for delivery		
Preservatives			

References

Balg A, He T. A novel dentifrice technology for advanced oral health protection. A review of technical and clinical data. *Compend Contin Educ Dent.* 2005;26:4–11.

Bergenholtz A, Bjorne A, Vikström B. The plaque removing ability of some common interdental aids. An intra-individual study. *J Clin Periodontol.* 1974;1:160–165.

Borkowska ED, Watts TLP, Weinman J. The relationship of health beliefs and psychological mood to patient adherence to oral hygiene behaviour. *J Clin Periodontol.* 1998;25:187–193.

Briner WW, Grossman E, Buckner RY, Rebitski GF, Sox TE, Setser RE, et al. Effect of chlorhexidine gluconate mouthrinse on plaque bacteria. *J Periodontal Res.* 1986;21(S16):44–52.

Christou V, Timmerman MF, Van der Velden U, Van der Weijden FA. Comparison of different approaches of interdental hygiene: interdental brushes versus dental floss. *J Periodontal.* 1998;69(7):759–764.

Cook SW, Ryan G, Fenn KM. Consolidation and transfer of learning after observing hand gestures. *Child Dev.* 2013;84:1863–1871.

Corbet EF, Davies WRI. The role of supragingival plaque in the control of progressive periodontal disease. A review. *J Clin Periodontol.* 1993;20:307–313.

Cronin M, Dembling W. An investigation of the efficacy and safety of a new electric interdental plaque remover for the reduction of interproximal plaque and gingivitis. *J Clin Dent.* 1996;7:74–77.

Drum Von W. Brushing and flossing. Patient instruction in toothbrushing. *Quintessence.* 1968;19:91.

Frandsen A. Mechanical oral hygiene practices. In: Loe H, Klienman DV, eds. *Dental Plaque Control Measures and Oral Hygiene Practices.* Oxford: IRL Press; 1985:93–116.

Goyal, C.R., Lyle D.M., Qaqish J.G., Schuller, R. Evaluation of the plaque removal efficacy of a water flosser compared to string floss in adults after a single use. *J. Clin. Dent.* 2013;24(2):37–42.

Honkala E, Nyyssonen V, Knuuttila M, Markkanen H. Effectiveness of children's habitual toothbrushing. *J Clin Periodontol.* 1986;13:81–85.

Hugoson A, Koch G. Oral health in 1000 individuals age 3–70 years in the community of Jönköping, Sweden. *Swed. Dent J.* 1986;3:69–87.

Hujoel PP, Cunha-Cruz J, Löeshe WJ, Robertson PB. Personal oral hygiene and chronic periodontitis: a systematic review. *Periodontol.* 2005;37:29–34. 2000.

Jenkins S, Addy M, Newcombe RJ. A dose-response study of triclosan mouthrinses on plaque growth. *J Clin Periodontol.* 1993;20:609–616.

Jonsson B, Ohrn K, Oscarson N, et al. The effectiveness of an individually tailored oral health education programme on oral hygiene behaviour in patients with periodontal disease: a blinded randomised-controlled clinical trial (one-year follow-up). *J Clin Periodontol.* 2009;36:1025–1034.

Goyal CR, Lyle DM, Qaqish JG, Schuller R. Evaluation of the plaque removal efficacy of a water flosser compared to string floss in adults after a single use. *J Clin Dent.* 2013;24(2):37–42.

Kashani H. Studies on fluoridated toothpicks. *Swed Dent J.* 1998;126:1–48.

Kinane DF. The role of interdental cleaning in effective plaque control: need for interdental cleaning in primary and secondary prevention. In: Lang NP, Attström R, Löe H, eds. *Proceedings of the European Workshop on Mechanical Plaque Control.* Berlin: Quintessenz; 1998:156–168.

Kyak HA, Persson RE, Persson RG. Influences on the perceptions of and responses to periodontal disease among older adults. *Periodontol.* 1998;16:34–43. 2000.

Lamberts DM, Winderlich RC, Caffese RG. The effect of waxed and un-waxed dental floss on gingival health. Part 1. Plaque removal and gingival response. *J Periodontol.* 1982;53:393–396.

Lang NP, Shatztle MA, Löe H. Gingivitis as a risk factor in periodontal disease. *J Clin Periodontol.* 2009;36(Suppl. 10):3–8.

Löe H, Theilade E, Jensen SB. Experimental gingivitis in man. *J Periodontol.* 1965;36:177–187.

MacKintosh JM. *Trends of Public Opinion About Public Health.* London: Oxford University Press; 1953:1901–1951.

Robinson P, Deacon SA, Deery C, et al. Manual versus powered toothbrushing for oral health. *Cochrane Database Syst Rev.* 2003. CD002281, updated in 2005.

Rogers R. Protection motivation and self-efficacy: a revised theory of fear appeals and attitude change. *J Exp Soc Psychol.* 1998;19:469–479.

Sbordonel L, Ramalglia L, Gulletta E, Iacanno V. Recolonisation of the sub gingival microflora after scaling and root planing in human periodontitis. *J Periodontol.* 1990;61:579–584.

Schou L. Behavioural aspects of dental plaque control: an oral health promotion perspective. In: Lang NP, Attström R, Löe H, eds. *Proceedings of the European Workshop on Mechanical Plaque Control.* Berlin: Quintessenz; 1998:297–299.

Slot DE, Valkenburg C, Van der Weijden FA. Mechanical plaque removal of periodontal maintenance patients – a systematic review and network meta-analysis. *J Clin Periodontol.* 2020;47(Suppl. 22):107–124.

Stamm JW. Multi-function toothpastes for better oral health: a behavioural perspective. *Int Dent J.* 2007;57:351–363.

Stephen KW, Saxton CA, Jones CL, et al. Control of gingivitis and calculus by a dentifrice containing zinc salt and triclosan. *J Periodontol.* 1990;61:674–679.

Waerhaug J. The interdental brush and its place in operative crown and bridge dentistry. *J Oral Rehabil.* 1976;3:107–113.

Wilson Jr TG. Compliance, A review of the literature with possible applications to periodontics. *J Periodontol.* 1987;58:706–714.

Worthington HV, MacDonald L, Pericic TP, Sambunjak D, Johnson TM, Imai P. Home use of interdental cleaning devices, in addition to toothbrushing, for preventing and controlling periodontal diseases and dental caries. *Cochrane Database of Systematic Reviews.* 2019;issue 4. Art. No.: CD012018. DOI: 10.1002/14651858. CD012018.pub2. Accessed 26 April 2022.

4.2

Clinical Imaging in Patient Assessment and Motivation

ULPEE DARBAR

CHAPTER OUTLINE

Introduction

Types of Imaging Systems

Factors to Consider

   1. Radiography
      Conventional Radiography
      Computerised Tomography

   2. Clinical Photography
   3. Videos
   4. Digital Scanning

Clinical Imaging to Enhance Adherence

OVERVIEW OF THE CHAPTER

Clinical imaging, which includes both photographic and radiographic techniques, can be used for diagnostic, educational and motivational purposes as well as patient involvement in making decisions about their treatment. Patient-centred decision-making is the cornerstone of managing patients with chronic diseases, including periodontal diseases, especially as behavioural change is understood to be essential in achieving successful outcomes when treating such conditions. This chapter provides the reader with an overview of the different types of imaging techniques that are available and how these can be used to help to assess periodontal conditions, to aid communication with the patient and to improve patient compliance and motivation, as well as driving patient-centred decision-making.

By the end of the chapter the reader should:

- Appreciate the various systems for recording different types of images
- Describe how clinical imaging can be used to improve patient understanding, motivation and adherence
- Understand the need for consent in relation to clinical imaging
- Explain how imaging can be used to drive patient-centred care.

The chapter covers the following topics:

- Types of imaging systems
- Applications of imaging in patient management and decision-making
- Improving patient adherence and engagement using clinical imaging
- Consent for clinical imaging.

Introduction

The successful management of periodontal diseases is largely dependent on patient involvement. The role that patients play in the management of their conditions is crucial to achieving a positive treatment outcome. This is particularly true for chronic periodontal diseases for which the bacterial biofilm is the key initiating factor. The role of the patient in the management of chronic periodontitis is well established (Sanz & Teughels 2008, Renz et al. 2007). Successful treatment outcomes, avoiding tooth loss, are only possible with the full involvement and cooperation of the patient. The use

of clinical imaging helps patients gain a better understanding of their condition and gives them the opportunity to initiate behaviour change, which is essential if treatment is to be successful.

KEY POINT 1

Successful periodontal treatment outcomes are dependent on patient involvement and acceptance of their role in disease management.

While a clinical assessment and discussion can enable patients to understand the disease process, it is well known that visual representation of a problem leads to improved compliance and understanding (Houts et al. 2006). The visualisation of a condition and the possible outcomes of treatment are often communicated to a patient more effectively and quickly using images rather than words, particularly when before and after images are shared. Clinical imaging can be used to explain the supporting structures of the teeth and gums, and this enables the clinician to discuss issues more effectively with the patient, thereby empowering a better understanding and encouraging improved adherence. This joint approach between patient and clinician enables more effective disease management by offering the patient the opportunity to lead the conversation about their disease. In terms of diagnosis it is important that clinical imaging systems are used in conjunction with the clinical assessment and should never be used in isolation to arrive at diagnoses (Figure 4.2.1). As the use of video-based clinics has increased, clinical imaging provides the opportunity to share information on a virtual platform. Clinical imaging systems have the following key benefits:

- add value to the clinical assessment made by the clinician
- enable sharing of information giving more clarity and reducing the risk of ambiguity
- underpin and strengthen the information collected as part of the history and clinical examination
- provide additional information about the condition to both the clinician and the patient, leading to improved understanding and treatment outcomes
- provide documented evidence of the condition, before, during and after treatment in the event of medico-legal challenge.

Imaging systems fall into two categories:
- invisible light imaging such as radiographic techniques
- visible light imaging which includes photographs and videos.

Both types of systems have been used extensively in medicine; radiography has been an essential diagnostic tool since its introduction in the early 20th century. Photography has also been widely used in dentistry both to monitor the progress of treatment and for educational purposes. The advent of digital technology in both photography and radiography has greatly broadened the scope of what can be achieved and how patients can be involved in decision-making. Most dental practices predominantly use digital technology as essential tools to aid with diagnosis, as adjuncts to history taking and physical examination and for patient engagement and communication. Clinical imaging thus allows clinicians to improve patient management in a variety of ways (Figure 4.2.2), such as:

- to aid clinical assessment
- to improve patient understanding by allowing visualisation of the disease
- to improve patient motivation and adherence
- to help monitor the treatment response
- to allow patients to see the progress and outcome of their treatment.

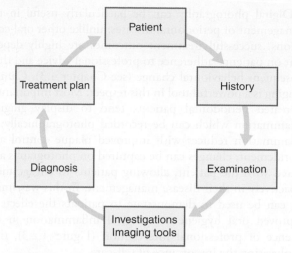

• **Figure 4.2.1** The place for imaging in patient management.

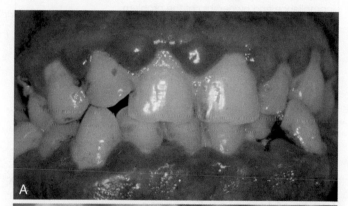

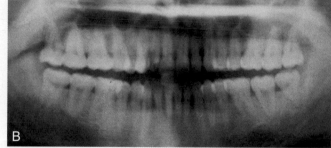

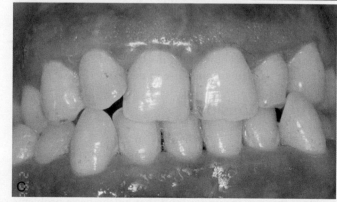

• **Figure 4.2.2** Images of a patient with initially poor plaque control, before and after treatment. (A) Clinical presentation; (B) radiographic presentation; (C) clinical response to improved oral hygiene and treatment.

Digital photography can be particularly useful in the management of periodontal diseases; unlike other oral conditions, successful treatment outcomes are highly dependent on patients' adherence to professional advice and their subsequent behavioural change (see Chapter 4.3). Clinical imaging is a powerful tool in this respect. Most importantly, untreated periodontal patients tend to display gingival inflammation which can be recorded photographically; as inflammation reduces with improved plaque control and debridement, changes can be captured on photographs and shared with the patient, allowing patients to engage more proactively in their disease management. In this way imaging can be used to demonstrate to patients the effects of improved oral hygiene on gingival inflammation in the absence of professional intervention (Figure 4.2.3), thus emphasising the importance of self-care.

KEY POINT 2

Early understanding of periodontal diseases improves patient compliance and ownership of the problem.

Several studies have reported on the strategic role patient compliance plays in the management of patients with chronic conditions such as periodontitis (Wilson 1987, Soolari 2002, Ng et al. 2011, Costa et al. 2012). While written information is valuable, imaging techniques improve patient engagement by providing the patient with a visual awareness of their problems both before and after treatment, thus providing a means of involving patients in their periodontal management (Figure 4.2.4).

Types of Imaging Systems

The imaging systems most often used as educational tools in dentistry are:
1. Radiography
2. Clinical photography
3. Videos
4. Digital Scanning

Other systems, such as ultrasound and magnetic resonance imaging, have more application in other branches of dentistry, such as oral and maxillofacial surgery and oral medicine, and are rarely indicated or used in general dentistry. Laser Doppler imagining (LDI) has been used as a tool for monitoring blood flow in gingival tissues in research studies but has only limited use in dentistry (Figure 4.2.5).

Factors to Consider

When clinical imaging is used as an educational tool, it is important to ensure that the appropriate imaging tools are used. Factors to consider include:
- What type of disease does this patient have?
- Does this patient understand that he/she has a problem?
- What do I want to do for this patient?
- What am I trying to explain to the patient?
- What do I want the patient to understand?

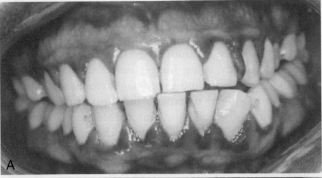

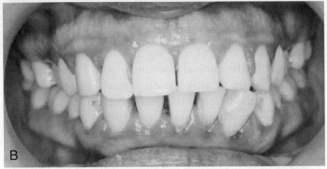

• **Figure 4.2.3** (A) Gingival inflammation in a patient with poor oral hygiene. (B) Reduction in the inflammation after oral hygiene improvement.

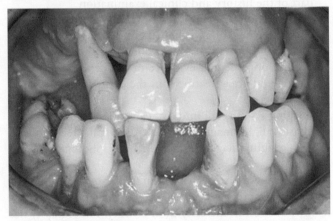

• **Figure 4.2.4** Patient with poor compliance. The image shows the severity of breakdown which can be shared with the patient during the explanation of the problem.

- What can I use to clarify the condition to the patient in the simplest way?
- How will I ensure that the patient has understood what I am trying to explain?

Radiographs, photographs and videos can be used alone or in combination to educate and inform the patient and sometimes together with written information (such as leaflets). This visual information can also be used in combination with periodontal charts, which record the bleeding scores and/or pocket depths, to enhance patients' understanding of their condition. With digital technology, images of possible treatment outcomes can be created to further enhance patient understanding and to improve patient ownership of their disease(s).

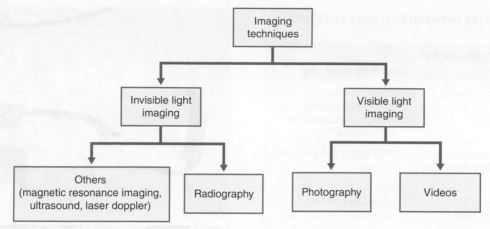

• **Figure 4.2.5** Types of imaging techniques.

1. Radiography

- Conventional radiographs (X-rays)
- Computerised tomography (CT scans).

Conventional Radiography

A. Analogue Radiographs

Conventional radiography aids diagnosis by displaying the underlying bone support for the teeth and, as previously mentioned, can also be used as a means of explaining disease processes to patients. In periodontology radiographic images are used to assess bone loss and, in conjunction with clinical data, to assess levels of disease and to aid diagnosis. The choice of radiographs to be taken will depend on the type of information needed; usually for periodontal assessment (when bone levels need to be determined), long cone periapical views are used. However, for patients with minimal bone loss, vertical bitewings can be an alternative, exposing the patient to less ionising radiation. Extra-oral views such as orthopantomogram (OPT) can be used for patients who cannot tolerate intra-oral films but, although such views provide an overview of the bone levels and are often useful as screening tools, the definition of the image can be inferior to the intra-oral view.

Radiography systems based on wet film processing are simple to use but they have the disadvantages of being slow and prone to operator errors during processing (Figure 4.2.6). The images produced (as films) also take up physical storage space.

B. Digital Radiographs

Modern radiography systems are based on digital technology and have largely superseded wet film processing. The main advantages of these are:

- No chemicals required
- Real-time applications
- Speed of image production
- Ease of storage
- Digital image enhancement and manipulation (brightness, contrast, etc.)

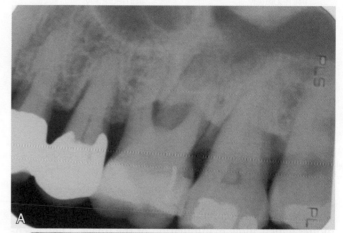

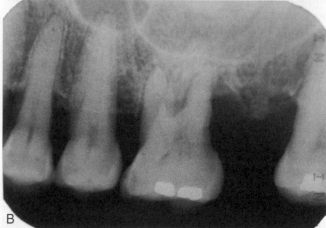

• **Figure 4.2.6** (A) Conventional wet film long cone periapical radiograph showing elongation of the image due to incorrect positioning of the film. (B) Image of a correctly positioned and processed film.

- Can be more easily shared with other clinicians and patients.

The main advantages and disadvantages of analogue and digital radiographs are shown in Table 4.2.1.

Digital radiographs are taken using a digital sensor which captures the image of the bone and the teeth instead of a film and, once captured, the image is digitally transferred.

TABLE 4.2.1	Differences between analogue and digital images	
Conventional radiography using wet films	**Digital radiography**	
More prone to processing errors	Because of image manipulation using sensors this aspect is eliminated	
Patients find these relatively easy to tolerate in their mouth	CMOS digital sensors can be bulky	
Physical handling of films necessary so can be cumbersome	Images can be shared with others easily	
Images are not available immediately	Images can be processed immediately	
Storage space needed	Physical storage space not needed	
Relatively low setup costs	Setup costs can be high depending on system selected	
Manipulation of images not possible	Digital manipulation of images (contrast, brightness, etc.)	
Limited training needs of staff	Training of staff needed	

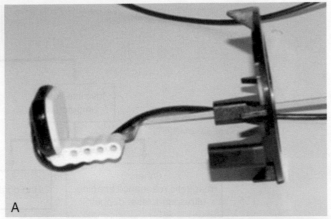

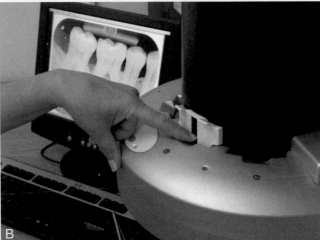

• **Figure 4.2.7** (A) CMOS sensor connected directly to the computer to produce the radiographic image. Note the size of the sensor. (B) PSP being processed in a digital scanner. Note the size of the film, which is similar to a wet film.

The image can be enhanced using digital processing techniques which allow manipulation of the image. Digital sensors may be direct or indirect types.

Direct sensors are solid state sensors which are either charged coupled devices (CCD) or complementary metal oxide semiconductors (CMOS) (Figure 4.2.7A). Both contain silicon crystals which covert photons to electrons, with the main difference being how the pixel conversion takes place. The CMOS devices convert at each pixel level, whereas with a CCD the pixel charges are transferred to a common output source. Both sensors tend to be thicker than indirect types and some have cable connections which result in a thicker sensor. With these systems the images generated digitally are transmitted directly from the detector to the computer.

Indirect sensors use photo-stimulated storage phosphor (PSP) plates as the sensors. These are extremely thin and are similar in size to conventional wet-processed intra-oral films. Once the plates have been exposed, they are processed in a digital scanner (see Figure 4.2.7B), producing a high-quality digital image (Figure 4.2.8). Patients tend to tolerate this type of sensor better because of the reduced bulk. The first-generation digital sensors performed suboptimally compared to conventional film. However, with improving detector technology, digital imaging is surpassing film in terms of contrast and resolution. Images generated using the PSP detect the X-rays and capture the image, which is then scanned into a PSP scanner that passes the image to the computer through a USB cable or network connection.

Computerised Tomography

Computerised tomography (CT) is an imaging technique that produces both two- and three-dimensional cross-sectional images of an object from a flat radiographic image. The internal structure of the object, such as the shape and severity of a bony defect, can be visualised to allow more precise and detailed assessment. However, because of the high radiation dose required, conventional CT has only limited use in periodontology. The implementation of the new volume-based cone beam CT scan (CBCT) (Figure 4.2.9) has enabled the radiation dosages to be reduced significantly, thus making this tool more valuable in the planning and assessment of complex bone defects. These images can be taken as sectional images exposing only the area in question, thus rendering their application to periodontology more appropriate (Figure 4.2.10). The images can be manipulated to show the bone and other structures in three dimensions, which aids both diagnosis and treatment planning. In the periodontally compromised patient, CBCT aids in the assessment of intra-bony defects and furcation involvements (Misch et al. 2006). The ability to manipulate such images and show patients bone defects around teeth and what could happen with treatment is useful in

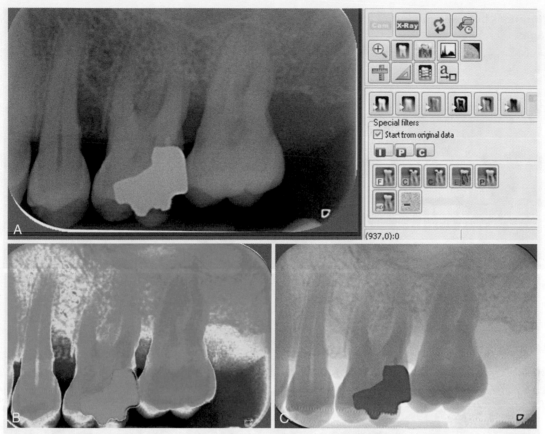

• **Figure 4.2.8** (A) Image produced using the PSP system. The ability to manipulate the images (B, C) enables the defects to be looked at with greater clarity and helps to explain disease to patients.

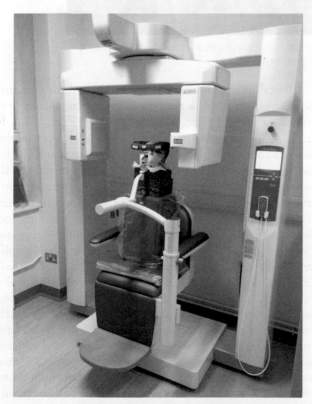

• **Figure 4.2.9** Cone beam CT scanner.

explaining the complex aetiology and treatment of such defects. It is important to remember that CBCT should only be used where the benefits of the investigation supplement the information already gathered. CBCT scans are also useful when discussing implant treatment plans with patients (see Chapter 7.3). The clinician should be aware of the guidelines on the use of CBCT published by the European commission in 2012. Because of the lack of a robust evidence base, the Faculty of General Dental Practitioners claim that "CBCT is not indicated as a routine method of imaging periodontal bone support" (2018).

2. Clinical Photography

Photographs enable the clinical manifestations of disease to be recorded at any point during the assessment and treatment of the disease. They are a vital tool for patient education, and a recent questionnaire-based study (Morse et al. 2010) showed that 84% of the respondents used photographs for treatment planning and 75% for patient instruction and motivation; 55.1% reported that they found photographs useful when giving patients instructions and improving their motivation and 56.2% reported their usefulness for medico-legal purposes. Prior to the use of clinical photographs, it was common for clinicians to draw

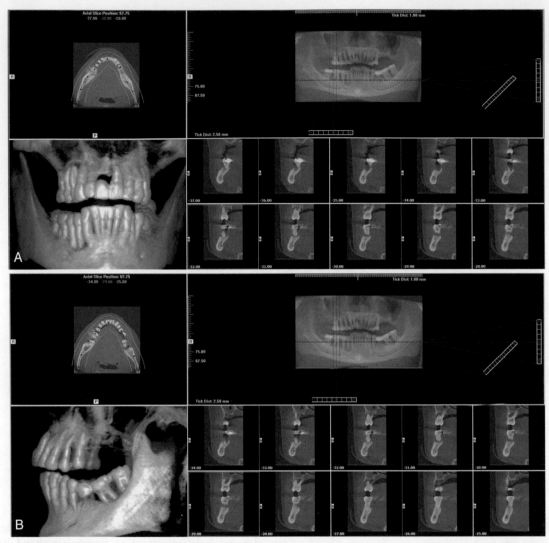

• **Figure 4.2.10** CBCT images showing the extent of information that can be seen from all angles. This information makes it easier for patients to understand their problems.

diagrams to explain to patients aspects of their condition which could not be explained verbally. Today, clinical photography has replaced this as a means of disease visualisation, using images of the patient's own condition. However, it is important to remember that:

- Photographs form part of the patient's clinical record
- The patient must have given their consent for the photographs to be taken. An example of a consent form is shown in Figure 4.2.11
- Consent should include a clear explanation of why the photographs are being taken, what they will be used for and where they will be stored
- If the photographs are to be used for publication, the patient must be informed about this, and a separate consent will be needed
- If the photographs are to be used for research, the patient must have consented to this as part of the process for enrolling into the research project
- If the patient is going to be identifiable in the photograph, they must be informed of this, and appropriate signed release of the photograph obtained.

Clinical photography is an invaluable tool for communicating information to patients and also for documentation of the clinical presentation of a patient's condition. It can assist in documenting the progressive changes in the patient's condition during a course of treatment and can be used to communicate to the patient changes in the condition, especially if there are issues with compliance and motivation. This visual involvement gives the patient the chance to directly observe what is happening in their mouth and allows the patient to become better aware of the progress (or otherwise) of their treatment. In the past, photographs were taken with films that had to be sent off to be processed, thus incurring an additional cost and inconvenience as the images could not be used immediately as part of the discussion. However, clinical photographs are currently taken with either a digital camera or an intra-oral camera and are immediately available and can be shown to the patient. A series of photographs will help convey messages where complexities of advanced treatments are often difficult to describe. Patients can thus get involved in making decisions about the management of the problems, thereby fostering

Consent/waiver for clinical photography

Patient name: .... Date of birth: ....

I consent that photographic images (including of x-rays, models and videos) of me
(or under 16 child of which I am parent or legal guardian) may be taken and used
in perpetuity for the following purpose(s) for which I understand that it may not be
possible for me to subsequently withdraw this consent:

Level 3 (open publication)

(a) Publication in a professional journal or textbook, and/or as part of a lecture,
display and/or information/marketing leaflet and:

(b) Publication on open access website (open access means making available and
communicating to anyone worldwide, including but not limited to clinical
professionals). The publication on open access websites may, but not necessarily,
form part of a course where users will download content onto any device for their
personal and non-commercial use.

Level 2 (Restricted educational use)

Clinical teaching and/or research, and shown only to appropriate clinical
staff and students and/or displayed for use by staff and students following
a course of study on a restricted access educational institutional website.

Level 1 (Confidential record only)

Storage as part of confidential patient dental records only.

Level of consent	Level 3	Level 2	Level 1
Please tick			

Image types	Images including face/eyes	Images except face/eyes
Please tick		

I confirm that I am over 16 years of age ....

I confirm that I am the parent/legal guardian of ....

(delete as applicable)

Signature: .... Date: ....

• **Figure 4.2.11** An example of a photographic consent form.

patient-centred decision-making. The use of clinical photographs along with the radiological images helps the clinician describe diagnosis and treatment with greater clarity. Generic photographs showing the disease at the beginning and after treatment are also useful tools in explaining treatment proposals and possible treatment outcomes (such as interdental recession).

There are several different camera systems that are available and the choice of which to use is largely clinician driven.

Intra-oral cameras are essentially small television cameras that can be connected to a hand-held device or a computer (Figure 4.2.12). Images are shown on the computer screen in "real time" but can also be captured and stored. These systems enable the information about the condition and the clinical findings to be shared with the patient as the assessment is taking place.

Digital camera systems can vary from simple compact digital cameras to more complex and expensive digital single lens reflex (DSLR) systems with macro lens and ring flash (Figure 4.2.13). Photographs taken with these systems also allow patient communication but only after the images have been uploaded to a computer.

The images taken, irrespective of the camera used, must be clear and relevant, with the focus being largely on the area of interest. The photographs should be standardised for accuracy and comparison and dated. Depending on

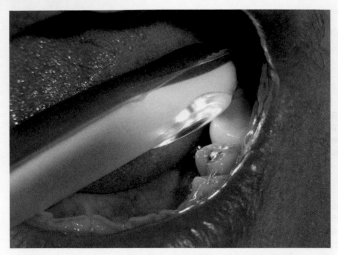

• **Figure 4.2.12** Intra-oral camera system. These devices are small and enable the patient to visualise their mouth as the examination is taking place.

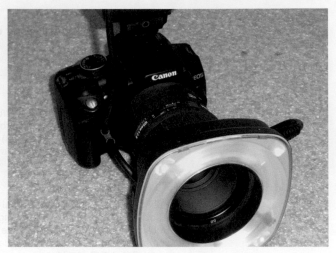

• **Figure 4.2.13** Digital SLR camera with a ring flash.

the sequence, the photographs can be used at the outset to communicate the issues with the patient and engage them in treatment decision-making. Photographs taken during treatment will help monitor how well the situation is improving and where there are ongoing challenges with motivation and compliance. Monitoring photographs can be used to highlight any issues with the patient, enabling the patient to better understand how and why the treatment may be compromised. For the photographs to be effective tools for patient education, they must be precise and clear and also demonstrate the clinical problems in question clearly. In addition to patient education, clinical photographs also have several other uses including:

- Monitoring the progression of disease
- Providing evidence to the patient of the need for certain treatments
- Before and after treatment effects
- Assessment of treatment outcomes
- Medico-legal purposes
- Communication with others, e.g. laboratory technicians, clinicians
- Enhancing patient referrals
- Long-term monitoring of oral status (useful in patients with suboptimal motivation and adherence)
- Providing evidence of treatment outcomes, especially in patients who have inconsistent oral hygiene.

The types of view will depend on the individual patient needs. The following views are standard views that should be taken at the start of treatment to form part of the clinical record (Figure 4.2.14):

- Smiling and at-rest view
- Intra-oral view with the teeth in occlusion
- Right and left buccal views
- Occlusal views of the upper and lower arches
- Any other views that are appropriate to the care of the patient and can include extra-oral views.

3. Videos

Videos may form part of the clinical photographic record and offer the patient a real-time presentation of the conditions in their mouth. Most digital camera equipment have a video-recording facility. Videos can be used to show patients treatment as it is being carried out, or they can be shown recordings of procedures that they may be considering. This can help the patient understand what is being proposed and also gives the patient the opportunity to ask questions about procedures. Videos may be used:

- To provide a realistic overview of what the patient may expect
- To provide a visual representation of a procedure that may otherwise be difficult to describe
- To give the patient an opportunity to ask questions about proposed procedures
- To demonstrate self-care such as oral hygiene.

Videos can also be a good resource to use if there are postoperative complications, as they help provide an easier means of giving an explanation and showing the patient why the complication has occurred.

4. Digital Scanning

As the digital era has evolved, different scanning systems enable direct images to be captured and manipulated to construct restorations. These systems can provide a means of explaining anticipated treatment outcomes to patients. Furthermore, study casts that have been taken using conventional impressions can also be scanned, converted into digital formats and used for discussion with patients. Depending on the software programmes, the images can be manipulated to show patients the end point of treatment, and if clinical photographs are also scanned, the side-by-side representation gives the patient a good opportunity of seeing the changes that can be achieved. Where the patient is expecting a change in the appearance or where tooth positions are to be modified, digital "wax-ups" have become a

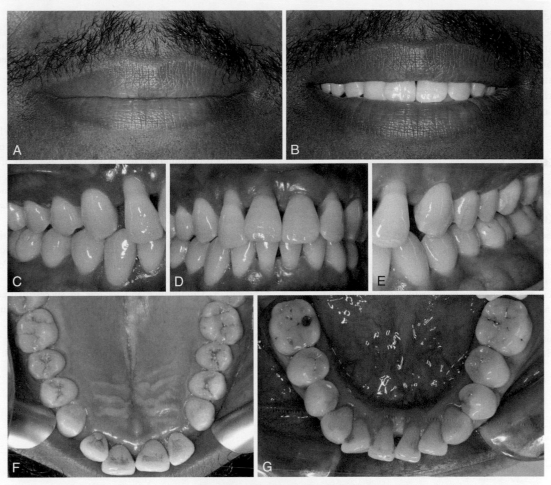

• **Figure 4.2.14** Standard clinical views.

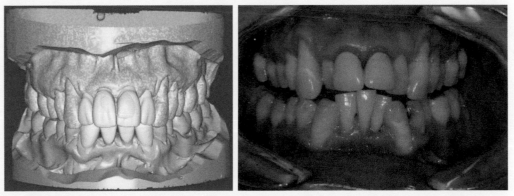

• **Figure 4.2.15** A digital "wax-up" of proposed treatment to upper and lower anterior teeth, with the pre-operative situation on the right.

powerful way of explaining to the patient the changes that can be achieved (see Figure 4.2.15).

Clinical Imaging to Enhance Adherence

Clinical images, such as pictures, photographs and videos, allow the clinician to convey information more effectively to patients about disease processes and treatment proposals. These tools are useful to help ensure that patients are fully engaged in the decision-making process about their own periodontal health and treatment planning. Patient adherence to professional advice is the cornerstone of long-term success in periodontal therapy, and images can be used to enhance this adherence, particularly when the patient can see that their efforts at home are having a positive effect on their oral condition. Before and after images can be invaluable in this respect (see Figure 4.2.3) and help patients appreciate the importance of home care. Untreated periodontal diseases often present as visible gingival inflammation, which can be imaged, and changes in inflammatory status can be recorded as treatment progresses. This can be shown to the patient and presents the clinician with a powerful motivational tool thus optimising patient compliance. Written information can be useful in this respect, but imaging has far more impact, particularly when the images are of the patient themselves.

Multiple choice questions on the contents of this chapter are available online at Elsevier eBooks+.

References

Costa FO, Cota LO, Lages EJ, Lima Oliveira AP, Cortelli SC, Cortelli JR, et al. Periodontal risk assessment model in a sample of regular and irregular compliers under maintenance therapy: a 3 year prospective study. *J Periodontol.* 2012;83:292–300.

European Commission. 2012. Radiation protection 172. Cone Beam CT for Dental and Maxillofacial Radiology: evidence-based guidelines; Luxembourg; European commission: 2012. Accessed from https://ec.europa.eu/energy/sites/ener/files/documents/172.

Faculty of General Dental Practitioners. *Selection Criteria for Dental Radiography 2018*; 2018. Recommendation 5.2.

Houts PS, Doak C, Matthew LG, Loscalzo A. The role of pictures in improving health communication: a review of research on attention, comprehension, recall and adherence. *Patient Educ Couns.* 2006;61:173–190.

Morse GA, Haque MS, Sharland MR, Burke FJT. The use of clinical photography by UK general dental practitioners. *Br Dent J.* 2010;208:E1.

Misch KA, Yi ES, Sarment DP. Accuracy of cone beam computerised tomography for periodontal defect measurements. *J Periodontol.* 2006;77:1261–1266.

Ng MC, Ong MM, Lim LP, Koh CG, Chan YH. Tooth loss in compliant and non-compliant periodontally treated patients: 7 years after active periodontal therapy. *J Clin Periodontol.* 2011;38:499–508.

Renz A, Ide M, Newton T, Robinson P, Smith D. Psychological interventions to improve adherence to oral hygiene instructions in adults with periodontal diseases. *Cochrane Database Syst Rev.* 2007;2:CD005097.

Sanz M, Teughels W. Innovations in non-surgical periodontal therapy: Consensus report of the 6th European Workshop on Periodontology. Group A of European Workshop on Periodontology. *J Clin Periodontol.* 2008;35(Suppl. 8):3–7.

Soolari A. Compliance and its role in successful treatment of an advanced periodontal case: review of the literature and a case report. *Quintessence Int (Berlin).* 2002;33:389–396.

Wilson TG. Compliance. A review of the literature with possible applications to periodontics. *J Periodontol.* 1987;58:706–714.

4.3

Patient Adherence

PHILIP OWER

CHAPTER OUTLINE

OVERVIEW OF THE CHAPTER

A high standard of biofilm control and self-care are essential for achieving and maintaining periodontal health. This chapter will describe the principles of improving patients' adherence to healthcare advice and highlight some of the difficulties that are often encountered when the clinician attempts to motivate patients to clean to a higher standard and to influence some of the lifestyle habits that may be contributing to their levels of periodontal breakdown. Strategies will be presented for overcoming these difficulties and practical advice will be given for improving patients' levels of biofilm and risk-factor control and assessing patients' response to this advice.

By the end of the chapter the reader should:

- Understand the need for a high level of adherence in periodontal patients
- Appreciate why patients can be resistant to healthcare advice
- Understand the principles of the stepwise approach to periodontal therapy
- Be able to provide plaque control and other advice more effectively

- Be able to motivate patients to improve their levels of self-care.

The chapter covers the following topics:

- Importance of adherence in periodontal care
- Improving adherence and affecting behaviour change
- Adherence to oral hygiene and other advice
- Assessing adherence in practice.

Importance of Adherence in Periodontal Care

Adherence to professional advice, often referred to as compliance, has become an increasingly important feature of many aspects of healthcare, as an increasing volume of research has shown that the behaviour of the individual can have a profound effect on a range of medical conditions. While a high standard of patient compliance is essential for successful periodontal therapy, absolute compliance is rare; one study (Umaki et al. 2012) showed that only 32% compliance was achieved on average. As far as terminology is concerned, the term "adherence" is preferable to "compliance" – the traditional term "compliance" denotes obedience, "following doctor's orders" – but the term "adherence"

infers a collaboration between clinician and patient, in which patients develop an understanding of their condition and the treatments required so that the patient has a collaborative involvement with the clinician and reaches "concordance" in consultations (Mullen 1997). Treatment failure is often the result of poor adherence to healthcare advice. One only has to think of heart disease and the effect of lifestyle and diet on this condition to realise the importance of patient behaviour in disease management. The same is equally true of periodontitis; there is abundant evidence that in periodontally susceptible individuals, a patient's periodontal condition is affected by their own behaviour, in particular the patient's ability to carry out daily oral hygiene to a high standard; the importance of the patient's oral hygiene in periodontitis management was shown in

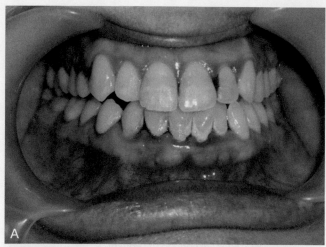

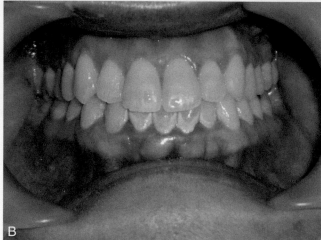

• **Figure 4.3.1** (A) A patient on presentation. (B) Patient after 1 month of oral hygiene alone with no professional intervention.

a randomised controlled trial by Preus et al. (2019). This study investigated the effect of a strict 3-month oral hygiene phase on plaque, bleeding on probing and pocket depth and found that these key periodontal parameters were reduced (by oral hygiene alone) to such an extent that therapy planning was affected. An example of how patient behaviour can have such profound effects is shown in Figure 4.3.1. In addition patient behaviour with respect to other risk factors in periodontal diseases (diet, obesity, exercise, smoking, stress and diabetic status) can also have profound effects on periodontal management.

> ### KEY POINT 1
> Treatment failure is often the result of poor adherence to healthcare advice.

It is appropriate to try to affect behavioural change in patients who have periodontitis to maximise the chances of treatment success. While advice to reduce lifestyle risk factors such as smoking, poor diet and lack of exercise are important, treatment of periodontitis is still based largely on reduction of the bacterial load through self-care, mainly in the form of effective oral hygiene. Some patients are more susceptible to periodontitis than others (see Chapter 1.4); the

more susceptible the patient the higher their level of biofilm disruption needs to be to control disease. Failure to maintain a sufficiently high standard of plaque control results in treatment failure in the long term (Axelsson & Lindhe 1981, Ramfjord et al. 1982, Listgarten et al. 1989, Sbordone et al. 1990, Rosen et al. 1999). It is therefore essential in periodontal management to adopt effective interventions to improve patients' adherence to oral hygiene advice (Wilson 1996). A consensus report of the 5th European Workshop in Periodontology (2005) concluded that removal of the bacterial biofilm by the patient and smoking cessation were the two most important subject-based measures to be established in the management of periodontitis (Ramseier 2005).

European Federation of Periodontology S3-Level Clinical Practice Guideline 2020

Following the introduction of the new classification system for periodontal and peri-implant diseases by the World Workshop in 2017 (see Chapter 2.1 for full details), the European Federation of Periodontology (EFP) published S3 clinical guidelines for the treatment of stages 1–3 periodontitis (Sanz et al. 2020), which was mapped to the new classification system. The EFP guideline combined assessment of 15 systematic reviews with a moderated consensus process of a group of representative stakeholders to arrive at a set of recommendations for the treatment of stages 1–3 periodontitis. The term S3 refers to the highest level (or step) of guideline development (see Table 4.3.1). When developing an S3 guideline the strength of consensus agreement is reported (see Table 4.3.2) and a formal "evidence-to-decision" process is followed to arrive at a clinical recommendation (see Table 4.3.3). Clinical recommendations (CRs) may be evidence based or consensus based or both (see Figures 4.3.3–4.3.5 for examples of CRs). For further details on the development of CRs the reader is referred to West et al. (2021) and Kebschull & Chapple (2020). The new EFP guideline thus established an evidence- and consensus-based *stepwise* approach to the management of periodontitis patients (Figure 4.3.2 and Appendix 3), central to which was patient adherence to advice on oral hygiene and risk-factor control. The British Society of Periodontology and Implant Dentistry (BSP) subsequently developed and published (West et al. 2021) a UK version of this guideline using a formal process known as the *Grade Adolopment* framework (readers are referred to Sanz et al. [2020] and West et al. [2021] for details of this process). The BSP UK Clinical Practice Guidelines for the Treatment of Periodontal Diseases, based on the EFP guidelines, can be found at Appendix 4.

Stepwise Approach to the Management of Stages 1–3 Periodontitis

The main principle of the stepwise approach to periodontal management (Figure 4.3.2) is that treatment is carried out in steps and that progression to the next step does not take

TABLE 4.3.1   Development of Clinical Guidelines

Level	Guideline description	Characteristics
S3	Evidence and consensus based	Systematic review, selection and analysis of evidence, grading of evidence and representative guideline group including stakeholders from other disciplines, moderated consensus process
S2e	Evidence based	Systematic review, selection and analysis of evidence, grading of evidence
S2c	Consensus based	Representative guideline group including stakeholders from other disciplines, moderated consensus process
S1	Recommendation of a panel of experts	Informal process to reach consensus

TABLE 4.3.2   Strength of Consensus

Strength of consensus	Necessary agreement (excluding abstentions due to potential conflicts of interest)
Unanimous consensus	Agreement of 100% of participants
Strong consensus	Agreement of >95% of participants
Consensus	Agreement of 75–95% of participants
Simple majority	Agreement of 50–74% of participants
No consensus	Agreement of <50% of participants

TABLE 4.3.3   Grades of Recommendation

Grade	Recommendation level	Wording
A	Strong	We recommend (↑) / we recommend not to (↓)
B	Recommendation	We suggest (↑) / we suggest not to (↓)
O	Open	May be considered (↔)

KEY POINT 2

Step 1 of the stepwise approach involves:
1. Supragingival biofilm control (OHI)
- Adjunctive therapies to control inflammation
- PMPR
- Risk-factor control (e.g. smoking cessation, improved diabetes control, exercise, dietary control and weight loss)

---

place until the requirements of the current step have been met; it can be seen that patient adherence is a key component of step 1, along with professional mechanical plaque reduction (PMPR). This approach ensures that the foundations for an optimal treatment response are in place at the start of patient management. PMPR involves not just professional plaque removal and removal of plaque retention factors but also efficient and consistent plaque removal by the patient; PMPR should not be thought of as another term for "scale and polish", which is an outdated term that should not be used in clinical records. Step 1 should be implemented in all periodontitis patients, regardless of the stage of their disease, and involves the following interventions – the aims of which are to guide behaviour change:
- supragingival biofilm control (OHI)
- adjunctive therapies to control inflammation
- PMPR
- risk-factor control (e.g. smoking cessation, improved diabetes control, exercise, dietary control and weight loss).

The EFP CR (2020) on oral hygiene and patient engagement was to emphasise the importance of these aspects of disease control to patients (Figure 4.3.3), based on the systematic review by Carra et al. (2020).

Improving Adherence and Affecting Behaviour Change

There are numerous barriers to achieving effective adherence to professional advice in periodontal management including:
- A belief that periodontitis is a chronic, non-threatening disease
- Poor understanding of the condition by the patient
- A belief that treatment is expensive
- Inherent dental phobias
- A perception of a lack of compassion on the part of the clinician (Wilson 1996).

Overcoming these barriers can be difficult, and improving patients' adherence to advice may indeed be one of the biggest challenges in modern dentistry. Over the years, several psychological models have been developed to try to understand the determinants of healthcare behaviour and to try to overcome these barriers. These models have included social cognition models which "consider individuals to be

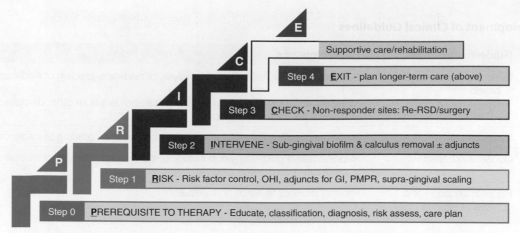

• **Figure 4.3.2** The European Federation of Periodontology S3-Level Clinical Practice Guideline 2020 *stepwise* approach for the treatment of stages 1–3 periodontitis (Sanz et al. 2020). (Reprinted by permission from Springer Nature: Br. Dent. J. Evidence-based, personalised and minimally invasive treatment for periodontitis patients - the new EFP S3-level clinical treatment guidelines, Kebschull, M., Chapple, I., Copyright 2020.)

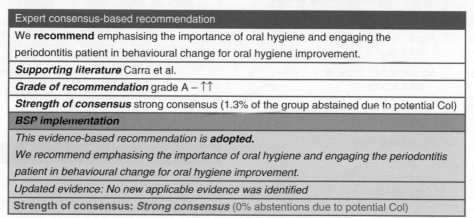

• **Figure 4.3.3** EFP Clinical Recommendation (BSP implementation) with respect to the importance of oral hygiene and patient engagement in periodontal management. *Col, Conflict of interest.* (Reprinted from J. Dent., 106, West, N., Chapple, I., Claydon, N., D'Aiuto, F., Donos, N., Ide, M., Needleman, I., Kebschull, M. [2021], with permission from Elsevier.)

processors of information and vary in the extent to which they address the individual's cognitions about their social world" (Ogden 2000). Such models include the Health Belief Model (Rosenstock 1974), the Theory of Planned Behaviour (Ajzen 1988), the Health Locus of Control (Wallston & Wallston 1982), the Self-Efficacy Model (Bandura 1977) and motivational interviewing (MI) (Rollnick et al. 2010). There is some evidence that such models could be used to improve oral hygiene, but there is little evidence that the use of such methods by clinicians would be beneficial in a dental practice setting. MI in particular has gained much popularity. However a systematic review by Carra et al. (2020) which examined two randomised controlled trials (RCTs) on MI and three RCTs on psychological interventions based on social cognitive theories found no significant additional benefit of implementing specific psychological interventions in conjunction with oral hygiene instruction. The CR developed by the EFP S3 guideline (BSP implementation) was therefore *not* to recommend such approaches (Figure

4.3.4, although the need for further research in this area was acknowledged. Although to date MI has not been shown to improve patient adherence, there are some basic principles of MI which can enhance a clinician's rapport with patients and thus, potentially, improve a patient's response to professional advice with respect to oral hygiene and risk-factor control.

Motivational Interviewing

MI involves helping patients say why and how they might change and is based on the use of a guiding style. It is a person-centred, goal-directed method of communication for eliciting and strengthening patients' intrinsic motivation for positive change. MI was developed in the 1980s by Miller et al. (1988) in response to their observations regarding treatment of patients with alcohol-related problems. The standard confrontational approach to such patients often failed because of denial, personality defect or a failure of

Expert consensus-based recommendation
We **recommend** that the same guidance on oral hygiene practices to control gingival inflammation is enforced throughout all the steps of periodontal therapy including supportive periodontal care.
Supporting literature Van der Weijden and Slot
Grade of recommendation grade A – ↑↑
Strength of consensus strong consensus (3.8% of the group abstained due to potential conflict of interest [CoI])
BSP implementation
This evidence-based recommendation is **adopted.** We recommend that the same oral hygiene guidance to control gingival inflammation is practised throughout steps 1–4 of periodontal therapy including supportive periodontal care.
Updated evidence: No new applicable evidence was identified
Strength of consensus: Unanimous consensus (0% abstentions due to potential CoI)

• **Figure 4.3.4** EFP Clinical Recommendation (BSP implementation) with respect to oral hygiene practices by the patient. (Reprinted from J. Dent., 106, West, N., Chapple, I., Claydon, N., D'Aiuto, F., Donos, N., Ide, M., Needleman, I., Kebschull, M. [2021], with permission from Elsevier.)

Evidence-based statement
To improve patient's behaviour towards compliance with oral hygiene practices, psychological methods such as motivational interviewing or cognitive behavioural therapy **have not** shown a significant impact
Supporting literature Carra et al.
Quality of evidence five randomised clinical trials (RCTs) (1718 subjects) with duration ≥ 6 months in untreated periodontitis patients (4 RCTs with high and 1 RCT with low risk of bias [RoB])
Grade of recommendation statement - unclear, additional research needed
Strength of consensus strong consensus (1.3% of the group abstained due to potential CoI)
BSP implementation
This evidence-based recommendation is **adopted.** Psychological methods such as motivational interviewing or cognitive behavioural therapy have not been shown to have a significant impact on patient's compliance with oral hygiene practices.
Updated evidence: No new applicable evidence was identified
Strength of consensus: Consensus (0% abstentions due to potential CoI)

• **Figure 4.3.5** EFP Clinical Recommendation (BSP implementation) with respect to psychological interventions in behaviour change. *CoI, Conflict of interest.* (Reprinted from J. Dent., 106, West, N., Chapple, I., Claydon, N., D'Aiuto, F., Donos, N., Ide, M., Needleman, I., Kebschull, M. (2021), with permission from Elsevier.)

engagement. This study found that a confrontational style and direct persuasion were likely to increase resistance but that positive change occurred more readily when the clinician connected the change with what was valued by the patient. MI is based on the concept that patient motivation is necessary for change to occur, that motivation resides within the individual and is achievable by eliciting personal values, desire and ability to change. It allows patients to perceive health behaviour information as being relevant to their own situation.

There are three steps necessary to develop an effective MI technique: using a "guiding" communication style, eliciting motivation to change and responding to the patient's language.

MI Step 1: Develop a "Guiding" Style

The main communication styles that clinicians can employ to impart healthcare advice are directing, guiding and following. Although each style has its own uses in different situations and with different patient personalities, a guiding style is best suited to discussions about change (Rollnick et al. 2010). There are three principles to follow when using a guiding style:

- Engage with and work in collaboration with a patient
- Emphasise the patient's autonomy over decision-making
- Elicit their motivation for change.

The clinician can still control the direction and structure of the consultation and provide all the information that is needed, but the patient retains the responsibility for change.

It is important for such an approach to be successful that an empathetic bond is established between clinician and patient. The three skills that a clinician needs to employ are asking, listening and informing:

- Ask: open-ended questions, invite the patient to consider how and why they might change
- Listen: to your patient's experience and encourage them to elaborate; this elicits empathy and is a good way to respond to resistance
- Inform: by asking permission to provide information and asking what the implications may be for the patient.

Much of this process involves *asking* the patient things rather than *telling* them.

MI Step 2: Elicit Motivation to Change

Various strategies can be used in a guiding style to establish motivation in a patient, but this usually involves the following, with examples in italics:

1. What would they like to change?
- *What bothers you the most? Bleeding gums? Tenderness?*
2. Why do they want to change?
- *Do you think it would be better if your gums didn't bleed? What do you think will happen if they continue to bleed?*
3. Assess the importance of the change
- *Is it important to you that your gums stop bleeding and feel more comfortable?*
4. Assess their confidence in achieving change
- *Do you think you would be able to spend longer on your cleaning if this reduced the bleeding and discomfort?*
5. Give them the information they need – elicit understanding, provide information and elicit their interpretation
- *Do you realise why your gums are bleeding? (Elicit) You are right that it is common, but it does show that there is a problem there. (Provide) Can you see that you can do something about this yourself? (Elicit)*
6. Set practical goals
- *Do you see any problems with spending longer on your cleaning? Do you see any difficulties in using floss? Would you rather try something else?*

The imparting of information to a patient is in itself a skill that needs to be developed, and there are a few key principles that need to be followed:

- Use layman's terms to ensure understanding
- Remove your mask
- Deliver advice when the patient is upright and relaxed rather than during treatment
- Encourage the patient to reiterate your advice to check understanding
- Repeat what they say to you, so they know you are listening
- Discuss specific goals with which they agree to encourage adherence.

MI Step 3: Respond to the Patient

Pay careful attention to the patient's responses; what you say to the patient should be in response to what they say to you so that you are working to their agenda, rather than imposing one of your own. This also increases empathy with your patient. This is referred to as "change talk". It is also important to remember how important body language is when undertaking these consultations. In the dental setting, this means having the patient sitting upright in the dental chair (or better still in an ordinary chair or in a different, non-clinical room altogether) and facing them rather than having the patient supine, and not imposing barriers like face masks and crossed arms. One set of guidelines that can be used is referred to with the acronym SOLER (Egan 1990):

*S*quare on to the patient, not turned away, patient sitting up
*O*pen posture, avoid crossed arms
*L*ean slightly forwards, look interested
*E*ye contact to establish rapport
*R*elaxed demeanour.

KEY POINT 3

Motivational interviewing principles:
- Respect patient autonomy
- Guide rather than direct
- Activate patient desires and motivations.

Adherence to Oral Hygiene and Other Advice

Oral Hygiene Advice

The EFP S3 guideline on oral hygiene practices (2020) strongly recommended the efficient use of oral hygiene practices by the patient at all stages of periodontal therapy (Figure 4.3.5), based on a systematic review by Van der Weijden and Slot (2015). In the management of periodontitis, once you have established with the patient what they need to do and why they need to do it, and that they are prepared to try to put your advice into action, discuss with them when, during the day, they might be able to devote the necessary time to the regimen. Thus a "concrete plan" is made with the patient (Schüz et al. 2006). This detail should be recorded and checked with patients at subsequent visits. If the patient thinks they may have difficulty in establishing the necessary routine on a daily basis, it is worth suggesting that they combine the new oral hygiene routine with a daily habit that is already established. This so-called event-based recall is more effective than "time-based recall" (Ellis 1998) when patients try to carry out a particular action at a specified time of day. In the case of oral hygiene, the event could be a mealtime, the daily shower, a radio programme or any established habit that could trigger recall to carry out the oral hygiene routine.

Oral hygiene advice is traditionally given verbally, usually using a "tell–show–do" approach (tell the patient about the technique, show what is needed then get the patient to do it themselves), but it has been shown that the provision of written information increases adherence (Ley 1988). This could be done with a locally produced leaflet, which

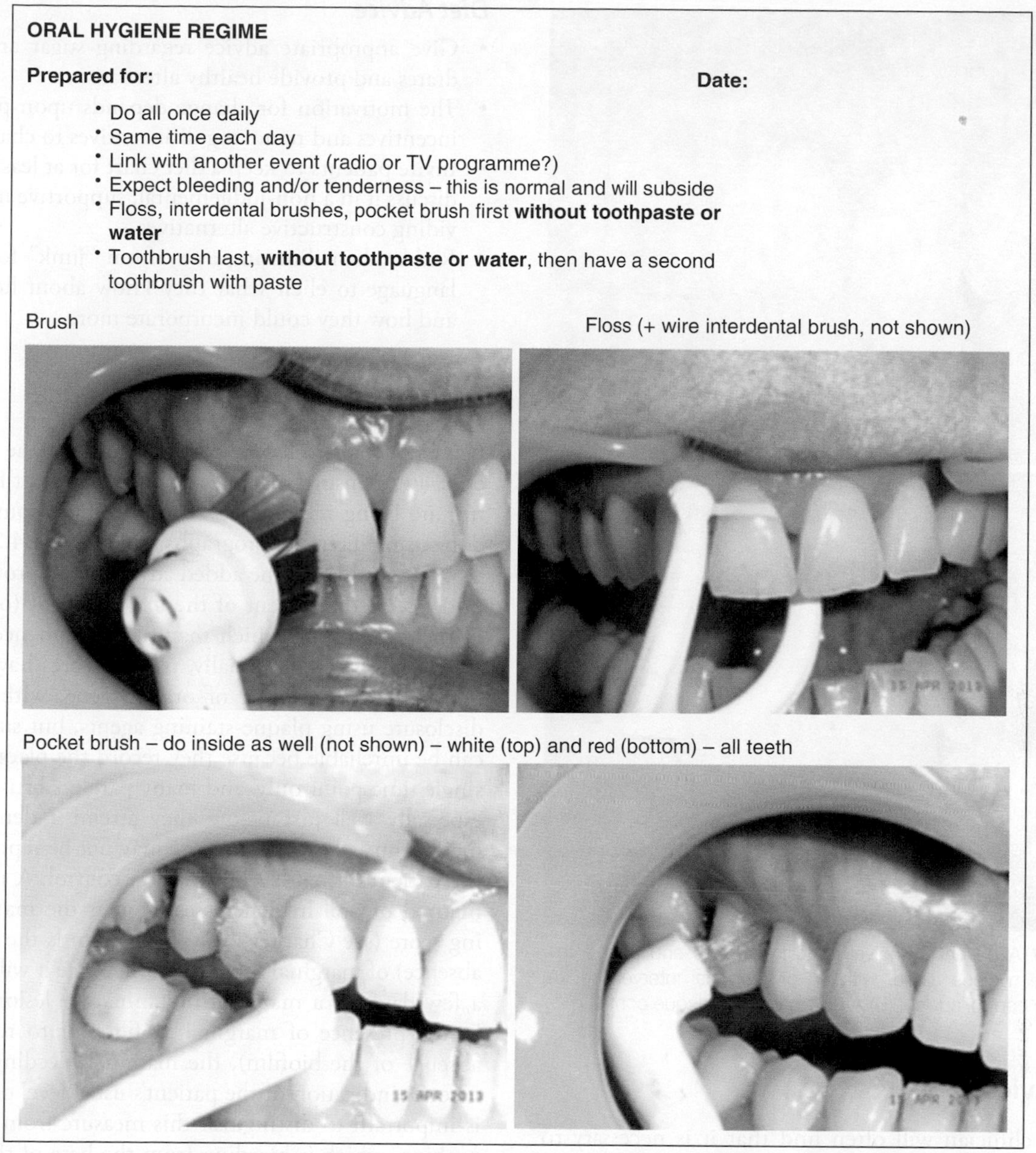

ORAL HYGIENE REGIME

Prepared for:

Date:

- Do all once daily
- Same time each day
- Link with another event (radio or TV programme?)
- Expect bleeding and/or tenderness – this is normal and will subside
- Floss, interdental brushes, pocket brush first **without toothpaste or water**
- Toothbrush last, **without toothpaste or water**, then have a second toothbrush with paste

Brush

Floss (+ wire interdental brush, not shown)

Pocket brush – do inside as well (not shown) – white (top) and red (bottom) – all teeth

• **Figure 4.3.6** Oral hygiene regimen instruction sheet, customised for a patient.

is probably more effective than a generic, commercially produced document, but an alternative is to produce a customised instruction sheet utilising digital photographs of the patient themselves (Figure 4.3.6). It has also been suggested that if a patient has a smartphone with video recording capabilities (many patients have such devices) then a short personalised oral hygiene training video can easily be made for the patient to view. An individualised approach to oral hygiene advice, of which these are examples, has been shown to improve adherence (Harnacke et al. 2012).

Perhaps most importantly, the patient's level of self-efficacy can be developed by withholding any form of professional intervention during the initial (oral hygiene) phase of therapy, so that they can observe that what they do themselves can improve their condition. Self-efficacy is a patient's belief about their capability to produce designated levels of performance that exercise influence over events that affect

their lives (Bandura 1994). Philippot et al. (2005) showed that patients' sense of self-efficacy can be developed through their own direct experience by observing the effects of their behaviour on their periodontitis symptoms. In the context of periodontal management, this is most readily achieved by taking photographs before and after a period of oral hygiene alone, usually a few weeks (Figure 4.3.7), so that patients can see that what they do, without professional intervention, can make a visible difference to levels of marginal inflammation.

One study (Mizutani et al. 2012) investigated the association between self-efficacy, oral health behaviour and gingival health and found that patients with a more developed sense of self-efficacy had better oral health behaviour and less gingivitis. Self-efficacy can be improved by using the techniques described above, and this will benefit patients' gingival and periodontal health.

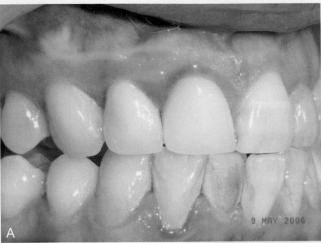

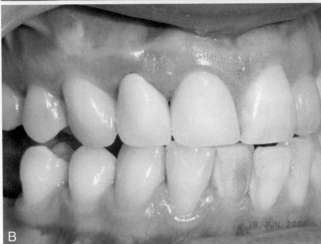

• **Figure 4.3.7** A patient's gingival condition before and after a few weeks of oral hygiene alone, with no professional intervention. (A) Before plaque control advice. (B) After 1 month of plaque control.

Other Advice

The dental clinician will often find that it is necessary to give advice with respect to other health issues, such as diet and smoking, when treating a patient who has periodontitis. The principles outlined above still apply. Always try and highlight those risk factors that are specifically relevant to the individual patient. In addition the following points should be observed:

Smoking Cessation Advice

• The accepted method is the 5 As: ask, advise, assess, assist, arrange
• Affirm belief in cessation, keep dialogue open, accept it may take time
• Reflect back any comments which can be used to motivate, such as concerns about the cost of smoking and smelling of nicotine and in finding places to smoke in public, for example
• Use positive language
• Signpost the patient to smoking cessation support services.

Diet Advice

• Give appropriate advice regarding sugar and carbohydrates and provide healthy alternatives
• The motivation for change depends upon pointing out incentives and removing disincentives to change
• Invite patients to keep a diet chart for at least 3 days and discuss it in a non-judgemental, supportive manner, providing constructive alternatives
• Rather than directing away from "junk" food, use MI language to elicit what they know about healthy foods and how they could incorporate more.

Assessing Adherence in Practice

It is important to assess patients' oral hygiene efforts periodically to ensure that the necessary levels of biofilm control are being maintained. This can most conveniently be done using digital photographs (see Chapter 4.2 and Figure 4.3.7), and this has the added advantage of providing visual evidence to the patient of the improvement (or otherwise) in their condition, which may further enhance their sense of self-efficacy. Traditionally, plaque scores have been used to assess patients' level of oral hygiene, with or without disclosure using plaque-staining agents, but such measures can be unreliable because they record the plaque levels at a single time point only, and many patients brush their teeth especially well just before they attend a dental appointment. Thus a low plaque score may not be representative of the patient's usual level of biofilm control. A more reliable method of oral hygiene assessment is the marginal bleeding score (see Chapter 2.2) which records the presence (or absence) of marginal inflammation. Since it will always take a few days for a marginal inflammatory lesion to develop in the presence of marginal biofilm (or to resolve in the absence of the biofilm), the marginal bleeding score gives a better indication of the patient's usual level of cleaning. It is important to distinguish this measure from bleeding on probing, which is bleeding from the base of the periodontal pocket and is used to assess the response to professional treatment.

Conclusion

Motivating patients to improve their levels of self-care can be difficult, may be met with resistance and, at times, may be frustrating for the clinician. In periodontics, however, perhaps more so than in other dental disciplines, it is perhaps the most crucial part of the periodontal patient's disease management. However, developing a supportive and non-judgemental approach to oral hygiene and healthcare advice can be highly effective, and the techniques outlined in this chapter should be practiced until they become the clinician's routine way of communicating with patients.

Multiple choice questions on the contents of this chapter are available online at Elsevier eBooks+.

References

Ajzen I. *Attitude, Personality and Behaviour*. London: Open University Press; 1988.

Axelsson P, Lindhe J. Effect of controlled oral hygiene procedures on caries and periodontal disease in adults. Results after 6 years. *J Clin Periodontol*. 1981;8:239–248.

Bandura A. Self-efficacy: towards a unifying theory of behaviour change. *Psychol Rev*. 1977;84:191–215.

Bandura A. Self-efficacy. In: Ramachaudran VS, ed. *Encyclopedia of Human Behavior*. 1994;4:71–81.

Carra MC, Detzen L, Kitzmann J, Woelber JP, Ramseier CA, Bouchard P. Promoting behavioural changes to improve oral hygiene in patients with periodontal diseases: a systematic review. *J Clin Periodontol*. 2020;47(suppl 22):72–89.

Egan G. *The Skilled Helper*. 4th ed. Pacific Grove, CA: Brooks/Cole; 1990.

Ellis J. Prospective memory and medicine-taking. *Adherence to Treatment in Medical Conditions*. London: Harwood Academic; 1998.

Harnacke D, Beldoch M, Bohn GH, Seghaoui O, Hegel N, Deinzer R. Oral and written instruction of oral hygiene: a randomized trial. *J Periodontol*. 2012;83:1206–1212.

Ley P. *Communicating with the Patient*. London: Croom Helm; 1988.

Kebschull M, Chapple I. Evidence-based, personalised and minimally invasive treatment for periodontitis patients - the new EFP S3-level clinical treatment guidelines. *Br Dent J*. 2020;229(7):443–449.

Listgarten MA, Sullivan P, George C, Nitkin L, Rosenberg ES, Chilton NW. Comparative longitudinal study of 2 methods of scheduling maintenance visits: 4-year data. *J Clin Periodontol*. 1989;16:105–115.

Miller WR, Sovreign RG, Krege B. Motivational interviewing with problem drinkers: II. The drinker's check-up as a preventive intervention. *Behavioral Psychotherapy*. 1988;16:251.

Mizutani S, Ekuni D, Furuta M, Tomofuji T, Irie K, Azuma T, et al. Effects of self-efficacy on oral health behaviours and gingival health in university students aged 18- or 19-years-old. *J Clin Periodontol*. 2012;39:844–849.

Mullen PD. Compliance becomes concordance. *Br Med J*. 1997;314:691–692.

Ogden J. *Health Psychology*. 2nd ed. Buckingham: Open University; 2000.

Philippot P, Lenoir N, D'Hoore W, Bercy P. Improving patients' compliance with the treatment of periodontitis: a controlled study of behavioural intervention. *J Clin Periodontol*. 2005;32:653–658.

Preus HR, Al-Lami Q, Baelim V. Oral hygiene revisited. The clinical effect of a prolonged oral hygiene phase prior to periodontal therapy in periodontitis patients. A randomised clinical study. *J Clin Periodontol*. 2019;47(1):36–42.

Ramfjord SP, Morrison EC, Burgett FG, Nissle RR, Shick RA, Zann GJ. Oral hygiene and maintenance of periodontal support. *J Periodontol*. 1982;53:26–30.

Ramseier CA. Potential impact of subject-based risk factor control on periodontitis. *J Clin Periodontol*. 2005;32(suppl 6):283–290.

Rollnick S, Butler CC, Kinnersley P, Gregory J, Mash B. Motivational interviewing. *Br Med J*. 2010;340:c1900.

Rosen B, Olavi G, Badersten A, Ronstrom A, Soderholm G, Egelberg J. Effect of different frequencies of preventive maintenance treatment on periodontal conditions. 5-year observations in general dentistry patients. *J Clin Periodontol*. 1999;26:225–233.

Rosenstock I. Historical origins of the health belief model. *Health Educ Monogr*. 1974;2:328–335.

Sanz M, Herrera D, Kebschull M, Chapple I, Jepsen S, Beglundh T, et al. Treatment of stage I-III periodontitis-The EFP S3 level clinical practice guideline. *J Clin Periodontol*. 2020;47(suppl 22):4–60.

Sbordone L, Ramaglia L, Gulletta E, Iacono V. Recolonization of the subgingival microflora after scaling and root planing in human periodontitis. *J Periodontol*. 1990;61:579–584.

Schüz B, Sniehotta FF, Wiedemann A, Seemann R. Adherence to a daily flossing regimen in university students: effects of planning when, where, how and what to do in the face of barriers. *J Clin Periodontol*. 2006;33:612–619.

Umaki TM, Umaki MR, Cobb CM. The psychology of patient compliance: a focused review of the literature. *J Periodontol*. 2012;83:395–400.

Van der Weijden FA, Slot DE. Efficacy of homecare regimens for mechanical plaque removal in managing gingivitis: a metareview. *J Clin Periodontol*. 2015;42(suppl 16):S77–S91.

Wallston KA, Wallston BS. Who is responsible for your health? The construct of health locus of control. In: Sanders G, Suls J, eds. *Social Psychology of Health and Illness*. Hillsdale, NJ: Lawrence Erlbaum & Associates; 1982:65–95.

West N, Chapple I, Claydon N, D'Aiuto F, Donos N, Ide M, Needleman I, Kebschull M. BSP implementation of European S3 - level evidence-based treatment guidelines for stage I-III periodontitis in UK clinical practice. *J Dent*. 2021;106:103562.

Wilson Jr TG. Compliance and its role in periodontal therapy. *Periodontol 2000*. 1996;12:16–23.

Non-surgical Periodontal Management

5.1

The Diseased Root Surface in Periodontitis

PHILIP OWER

CHAPTER OUTLINE

The Clinical Presentation of Periodontitis

    Features of Periodontitis

    The Role of Bacteria

    Current Concepts of the Aetiology of Periodontitis

Treating the Diseased Root Surface

Non-Surgical vs Surgical Treatment

The Role of the Biofilm

Calculus in Disease

Contaminated Cementum

OVERVIEW OF THE CHAPTER

This chapter describes the nature of the diseased root surface in periodontitis and will examine the relative roles of the bacterial biofilm, dental calculus and contaminated cementum in the disease process.

By the end of the chapter the reader should:

- Understand the nature of the diseased root surface
- Appreciate the relative roles of biofilm, calculus and contaminated cementum in periodontitis
- Be able to differentiate between various methods for treating diseased root surfaces

- Be able to appreciate the importance of biofilm removal in disease control
- Be able to select appropriate treatments for patients with periodontitis.

This chapter covers the following topics:

- Clinical presentation of periodontitis
- Treating the diseased root surface.

The Clinical Presentation of Periodontitis

Features of Periodontitis

Periodontitis is observed clinically as the apical migration of the junctional epithelial attachment and progressive loss of the connective tissue attachment to the tooth surface, with increasing clinical pocket depth and inflammatory change in the soft tissues. Increasing levels of soft tissue inflammation result in redness, swelling, bleeding and tenderness. Radiographically, alveolar bone loss is seen as the bone is resorbed (by the host) to prevent its infection by the encroaching bacterial biofilm which colonises the root surface of the periodontal pocket. Although it is widely accepted that periodontitis has a microbial aetiology and that bacteria and other microbes are essential for disease to occur, there is now a clearer understanding of the multiple host factors that play a major part in this disease process.

Periodontitis is now recognised as one of the most complex of human diseases, and it is a major cause of tooth loss in all populations throughout the world. In addition, there is also mounting evidence that periodontitis may play a significant role in general health, so the effective treatment of periodontitis may be even more important than was once thought.

The Role of Bacteria

It was thought in the past that the release of bacterial toxins from dental plaque caused most of the tissue damage seen in periodontitis, and that only a small amount of damage was caused by the host response (inflammatory and immune) to these toxins. Periodontitis was then frequently, and erroneously, referred to as an infection and various explanations were proposed for the bacterially mediated destructive mechanisms involved; these have been referred to in the literature as *plaque hypotheses*. Initially, it was thought that it was the total plaque mass that was responsible for disease, the *non-specific plaque hypothesis (NSPH)*, and that the more plaque a patient had the more periodontitis they would get. This clearly does not fit with what is seen in practice, where some patients have a lot of plaque and little periodontitis and others have little plaque but significant bone and attachment loss, and is not supported by research findings. For example Löe et al. (1986) investigated a population of tea workers in Sri Lanka over a 15-year period who had no access to dental care and did not carry out any form of conventional oral hygiene. Despite having large deposits of both plaque and calculus, they did not all have periodontitis – about 10% had no disease beyond gingivitis, about 80% had moderate progression of periodontitis and about 10% had a form of rapidly progressing periodontitis. As advances in microbiological investigation allowed the examination of dental plaque in more detail and the identification of the individual species of bacteria that predominated in plaque, both in health and disease, a second theory was developed – the *specific plaque hypothesis (SPH)*. This suggested that specific microorganisms in plaque were responsible for disease and that only plaque that contained these organisms was capable of producing disease (Loesche 1976). This concept was supported by the fact that the microbial composition of plaque was different in diseased and healthy sites (Socransky & Haffajee 1992), and researchers started compiling lists of bacteria (which were colour-coded by level of pathogenicity, the "red complex" organisms being the most pathogenic) that were found in the most diseased sites (Socransky et al. 1998). Whether these bacteria were causative (responsible for disease) or opportunistic (taking advantage of the living conditions at deep sites) could not be established. This research, which appeared to support the concept of a SPH, also coincided with increasing interest in and research into the use of antimicrobials in periodontal treatment, specifically locally applied drugs, which could target certain bacteria as a means of disease control. However, at the same time, there was a developing realisation that the host response might have a larger role in the disease process than was previously thought.

Current Concepts of the Aetiology of Periodontitis

The recognition that host factors play a major role in periodontitis has led to the concept of the *ecological plaque hypothesis* which incorporates elements of both the non-specific and specific plaque hypotheses but also takes into account the role that various host factors play in the development and organisation of the dental biofilm. Indeed, the use of the term *biofilm* is preferable to the use of the term *plaque* because it better reflects the highly complex nature of the growth, development and behaviour of bacteria (and other microbes) on diseased root surfaces. Biofilms are described in detail in Chapter 1.5.

> **KEY POINT 1**
>
> The ecological plaque hypothesis incorporates elements of both the non-specific and specific plaque hypotheses but also takes into account the role that various host factors play in the development and organisation of the dental biofilm.

The *ecological plaque hypothesis* was proposed (Marsh 1994) to explain how the host interacts with the microbial biofilm; this incorporates elements of both the NSPH and the SPH but also considers the role of host response factors in the development of disease. Thus, in health, there is *symbiosis* – a balance between the microbial composition of the biofilm and the host response. In disease, there is a disturbance of this balance (think about the word "disease" – a combination of "dis" and "ease") caused by a change in the microbial threat or a change in the host response, or often a change in both (Figure 5.1.1). This is referred to as *dysbiosis*. The microbial threat may increase due to an increase in the bacterial mass – NSPH – which may result in an increased host inflammatory response, resulting in host-mediated tissue damage. Given that the host response is largely genetically determined, this explains why periodontitis can be seen to run in families and why some patients are more susceptible than others to periodontal breakdown – in these individuals, relatively small changes in biofilm mass may result in a greater, and more damaging, host response. The increased inflammatory response, if sustained, results in increased gingival crevicular fluid (GCF) flow, which contains host proteins and glycoproteins that can be exploited as substrates by subgingival anaerobic bacteria. This leads to a gradual shift in the microbial composition of the biofilm which can disrupt the natural balance of organisms within the biofilm community – SPH – and increase the risk of disease (Marsh et al. 2011). The host response may also change because of environmental factors (such as smoking, stress, systemic disease or diet) which may also favour a shift in the microbial composition of the biofilm towards greater numbers of more pathogenic (predominantly anaerobic) bacterial species.

> **KEY POINT 2**
>
> It is thought that the majority (an estimate of 80% has been suggested) of the damage observed in periodontitis is due to the inflammatory host response to the bacterial biofilm, rather than direct bacterial activity.

Currently, it is thought that the majority (an estimate of 80% has been suggested) of the damage observed in periodontitis is due to the inflammatory host response to the bacterial biofilm rather than direct bacterial activity. Thus, bacteria are necessary as a trigger for the host response, but it is the host response that causes most of the damage. Periodontitis should therefore be thought of as an inflammatory disease rather than an infection; because most of the damage is host mediated, the bacteria involved are commensal organisms and they do not usually invade the host tissues but remain on the root surface in the biofilm. Current thinking

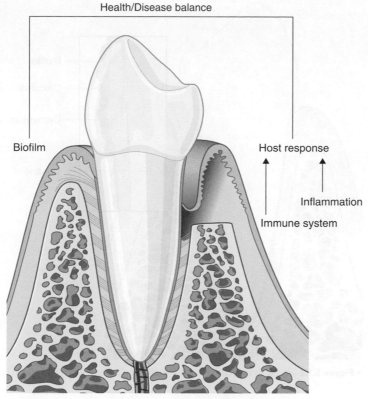

• **Figure 5.1.1** Health/disease balance.

has been encapsulated in this statement from the 2008 *Workshop on Inflammation and Periodontal Disease: A Reappraisal*: "Periodontitis is an inflammatory disease initiated by the oral microbial biofilm . . . it is the host response to the biofilm that destroys the periodontium" (Van Dyke 2008).

So if the trigger for the damaging host response is the bacterial presence on the root surface, effective treatments need to reduce this presence to a level that does not initiate a damaging host response.

Treating the Diseased Root Surface

The diseased root surface in a periodontal pocket comprises several layers of potential contamination that could harbour sufficient microbes to trigger the disease process (Figure 5.1.2).

The outermost layer of contamination will always be the microbial biofilm, but there is also the potential for contamination from subgingival calculus and from any microbes that may have invaded the cemental layer of the root. Most periodontal therapies involve the removal of these sources of contamination, and it has been stated (Lindhe & Echeverria 1993) that root surface disinfection is the primary objective of therapy. This objective may be achieved by both non-surgical and surgical means.

Non-Surgical vs Surgical Treatment

In the past, much periodontal therapy has involved the surgical excision of soft tissue as a means of removing "infected" soft tissue and reducing pocket depths to facilitate the maintenance of a healthy subgingival environment by both the patient and clinician. However, with the increasing understanding of the inflammatory nature of the periodontitis process and the fact that the soft tissues are only rarely invaded by bacteria and other microbes, there has been a shift towards more conservative, non-surgically based therapies as a means of controlling inflammation. That non-surgical treatment is an effective method for treating chronic periodontitis (or indeed the less common aggressive form of disease) is not in doubt; a systematic review and meta-analysis published in 2005 (Heitz-Mayfield 2005) looked at the findings of three previous systematic reviews, published between 1993 and 2002, confirming that better treatment outcomes can be achieved by non-surgical means, when compared to surgical treatment, for moderate pockets (up to 6 mm), whereas surgical treatment is only of greater benefit for deeper pockets in excess of 6 mm. Although this appeared to show that deep pockets should be treated surgically, the authors pointed out that this latter finding is only applicable to 12-month post-treatment results, and those studies that followed patients for 5 years or more found that, even for deep pockets, non-surgical therapy was as effective as surgical treatment.

> ### KEY POINT 3
> Non-surgical treatment is an effective method for treating chronic periodontitis.

Many of the non-surgical methods commonly used today to treat periodontal diseases have remained largely

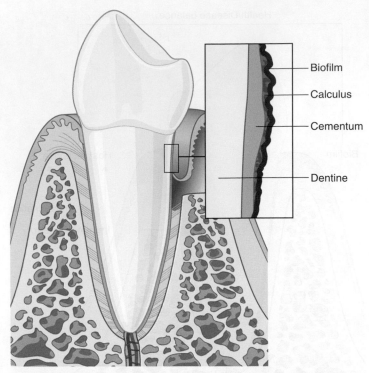

• **Figure 5.1.2** Possible sources of contamination on a diseased root surface.

unchanged for decades. In non-surgical periodontal therapy, for example, the process of root planing is still practised, but it was illustrated in Egyptian hieroglyphics 4000 years ago and was described, and named, in the dental literature a century ago (Hartzell 1913). More recently, the term "root surface debridement" has been used to describe the instrumentation of the diseased root surface. Some confusion has arisen surrounding the terminology used to describe these different instrumentation techniques, and definitions of the various terms used will be considered in Chapter 5.2 on periodontal instrumentation. The current chapter will now consider the relative roles of the bacterial biofilm, calculus and cementum in periodontitis.

The Role of the Biofilm

It may seem obvious that the biofilm on the root surface needs to be removed or disrupted for treatment to be effective. However, fundamental to the successful management of disease by non-surgical means (or indeed surgical means for that matter) is the establishment, before any treatment is carried out, of optimal self-performed biofilm (plaque) control. Although the evidence base for an association between personal oral hygiene and the control or prevention of chronic periodontitis is surprisingly weak (there are no randomised controlled trials to show such an association; Hujoel et al. 2005), it is assumed that an adequate level of daily plaque control is a prerequisite for successful periodontal therapy of any form. For example, the Sixth European Workshop in Periodontology in 2008 stated that: "It should be noted that the performance of optimal oral hygiene practices is an inseparable principle to be observed

with any protocol of mechanical debridement" (Sanz & Teughels 2008).

The effects of good biofilm control before starting treatment can be dramatic (Figure 5.1.3), the goal being to establish an optimal supragingival environment prior to starting subgingival instrumentation. Patient self-care is considered in detail in Chapter 4.1.

> ### KEY POINT 4
> "It should be noted that the performance of optimal oral hygiene practices is an inseparable principle to be observed with any protocol of mechanical debridement" (Sanz and Teughels 2008).

As far as therapy is concerned, it is now universally accepted that mechanical biofilm removal forms the cornerstone of successful periodontal therapy (Guentsch & Preshaw 2008, Chapple 2009, van der Weijden & Slot 2011) and that a reduction in subgingival biofilm mass is essential for successful therapy (Mombelli et al. 1995).

> ### KEY POINT 5
> Mechanical biofilm removal forms the cornerstone of successful periodontal therapy.

Calculus in Disease

Calculus is the result of the mineralisation of biofilm by salivary mineral components (Lang et al. 2008), which is why supragingival calculus is mostly found adjacent to the opening of the ducts of the major salivary glands that are buccal to the upper first molars and lingual to the lower

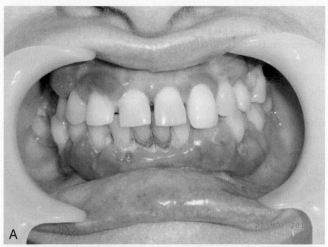

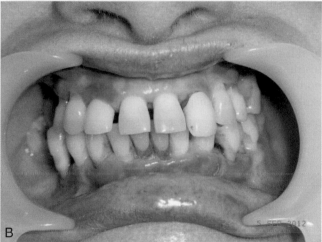

• **Figure 5.1.3** Effects of self-performed plaque control. (A) The patient on presentation. (B) The same patient after 3 months of self-performed oral hygiene measures only with no professional intervention.

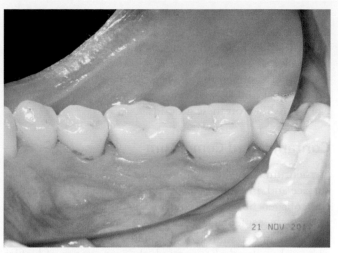

• **Figure 5.1.4** Exposed subgingival calculus after oral hygiene measures alone.

anterior teeth. Subgingival calculus is found in periodontal pockets and is a darker colour than supragingival calculus as a result of incorporation of blood products from subgingival inflammation. Calculus is porous in nature; although some studies have identified viable organisms within the lacunae of supragingival calculus (Tan et al. 2004), others have suggested that most of the bacteria contained within calculus have been killed by the mineralisation process and are therefore incapable of producing harmful toxins (Sidaway 1980). It is also worth remembering that individual bacteria that survive in calculus are not part of a biofilm and thus have little pathogenic potential. Traditionally, it has been thought essential to remove all such calcified deposits from the root surface in order to achieve root surface decontamination and promote resolution of periodontal inflammation. Indeed, in the past, treatment seems to have focused entirely on the meticulous removal of all calculus deposits, and much dental hygienist training has centred on developing efficient and effective calculus-removal skills. However, it is now understood that the importance of biofilm removal in therapy far outweighs the need to remove the mineralised calculus deposits or potentially contaminated tooth

structure (Mombelli et al. 1995). In addition, the concept of removing all subgingival calculus has been shown to be both unrealistic and unnecessary (Cobb 2002) and that clinical healing occurs in the presence of residual subgingival calculus (Nyman et al. 1986, Blomlöf et al. 1987, Buchanan & Robertson 1987) providing the surface of the calculus is biofilm-free (Mombelli et al. 1995, Jepsen et al. 2011). This is just as well because clinicians rarely remove all subgingival calculus deposits even when they try to do so, whether by non-surgical or surgical means and whether using hand or machine-driven instrumentation techniques (Eaton et al. 1985, Caffesse et al. 1986, Kepic et al. 1990). One review (Robertson 1990) showed that, even after 12–15 minutes of treatment per tooth, 63% of root surfaces still harboured residual calculus. However, it is now understood that calculus does not contain significant quantities of bacterial lipopolysaccharide (Chiew et al. 1991), and it has been concluded that calculus is the result of the periodontal lesion and not its cause (Corbet et al. 1993, Jepsen et al. 2011). Calculus is therefore another surface on which biofilm can form, but the biofilm can be as easily removed from the calculus surface as it can from other intraoral surfaces. Thus when patients achieve high standards of self-performed biofilm control, periodontal lesions can heal, even in the absence of professional intervention, and previously subgingival calculus can become supragingival (Figure 5.1.4), supporting the concept of calculus being the result of the disease process and not its cause.

KEY POINT 6

The importance of biofilm removal in therapy far outweighs the need to remove the mineralised calculus deposits or potentially contaminated tooth structure.

KEY POINT 7

Calculus is the result of the periodontal lesion and not its cause.

Calculus is sometimes described as a plaque-retention factor, but there is no evidence to support the concept of biofilm being more adherent to the surface of the calculus than it is to other surfaces. However, calculus may be thought of as presenting an obstacle to optimal personal and professional care, as well as being unsightly, and its removal can be justified on these grounds.

Contaminated Cementum

Cementum is the highly mineralised outer layer of the root surface and, in health, it provides a means of attachment for the collagen fibres of the normal periodontal ligament. In disease, the cemental layer becomes exposed and can potentially become a source of bacterial contamination. However, as has already been stated, the importance of biofilm removal in therapy far outweighs the need to remove mineralised deposits (calculus) or tooth structure (Mombelli et al. 1995). So how important is the exposed cemental layer in the disease process?

For at least the last century, it has been assumed (with no clinical evidence to support the concept) that the surface layer of the cementum of the diseased root surface became contaminated with both bacteria and their toxins. In vitro research had suggested that bacteria and bacterial endotoxins could penetrate and be bound to root cementum (Aleo et al. 1974, 1975, Daly et al. 1982, Adriaens et al. 1988) and that this could act as a potential reservoir of toxins that could lead to re-infection after therapy. This apparently justified the concept of "root planing", a treatment technique that involved the use of highly sharpened (and therefore highly damaging) hand instruments to "plane" away the apparently contaminated surface cementum of the root to achieve a biocompatible root surface that would allow periodontal healing. Although such a treatment approach could be shown to be effective (because the treatment also resulted in the removal of the biofilm), disease control was achieved at considerable cost to both patient and clinician; the treatment was time consuming, caused considerable postoperative discomfort, was difficult to perform and thus required a high degree of clinical skill. It also had to be performed under local anaesthesia and could only be realistically achieved on a quadrant-by-quadrant basis. The concept of quadrant-by-quadrant, scaling and root planing (QSRP) under local anaesthesia became, for decades, the mainstay of non-surgical periodontal therapy. Each quadrant would usually require at least 45 minutes of treatment to achieve the goal of a "hard" and "smooth" root surface (Palmer & Floyd 2006). In the 1980s, it was suggested that the rationale for root planing was not evidence based and was based "on clinical impression rather than scientific investigation" (Daly et al. 1982). It was subsequently shown that the majority of the bacterial contaminants were only loosely adherent to the root surface and did not penetrate the root cementum to any significant degree (Nakib et al. 1982, Ito et al. 1985, Hughes & Smales 1986, 1990, Moore et al. 1986), and that

the root surface could be easily decontaminated by much lighter and quicker instrumentation techniques than had previously been thought. One in vitro study (Moore et al. 1986) showed that over 99% of the bacterial contaminants could be removed by light instrumentation alone, without the need for cementum removal by root planing. This led to the concept of "root surface debridement" that involved ultrasonic instruments used with light and overlapping strokes for a limited time period (Smart et al. 1990). Often such treatments do not require the use of local anaesthesia, and there is a much-reduced risk of iatrogenic root surface damage. The differences between traditional root planing and root surface debridement should therefore now be apparent to the reader. However, following publication of the European Federation of Periodontology (EFP) S3 clinical guideline for the treatment of stages I– III periodontitis (Sanz et al. 2020), and the subsequent British Society of Periodontology and Implant Dentistry (BSP) UK version of this guideline (West et al. 2021), the term "subgingival instrumentation" is now proposed as a universal term for non-surgical treatment of the root surface. These issues are explored further in Chapter 5.2.

> ### KEY POINT 8
> Bacterial contaminants are only loosely adherent to the root surface and do not penetrate the root cementum to any significant degree.

Multiple choice questions on the contents of this chapter are available online at Elsevier eBooks+.

References

Adriaens PA, Edwards CA, De Boever JA, Loesche WJ. Ultrastructural observations on bacterial invasion in cementum and radicular dentin of periodontally-diseased human teeth. *J Periodontol.* 1988;59:493–503.

Aleo JJ, De Renzis FA, Farber PA, Varboncoeur AP. The presence and biologic activity of cementum-bound endotoxin. *J Periodontol.* 1974;45:672–675.

Aleo JJ, De Renzis FA, Farber PA. *In vitro* attachment of human gingival fibroblasts to root surfaces. *J Periodontol.* 1975;46:639–645.

Blomlöf L, Lindskog S, Appelgren R, Jonsson B, Weintraub A, Hammarström L. New attachment in monkeys with experimental periodontitis with and without removal of the cementum. *J Clin Periodontol.* 1987;14:136–143.

Buchanan SA, Robertson PB. Calculus removal by scaling/root planing with and without surgical access. *J Periodontol.* 1987;58:159–163.

Caffesse RG, Sweeney PL, Smith BA. Scaling and root planing with and without periodontal flap surgery. *J Clin Periodontol.* 1986;13:205–210.

Chapple ILC. Periodontal diagnosis and treatment – where does the future lie? *Periodontol.* 2009; 2000, 51:9–24.

Chiew SY, Wilson M, Davies EH, Kieser JB. Assessment of ultrasonic debridement of calculus-associated periodontally-involved root surfaces by the limulus amoebocyte lysate assay. An in vitro study. *J Clin Periodontol.* 1991;18(4):240–244.

Cobb CM. Clinical significance of non-surgical periodontal therapy: an evidence-based perspective of scaling and root planing. *J Clin Periodontol.* 2002;29(suppl 2):22–32.

Corbet EF, Vaughan AJ, Kieser JB. The periodontally-involved root surface. *J Clin Periodontol.* 1993;20:402–410.

Daly CG, Seymour GJ, Kieser JB, Corbet EF. Histological assessment of periodontally-involved cementum. *J Clin Periodontol.* 1982;9:266–274.

Eaton KA, Kieser JB, Davies RM. The removal of root surface deposits. *J Clin Periodontol.* 1985;12:141–152.

Guentsch A, Preshaw PM. The use of a linear oscillating device in periodontal treatment: a review. *J Clin Periodontol.* 2008;35:514–524.

Hartzell TB. The operative and post-operative treatment of pyorrhea. *Dental Cosmos.* 1913;55:1094–1101.

Heitz-Mayfield LJ. How effective is surgical therapy compared with non-surgical debridement? *Periodontol 2000.* 2005;37:72–87.

Hughes FJ, Smales FC. Immunohistochemical investigation of the presence and distribution of cementum-associated lipopolysaccharides in periodontal disease. *J Periodontal Res.* 1986;21:660–667.

Hughes FJ, Smales FC. The distribution and quantitation of cementum-bound lipopolysaccharide on periodontally diseased root surfaces of human teeth. *Arch Oral Biol.* 1990;35:295–299.

Hujoel PP, Cunha-Cruz J, Loesche W, Robertson PB. Personal oral hygiene and chronic periodontitis: a systematic review. *Periodontol 2000.* 2005;37:29–34.

Ito K, Hindman RE, O'Leary TJ, Kafrawy AH. Determination of the presence of root-bound endotoxin using the local Shwartzman phenomenon (LSP). *J Periodontol.* 1985;56:8–17.

Jepsen S, Deschner J, Braun A, Schwarz F, Eberhard J. Calculus removal and the prevention of its formation. *Periodontol 2000.* 2011;55:167–188.

Kepic TJ, O'Leary TJ, Kafrawy AH. Total calculus removal: an attainable objective? *J Periodontol.* 1990;61:16–20.

Lang NP, Mombelli A, Attstrom R. Oral biofilms and calculus. In: *Clinical Periodontology and Implant Dentistry.* 5th ed. Blackwell Munksgaard *Copenhagen;* 2008:197.

Lindhe J, Echeverria J. Consensus report of session II. In: *Proceedings of the 1st European Workshop on Periodontology.* London: Quintessence; 1993:212.

Löe H, Anerud A, Boysen H, Morrison E. Natural history of periodontal disease in man. Rapid, moderate and no loss of attachment in Sri Lankan laborers 14 to 46 years of age. *J Clin Periodontol.* 1986;13:431–445.

Loesche WJ. Chemotherapy of dental plaque infections. *Oral Sci Rev.* 1976;9:63–195.

Marsh PD. Microbial ecology of dental plaque and its significance in health and disease. *Adv Dent Res.* 1994;8:263–271.

Marsh PD, Moter A, Devine DA. Dental plaque biofilms: communities, conflict and control. *Periodontol 2000.* 2011;38(suppl 11):28–35.

Mombelli A, Nyman S, Bragger U, Wennstrom J, Lang NP. Clinical and microbiological changes associated with an altered subgingival environment induced by periodontal pocket reduction. *J Clin Periodontol.* 1995;22:780–787.

Moore J, Wilson M, Kieser JB. The distribution of bacterial lipopolysaccharide (endotoxin) in relation to periodontally involved root surfaces. *J Clin Periodontol.* 1986;13:748–751.

Nakib NM, Bissada NF, Simmelink JW, Goldstine SN. Endotoxin penetration into root cementum of periodontally healthy and diseased teeth. *J Periodontol.* 1982;53:368–378.

Nyman S, Westfelt E, Sarhed G, Karring T. Role of "diseased" root cementum in healing following treatment of periodontal disease. *J Clin Periodontol.* 1986;13:464–468.

Palmer RM, Floyd PD. Non-surgical treatment and maintenance. In: *A Clinical Guide to Periodontology.* 2nd ed. British Dental Association *London;* 2006:30.

Robertson PB. The residual calculus paradox. *J Periodontol.* 1990;61:65–66.

Sanz M, Teughels W. Innovations in non-surgical periodontal therapy: Consensus Report of the Sixth European Workshop on Periodontology. *J Clin Periodontol.* 2008;35(suppl 8):3–7.

Sanz M, Herrera D, Kebschull M, Chapple I, Jepsen S, Beglundh T, Sculean A, Tonetti M. Treatment of stage I-III periodontitis-The EFP S3 level clinical practice guideline. *J Clin Periodontol.* 2020;47(suppl 22):4–60.

Sidaway DA. A microbiological study of dental calculus IV. An electron microscope study of in vitro calcified micro-organisms. *J Periodontal Res.* 1980;15:240–254.

Smart GJ, Wilson M, Kieser JB. The assessment of ultrasonic root surface debridement by determination of residual endotoxin levels. *J Clin Periodontol.* 1990;17:174–178.

Socransky SS, Haffajee AD. The bacterial etiology of destructive periodontal disease: current concepts. *J Periodontol.* 1992;63(suppl 4):322–331.

Socransky SS, Haffajee AD, Cugini MA, Smith C, Kent Jr RL. Microbial complexes in subgingival plaque. *J Clin Periodontol.* 1998;25(2):134–144.

Tan BTK, Mordan NJ, Embleton J, Pratten J, Galgut PN. Study of bacterial viability within human supragingival dental calculus. *J Periodontol.* 2004;75:23–29.

van der Weijden F, Slot DE. Oral hygiene in the prevention of periodontal diseases: the evidence. *Periodontol 2000.* 2011;55:104–123.

Van Dyke TE. Inflammation and periodontal diseases: a reappraisal. *J Periodontol.* 2008;79(suppl 8):1503–1507.

West N, Chapple I, Claydon N, D'Aiuto F, Donos N, Ide M, Needleman I, Kebschull M. BSP implementation of European S3 - level evidence-based treatment guidelines for stage I-III periodontitis in UK clinical practice. *J Dent.* 2021;106:1–72:103562. https://doi.org/10.1016/j.jdent.2020.103562.

5.2

Periodontal Instrumentation

PHILIP OWER

CHAPTER OUTLINE

OVERVIEW OF THE CHAPTER

This chapter will examine the methods that are available to instrument diseased root surfaces during both non-surgical and surgical therapy. This chapter should be read in conjunction with Chapter 5.1.

By the end of the chapter the reader should:

- Understand treatment objectives in periodontal therapy
- Understand the terminology that is used to describe instrumentation techniques
- Understand the choice of instruments that are available
- Understand the effects of different types of instrumentation
- Be able to outline the different strategies that can be employed to instrument diseased root surfaces
- Be able to select appropriate instruments to meet treatment objectives.

The chapter covers the following topics:

- Introduction
- Treatment objectives
- Terminology and definitions
- Types of instruments
- Instrumentation strategies
- Adjuncts to periodontal instrumentation
- Conclusions.

Introduction

Decontamination of the teeth, and in a diseased state the roots of teeth, by various methods of instrumentation has been a fundamental aspect of dental treatment for hundreds, and possibly thousands, of years. Many different methods, techniques and instruments to achieve a level of decontamination compatible with dental health have been proposed in the past, and extensive research over the last century or so has resulted in a number of these techniques

being used in current dental practice. Research has shown that many of these treatment modalities achieve broadly similar results. The purpose of this chapter is to highlight the most commonly used techniques and instruments in practice today. The use of chemicals and host-modulating agents as adjuncts to periodontal instrumentation will also be examined. In 2021 the European Federation of Periodontology (EFP) published S3 clinical guidelines for the treatment of stages I–III periodontitis (Sanz et al. 2020) which introduced a series of consensus- and evidence-based

Evidence-based recommendation
We **recommend** that sub-gingival instrumentation **be employed** to treat periodontitis in order to reduce probing pocket depths, gingival inflammation and the number of diseased sites.
Supporting literature Suvan et al.
Quality of evidence: One 3-month RCT (n = 169 patients); 11 prospective studies (n = 258) ≥6 months
Grade of recommendation grade A – ↑↑
Strength of consensus unanimous consensus (2.6% of the group abstained due to potential CoI)
BSP implementation
*This evidence-based recommendation is **adopted.***
We recommend that sub-gingival instrumentation be employed to treat periodontitis in order to reduce gingival inflammation, the number of diseased sites and probing pocket depths.
Updated evidence: No new applicable evidence was identified
Strength of consensus: *unanimous Consensus* (0% abstentions due to potential CoI)

• **Figure 5.2.1** EFP Clinical Recommendation (British Society of Periodontology and Implant Dentistry (BSP) implementation) with respect to the benefits of subgingival instrumentation in the treatment of periodontitis. *CoI, conflict of interest.* (image courtesy of BSP).

clinical recommendations (CRs) and included the introduction of a *stepwise* approach to the management of periodontitis patients. The process is explained in more detail in Chapter 4.3, and the CRs relevant to periodontal instrumentation will be described in this chapter.

Treatment Objectives

As we have seen in the previous chapter (Chapter 5.1), the principal objective of all forms of periodontal therapy is the decontamination of the diseased root surface and the prevention of its bacterial recolonisation (Lindhe & Echeverria 1993) to allow resolution of the inflammatory lesion in the soft tissues and arrest the destructive disease process. In the 2021 EFP S3 clinical guideline the second step of therapy in the stepwise approach (also referred to as "cause-related therapy") centres on periodontal instrumentation as a means of reducing the bacterial load on the root surface that is responsible for triggering the periodontal disease process. The EFP S3 clinical guideline considered a systematic review carried out by Suvan et al. (2020) which had examined whether subgingival instrumentation (SI) was beneficial for the treatment of periodontitis, and this resulted in a CR which strongly recommended the use of SI to reduce gingival inflammation, the number of diseased sites and probing pocket depths (see Figure 5.2.1).

KEY POINT 1

The principal objective of all forms of periodontal therapy is the decontamination of the diseased root surface.

The main source of bacterial contaminants on the root surface is the bacterial biofilm. It is therefore widely accepted that mechanical biofilm removal is the cornerstone of successful periodontal therapy (Chapple 2009, Guentsch & Preshaw 2008). In the past, emphasis has been placed on the removal of all subgingival calculus deposits. The association of subgingival calculus with periodontal lesions has led to the assumption that there is a cause and effect relationship between the two; a review of the evidence, however (Jepsen et al. 2011), has shown that calculus is the result of disease and not its cause and that healing can occur in the presence of calculus as long as the overlying bacterial biofilm is removed. Calculus can be thought of as an inert material and, clinically, it can be observed that healing of the periodontal lesion can take place and gingival shrinkage exposes previously subgingival calculus in the absence of subgingival calculus removal, providing there is optimal biofilm control by the patient during the oral hygiene phase of treatment (see Chapter 5.1). The removal of calculus then becomes necessary for better access to the subgingival biofilm and for aesthetics. Biofilm removal is therefore more important than calculus removal (Kocher et al. 2001).

KEY POINT 2

Biofilm removal is more important than calculus removal.

Similarly, the original concept of the need to remove the outer layer of root cementum, which was assumed to retain bacteria and their toxins, by means of planing the root surface with highly sharpened hand instruments, as was advocated in the dental literature in 1913 (Hartzell 1913) and has remained largely unchanged over the last century, has been shown by more recent evidence to be both harmful and unnecessary. The World Workshop in Periodontology (Cobb 1996) stated: "Aggressive root planing to remove cementum does not seem to be warranted".

Although such techniques have persisted, largely because they have been found to be effective because the biofilm is also removed during these procedures, there has been an increasing acceptance over recent years, in light of new evidence, that such treatment is overly destructive to the dental tissues, is excessively time consuming and causes unnecessary discomfort for the patient. Thus it has been found that equally effective clinical outcomes can be achieved by less invasive approaches in a shorter time by using different forms of instrumentation which are less technically demanding than traditional hand instrumentation techniques.

From the early 1980s onwards, studies have shown that bacterial toxins were only loosely adherent to the root surface and could be removed by much lighter instrumentation which did not damage the root surface to the same extent as root planing (Nakib et al. 1982, Ito et al. 1985, Hughes & Smales 1986, 1990, Moore et al. 1986, Nyman et al. 1988). One in vitro study (Moore et al. 1986) showed that over 99% of the bacterial contaminants could be removed by light instrumentation alone without the need for cementum removal by root planing. This led to the concept of root surface debridement (RSD) (Cheetham et al. 1988, Smart et al. 1990) as an alternative to root planing, the goal being the achievement of a biocompatible root surface without the removal of tooth structure. It was shown that RSD had the potential to achieve the same level of root surface decontamination as root planing but with the advantages of conservation of tooth structure, shorter treatment time and greater patient comfort. The study by Smart et al. (1990) showed that less than 1 second per mm^2 of debridement of the root surface, using ultrasonics alone, was required to render the root surface entirely toxin free. This amounted to a mean of 17 seconds instrumentation per diseased root surface. In addition, the concept of RSD allowed for the exclusive use of ultrasonic instrumentation, because there was no need to remove cementum by hand planing.

However there is some confusion about the meaning of the terminology used to describe different non-surgical treatment techniques, and this will be addressed in the next section.

Terminology and Definitions

The following terms will be found in the dental literature and they have different meanings, so they should not be used synonymously. Where appropriate, the definitions given here have been taken from the Medical Subject Headings (MeSH) pages of the National Library of Medicine website.

Dental Scaling

Dental scaling is instrumentation to "remove dental plaque and dental calculus from the surface of a tooth, from the surface of a tooth apical to the gingival margin accumulated in periodontal pockets, or from the surface coronal to the gingival margin" (MeSH, introduced 1991).

Root Planing (RP)

Root planing is "a procedure for smoothing of the roughened surface or cementum of a tooth after subgingival curettage or scaling, as part of periodontal therapy" (MeSH, introduced 1992). It is a technique of instrumentation by which cementum is removed and the root surface is made hard and smooth. This is usually done by hand instrumentation using sharpened blades. Because of the length of time involved in achieving the goal of a hard and smooth root surface, the treatment is usually carried out by quadrant, typically 45–60 minutes per quadrant (Palmer & Floyd 2006), using local anaesthesia. It is sometimes referred to as scaling and root planing (SRP) or quadrant scaling and root planing (QSRP).

Periodontal Debridement (PD)

Periodontal debridement (PD) is the term that has now replaced the original term root surface debridement (RSD), and it is defined as "the removal or disruption of dental deposits and plaque-retentive dental calculus from tooth surfaces and within the periodontal pocket space without deliberate removal of cementum as done in RP and often in dental scaling. The goal is to conserve dental cementum to help maintain or re-establish a healthy periodontal environment and eliminate periodontitis by using light instrumentation strokes and non-surgical techniques (e.g. ultrasonic, laser instruments)" (MeSH, introduced 2011).

KEY POINT 3

Periodontal debridement (PD) is the removal or disruption of dental deposits and plaque-retentive dental calculus from tooth surfaces and within the periodontal pocket space without deliberate removal of cementum.

Subgingival Instrumentation (SI)

In view of the confusion that was inevitably caused using so many different terms in the scientific literature to describe decontamination of the root surface, the 2021 EFP S3 clinical guideline agreed to use the term subgingival instrumentation (SI) for all non-surgical procedures performed by hand (i.e. curettes) or power-driven (i.e. sonic/ultrasonic devices) instruments that are specifically designed to gain access to the root surfaces in the subgingival environment.

Full-Mouth Disinfection (FMD)

Full-mouth disinfection (FMD) is a specific technique that was proposed by a group of researchers who compared full-mouth instrumentation (all diseased root surfaces treated within a 24-hour period) and quadrant-by-quadrant instrumentation, using chlorhexidine gluconate extensively in the full-mouth test groups (Bollen et al. 1998, Mongardini et al. 1999, Quirynen et al. 1999).

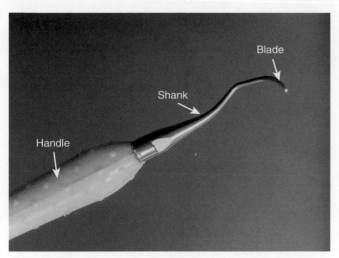

• **Figure 5.2.2** Hand instrument – handle, shank, blade.

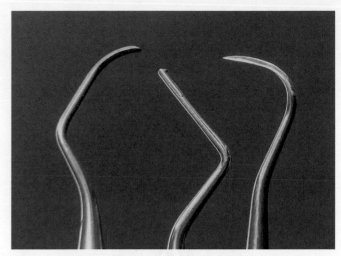

• **Figure 5.2.3** Curette, hoe, scaler from left to right.

Full-Mouth Ultrasonic Debridement (FMUD)

Full-mouth ultrasonic debridement (FMUD) is a full-mouth treatment carried out in one session, using ultrasonic instrumentation alone and a debridement (conserving tooth structure) technique.

Types of Instruments

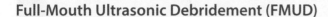

Hand Instruments

Hand instruments usually take the form of scalers, curettes and hoes which have sharpened blades that permit the removal of the root surface. All hand instruments consist of a handle, shank and blade (Figure 5.2.2).

Types

Scalers
Scalers, sometimes referred to as sickle scalers, have a curved or straight blade with a triangular cross-section and two cutting edges. They are usually used for supragingival instrumentation or instrumentation in shallow pockets (Figure 5.2.3).

Curettes
Curettes have a curved blade with curved cutting edges. They are usually double-ended with mirrored angles to the blades and come in a variety of shank lengths and angles and a variety of blade sizes. They are mostly used for subgingival root instrumentation (see Figure 5.2.3).

Hoes
The hoe has only one cutting edge, which is angled at over 90 degrees to the shank. It is used mostly for supragingival scaling (see Figure 5.2.3).

Methods
The methods used to hand instrument the root surface are analogous to those used to plane a piece of wood using a

carpenter's wood plane. Thus, the blade is maintained at an approximately 45-degree angle to the root surface and drawn along the root surface using pressure against the root surface to remove the surface layer, along with calcified (calculus) and uncalcified (biofilm) dental deposits (Figure 5.2.4). A pen grip and finger rest should be used.

This is a technically demanding process which requires a high degree of clinical skill in order to be effective, and the instruments need to be repeatedly sharpened (using a sterilised sharpening stone chairside) during the treatment because of the rapid blunting of the blades. Repeated overlapping strokes are performed to cover the entire root surface of the periodontal pocket, starting at the base of the pocket and proceeding coronally with each stroke. Local anaesthesia is usually required for such procedures, hence the need to treat the mouth quadrant by quadrant in most cases.

Machine-Driven Instruments

Machine-driven instruments take the form of a metal tip vibrating at sonic or ultrasonic frequencies, thereby disrupting both hard (calculus) and soft (biofilm) deposits from the root surface, if used correctly, without causing any loss of tooth structure. In all forms of machine-driven instrumentation, the vibrating tip is cooled by a water supply. Ultrasonic devices for non-surgical periodontal therapy were introduced in the 1950s.

Types

Sonic Scalers
Sonic scalers (Figure 5.2.5) use air pressure to create a mechanically vibrating tip at 2–6 kHz (Gankerseer & Walmsley 1987) which disrupts biofilm and removes calculus deposits from the tooth surface.

Ultrasonic Scalers
Ultrasonic scalers (Figure 5.2.6) have vibrating tips which operate at frequencies of between 18 and 45 kHz by using

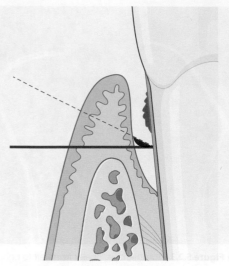

• **Figure 5.2.4** Curette against a root surface.

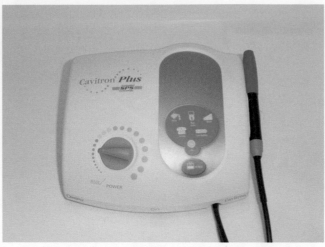

• **Figure 5.2.6** Magnetostrictive ultrasonic scaler.

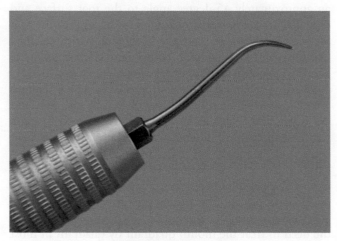

• **Figure 5.2.5** Sonic scaler.

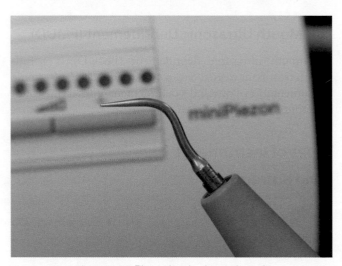

• **Figure 5.2.7** Piezo-electric ultrasonic scaler.

the conversion of electrical energy to mechanical energy. There are two main types of ultrasonic scalers – magnetostrictive and piezo-electric. As the physical action of the tip on the biofilm and calculus deposits on the root surface, ultrasonic instrumentation may also have cavitational and acoustic microstreaming effects that may also cause disruption of surface deposits.

Magnetostrictive

In this type of ultrasonic scaler, the electrical current produces a magnetic field in the handpiece that causes the insert to expand and contract and thus lead to vibration of the metal tip. The movement of the vibrating tip has an elliptical pattern.

Piezo-Electric

In piezo-electric scalers (Figure 5.2.7), the electric current leads to a dimensional change in the hand piece which is translated into vibration of the metal tip of the instrument. The tip movement is also elliptical (Lea et al. 2009).

Methods

All forms of machine-driven instruments should be used in the same way, with the metal tip of the instrument used parallel to the root surface and the entire root surface debrided using a series of light, overlapping strokes, usually in a "cross-hatching" form. The objective is to disrupt the entire biofilm and remove as much subgingival calculus as possible but without causing any damage to the root surface.

Other Types of Power-Driven Instruments

Vector

The Vector ultrasonic instrumentation system is a unique form of ultrasonic instrument that uses a resonating ring around a fine tip to deflect the horizontal oscillations vertically, producing a linear oscillating movement of the tip. The frequency used is 25 kHz. The system must be used in conjunction with a suspension of hydroxyapatite particles in water. This is capable of removing or disrupting the biofilm and removing subgingival calculus and causes no damage to the root surface. The main advantages are little heat development at the tip, no pathogenic aerosol and improved tactile sensation (Sculean et al. 2004). A review of studies that have investigated this system has shown that it is an effective method of treatment for periodontitis and results in similar clinical improvements to those achieved by other methods of periodontal therapy (Guentsch & Preshaw 2008).

Lasers

Dental laser systems are available in a number of forms (carbon dioxide, Er:YAG, Nd:YAG) and are used in a variety of clinical situations for treating both hard and soft tissues. Soft tissue lasers can be used for simple forms of periodontal surgery where the bone is not exposed. In non-surgical periodontal therapy, the system with the most promising potential use is the Er:YAG system which is a hard tissue laser, the goal being biofilm and calculus removal. However, there is the potential for damage to the root surface using this type of system. A review of the literature on lasers in periodontal therapy (Cobb 2006) concluded that there was insufficient evidence to suggest that lasers were superior to conventional therapy, either alone or as an adjunct. A statement issued by the American Academy of Periodontology in 2011, on the efficacy of lasers in the non-surgical treatment of chronic inflammatory periodontal diseases, concluded: "Current evidence shows lasers, as a group, to be unpredictable and inconsistent in their ability to reduce subgingival microbial loads beyond that achieved by SRP alone."

Furthermore, the statement highlighted the potential for root surface damage because the root surface is being debrided without being visualised. A prospective randomised controlled trial in 2012 that compared the Er:YAG laser and mechanical debridement found better clinical outcomes for the conventional mechanical debridement approach (Soo et al. 2012). A systematic review by Salvi et al. (2020) found insufficient evidence to recommend adjunctive application of lasers to SI, and the EFP S3 guideline CR (Sanz et al. 2020) was to suggest *not* to use lasers as adjuncts to SI.

Photodynamic Disinfection

Photodynamic disinfection therapy (PDT) is a laser-based treatment that involves the sensitisation of subgingival bacteria with a variety of dyes (for example methylene blue). The dye is taken up by the bacterial cell walls and when the sensitised bacteria are exposed to low energy laser light the dye molecules are dissociated with the subsequent release of oxygen-free radicals that destroy the bacterial cell walls and thus destroy the bacteria (Figure 5.2.8). Although such systems have been shown to be effective in vitro, results from clinical studies have been less convincing. A 2010 systematic review of the studies that have investigated the use of such systems, both as a stand-alone treatment or as an adjunct to conventional instrumentation, found that there was no evidence of the efficacy of PDT in periodontal therapy and concluded that the routine use of such systems could not be recommended (Azarpazhooh et al. 2010). A systematic review by Salvi et al. (2020) found insufficient evidence to recommend the use of PDT as an adjunct to SI, and the EFP S3 guideline CR (Sanz et al. 2020) suggested *not* to use PDT as adjuncts to SI.

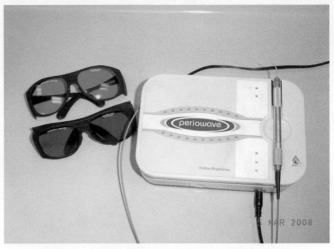

• **Figure 5.2.8** PerioWave system.

Subgingival Air Polishing

Subgingival air polishing has been developed from the concept of supragingival stain removal using sodium bicarbonate powder sprayed under pressure. In subgingival use, such systems would damage the root surface so a much finer glycine powder (20 μm particles) has replaced sodium bicarbonate and the pressure reduced by a disposable nozzle design (Figure 5.2.9). This system is not capable of removing calculus, simply of disrupting the bacterial biofilm and, to date, it has not been evaluated as a means of initial therapy but as an alternative to supportive therapy using conventional forms of instrumentation. In this context, it has been shown to be safe, more acceptable to patients and more time efficient (Moëne et al. 2010) and as effective as ultrasonic debridement (Wennström et al. 2011).

Instrumentation Strategies

Several decisions about the instrumentation strategy need to be made before commencing treatment:
1. Whether a PD or RP technique is to be used
2. Which is the most suitable instrument to use
3. Whether local anaesthesia is required
4. Whether a full-mouth or quadrant-by-quadrant approach is to be taken.

RP or PD – Choice of Instruments

The clinician needs to decide at the outset exactly what the therapeutic objectives are; if it is the intention to debride the root surface but preserve tooth structure, then a suitable debridement instrument should be chosen, but if it is intended to remove the outer layer of cementum, then a planing instrument should be chosen. Used correctly the ultrasonic tip is the most suitable debridement instrument because it does not damage or remove any root surface. If RP is the goal, then a variety of sharpened hand instruments should be used. It is not logical to attempt debridement with a sharpened hand instrument because removal of some tooth structure is inevitable, nor is it possible to plane roots with

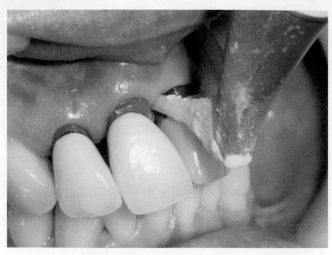

• **Figure 5.2.9** PerioFlow tip in use.

an ultrasonic tip. An analogy would be to attempt to clean a wood surface with a wood plane but without removing any of the wood surface. The choice of instrumentation for non-surgical therapy is therefore determined by the choice of RP or PD as a treatment strategy. Given that the main objective of therapy is biofilm disruption, with calculus removal where possible and conservation of tooth structure, the instrument of choice would appear to be the ultrasonic tip, and it is difficult, if not impossible, to justify the use of hand instruments in modern non-surgical periodontal therapy. However, it is worth considering whether any clinical studies have shown any benefits of hand instrumentation.

KEY POINT 4
Used correctly, the ultrasonic tip is the most suitable debridement instrument because it does not damage the root surface.

Hand vs Ultrasonic Instrumentation

Several studies have directly compared hand and machine-driven instruments in non-surgical periodontal therapy. In all such studies, ultrasonic or sonic instrumentation has been shown to produce equal or superior clinical outcomes (e.g. Lie & Meyer 1977, Iouanniou et al. 2009). Several studies have reported on the increased time savings and therefore cost-effectiveness of ultrasonic instrumentation, showing 20–50% time savings (Checchi & Pelliconi 1988, Dragoo 1992, Copulos et al. 1993, Drisko 1995). A systematic review of the literature in 2002 (Tunkel et al. 2002) found no difference in the efficacy of subgingival debridement whether using hand or machine-driven instruments, a finding that was repeated in the systematic review by Suvan et al. (2020). Greater comfort of ultrasonic devices for patients, with less postoperative pain, has also been noted (Iouanniou et al. 2009). One of the arguments for using hand instruments has been the production of greater root surface smoothness; although hand instruments have been shown to produce smoother root surfaces than ultrasonic instruments (Schmidlin et al. 2001), there is no

evidence that a smooth surface is necessarily a clean surface or that a smooth surface is a necessary end point for successful therapy (Cobb 2002). It has therefore been stated that: "When one considers the demands of clinical skill, time and stamina, the instrument of choice for universal application would appear to be either a sonic or ultrasonic scaler" (Cobb 2002).

KEY POINT 5
"When one considers the demands of clinical skill, time and stamina, the instrument of choice for universal application would appear to be either a sonic or ultrasonic scaler" (Cobb 2002).

Use of Anaesthesia

Traditionally, local anaesthesia has been used to carry out root surface instrumentation, but this has been based on the traditional use of sharpened hand instruments to carry out a RP technique which, being an invasive and tooth-destructive procedure, has necessitated some form of anaesthesia. Although the use of local anaesthesia improves patient comfort, under these circumstances there are a number of disadvantages relating to its use: first, the use of local anaesthesia has forced clinicians into partial mouth treatment strategies (since it is impractical to anaesthetise the entire mouth in a single session) which has resulted in the traditional QSRP approach. Thus the mouth is treated by quadrant over four visits, under local anaesthesia, with 45–60 minutes treatment time per visit. Second, there is a risk of greater iatrogenic damage to the root surface and soft tissues if the area is anaesthetised. As a result, patients often experience pain of significant duration and magnitude following scaling and RP (Pihlstrom et al. 1999). However, machine-driven instrumentation is non-invasive, as tooth structure is preserved, and local anaesthesia is usually not needed. Some patients may have individual teeth where there is some dentinal sensitivity, but this can usually be alleviated with desensitising agents and dietary control and by using the instrument at lower power and with a reduced water supply. The shorter treatment time needed for machine-driven instrumentation and the reduced need for anaesthesia also permits the use of full-mouth treatment strategies, where all diseased sites are treated at a single clinical session.

Full-Mouth or Quadrant Approaches?

A series of studies carried out in the late 1990s questioned the biological rationale of the quadrant approach to non-surgical periodontal therapy, suggesting that there was a risk of reinfection of treated sites by microorganisms from untreated sites, and proposed a "full-mouth approach" as an alternative, the object being to instrument all pathological pockets at a single session, or within a 24-hour period (Quirynen et al. 1995, 1999, Bollen et al. 1996, 1998, Vandekerckhove et al. 1996, Mongardini et al. 1999). The results of these studies showed that the full-mouth-treated patients achieved better clinical and microbiological treatment outcomes. The patients in these studies were treated using a RP instrumentation technique, and the full-mouth-treated groups also received extensive chlorhexidine gluconate application as an adjunct, both during and after treatment. The test treatment was referred to as FMD. Later studies showed that the benefits of the test treatments were because of the full-mouth approach and not because of the use of chemical adjuncts (Quirynen et al. 2000). Subsequent studies (Koshy et al. 2005) used a full-mouth debridement technique with ultrasonics exclusively for both test and control groups (FMUD vs QUD) and achieved the same results. The efficacy of the full-mouth approach was confirmed in a 2008 Cochrane systematic review (Eberhard et al. 2008). Several studies have directly compared FMUD with QSRP (Wennström et al. 2005, Zanatta et al. 2006, Del Peloso Ribiero et al. 2008) and have found that an hour (or less) of the FMUD treatment is as effective (clinically, microbiologically and immunologically) as 4 hours of QSRP and "offers tangible benefits for the chronic periodontitis patient" (Wennstrom et al. 2005). However in terms of clinical treatment outcomes (reduction in inflammation, pocket depth and number of diseased sites) there would appear to be little or no difference between quadrant or full-mouth approaches, and the EFP S3 clinical guideline (Sanz et al. 2020, West et al. 2021) suggested that SI can be carried out with either approach, based on the systematic review by Suvan et al. (2020). One argument against the full-mouth approach has been the possibility that this treatment strategy may produce a systemic acute-phase inflammatory response that may have the potential to be harmful to patients, especially those with vascular co-morbidities. One study (Graziani et al. 2015) has shown that full-mouth treatment may trigger a moderate acute-phase response compared to a quadrant approach. The significance of this finding is unclear at this time.

KEY POINT 6
An hour (or less) of FMUD treatment is as effective (clinically, microbiologically and immunologically) as 4 hours of QSRP.

Adjuncts to Periodontal Instrumentation

A number of chemical and host-modulating agents have been investigated as adjuncts to enhance the effects of SI. These agents have included:

- antiseptics such as chlorhexidine gluconate
- statin gels
- probiotics
- sub-antimicrobial dose doxycycline (SDD)
- locally delivered bisphosphonate (BP) gels or systemic BPs
- local or systemic non-steroidal anti-inflammatory drugs (NSAIDs)
- omega-3 polyunsaturated fatty acids (PUFA)
- metformin gel

An extensive systematic review by Donos et al. (2019) found that, with the exception of chlorhexidine gluconate

(CHX) in various formulations, none of these putative adjuncts to SI offered any benefits as adjuncts to SI and none was recommended as such by the EFP S3 clinical guideline (Sanz et al. 2020). With respect to CHX, the EFP S3 clinical guideline considered that CHX mouth rinse, used for a limited time period, could be considered as an adjunct to SI in specific cases (da Costa et al. 2017). An example of such a case might be a patient who presented with extensive marginal inflammation that prevented them from carrying out adequate self-care at home. The EFP guideline also found that locally delivered sustained-release CHX could be considered in patients with periodontitis (Herrera et al. 2020), although the clinical benefits remained small, amounting to a pocket reduction effect of only about 10%.

Conclusions

The principal objective of non-surgical therapy (or surgical therapy for that matter) is the disinfection of the periodontally involved root surface (Lindhe & Echeverria 1993). The main source of microbial contamination on the root surface is the bacterial biofilm, and it is biofilm disruption/removal that is the treatment goal. Removal of root surface calculus can enhance biofilm removal, but subgingival calculus does not per se have pathogenic potential. It is no longer justified to remove root surface cementum. The choice of instrumentation should reflect these treatment objectives, and there is a strong case for not treating root surfaces with potentially damaging hand instruments but instead to use lighter forms of instrumentation such as ultrasonic devices.

KEY POINT 7
The main source of microbial contamination on the root surface is the bacterial biofilm, and it is biofilm disruption/removal that is the treatment goal.

Multiple choice questions on the contents of this chapter are available online at Elsevier eBooks+.

References

American Academy of Periodontology. Statement on the efficacy of lasers in the non-surgical treatment of inflammatory periodontal disease (2011). *J Periodontol.* 2011;82:513–514.

Azarpazhooh A, Shah PS, Tenenbaum HC, Goldberg MB. The effect of photodynamic therapy for periodontitis: a systematic review and meta-analysis. *J Periodontol.* 2010;61:4–14.

Bollen CM, Vandekerckhove BN, Papaioannou W, Van Eldere J, Quirynen M. Full- versus partial-mouth disinfection in the treatment of periodontal infections. A pilot study: long-term microbiological observations. *J Clin Periodontol.* 1996;23:960–970.

Bollen CML, Mongardini C, Papaioannou W, van Steenberghe D, Quirynen M. The effect of a one-stage full-mouth disinfection on different intra-oral niches. Clinical and microbiological observations. *J Clin Periodontol.* 1998;25:56–66.

Chapple ILC. Periodontal diagnosis and treatment – where does the future lie?. *Periodontol 2000*. 2009;51:9–24.

Checchi L, Pelliconi GA. Hand versus ultrasonic instrumentation in the removal of endotoxins from root surfaces in vitro. *J Periodontol*. 1988;56:398–402.

Cheetham WA, Wilson M, Kieser JB. Root surface debridement – an in vitro assessment. *J Clin Periodontol*. 1988;15:288–292.

Cobb CM. Consensus report non-surgical pocket therapy: mechanical, pharmacotherapeutics and occlusion. *Ann Periodontol*. 1996;1:583.

Cobb CM. Clinical significance of non-surgical periodontal therapy: an evidence-based perspective of scaling and root planing. *J Clin Periodontol*. 2002;29(suppl 2):22–32.

Cobb CM. Lasers in periodontics: a review of the literature. *J Periodontol*. 2006;77(4):545–564.

Copulos TA, Low SB, Walker CB, Trebilcock YY, Hefti AF. Comparative analysis between a modified ultrasonic tip and hand instruments on clinical parameters of periodontal disease. *J Periodontol*. 1993;64:694–700.

da Costa L, Amaral C, Barbirato D, Leão A, Fogacci M. Chlorhexidine mouthwash as an adjunct to mechanical therapy in chronic periodontitis: a meta- analysis. *J Am Dent Assoc*. 2017;148(5):308–318.

Del Peloso Ribeiro É, Bittencourt S, Sallum EA, Nociti Jr FH, Goncalves RB, Casati MZ. Periodontal debridement as a therapeutic approach for severe chronic periodontitis: a clinical, microbiological and immunological study. *J Clin Periodontol*. 2008;35:789–798.

Donos N, Calciolari E, Brusselaers N, Goldoni M, Bostanci N, Belibasakis GN. The adjunctive use of host modulators in non-surgical periodontal therapy. A systematic review of randomized, placebo-controlled clinical studies. *Journal of Clinical Periodontology*. 2019;47(Suppl 22):116–238. https://doi.org/10.1111/jcpe.13232.

Dragoo MR. A clinical evaluation of hand and ultrasonic instruments on subgingival debridement. 1. With unmodified and modified ultrasonic inserts. *Int J Periodontics Restorative Dent*. 1992;12:310–323.

Drisko CL. Scaling and root planing without over instrumentation: hand versus power-driven scalers. *Curr Opin Periodontol*. 1995:78–88.

Eberhard J, Jervøe-Storm P-M, Needleman I, Worthington H, Jepsen S. Full-mouth treatment concepts for chronic periodontitis: a systematic review. *J Clin Periodontol*. 2008;35:591–604.

Gankerseer EJ, Walmsley AD. Preliminary investigation into the performance of sonic scalers. *J Periodontol*. 1987;58:780–784.

Graziani F, Cei S, Orlandi M, Gennai S, Gabriele M, Filice N, Nisi M, D'Aiuto F. Acute-phase response following full-mouth versus quadrant non-surgical periodontal treatment: a randomised clinical trial. *J Clin Periodontol*. 2015;42:843–852.

Guentsch A, Preshaw PM. The use of a linear oscillating device in periodontal treatment: a review. *J Clin Periodontol*. 2008;35:514–524.

Hartzell TB. The operative and post-operative treatment of pyorrhea. *Dental Cosmos*. 1913;55:1094–1101.

Herrera D, Matesanz P, Martin C, Oud V, Feres M, Teughels W. Adjunctive effect of locally delivered antimicrobials in periodontitis therapy. A systematic review and meta-analysis. *J Clin Periodontol*. 2020;47(suppl 22):239–256.

Hughes FJ, Smales FC. Immunohistochemical investigation of the presence and distribution of cementum-associated lipopolysaccharides in periodontal disease. *J Periodontal Res*. 1986;21:660–667.

Hughes FJ, Smales FC. The distribution and quantitation of cementum-bound lipopolysaccharide on periodontally diseased root surfaces of human teeth. *Arch Oral Biol*. 1990;35:295–299.

Iouanniou I, Dimitriadis N, Papadimitriou K, Sakellari D, Vouros I, Konstantinidis A. Hand instrumentation versus ultrasonic debridement in the treatment of chronic periodontitis: a randomized clinical and microbiological trial. *J Clin Periodontol*. 2009;36:132–141.

Ito K, Hindman RE, O'Leary TJ, Kafrawy AH. Determination of the presence of root-bound endotoxin using the local Shwartzman phenomenon (LSP). *J Periodontol*. 1985;56:8–17.

Jepsen S, Deschner J, Braun A, Schwarz F, Eberhard J. Calculus removal and the prevention of its formation. *Periodontol 2000*. 2011;55:167–188.

Kocher T, König J, Hansen P, Ruhling A. Subgingival polishing compared to scaling with steel curettes: a clinical pilot study. *J Clin Periodontol*. 2001;28:194–199.

Koshy G, Kawashima Y, Kiji M, Nitta H, Umeda M, Nagasawa T, et al. Effects of single-visit full-mouth ultrasonic debridement versus quadrant-wise ultrasonic debridement. *J Clin Periodontol*. 2005;32:734–743.

Lea SC, Felver B, Landini G, Walmsley AD. Three-dimensional analysis of ultrasonic scaler oscillations. *J Clin Periodontol*. 2009;36:44–50.

Lie T, Meyer K. Calculus removal and loss of tooth substance in response to different periodontal instruments. A scanning electron microscope study. *J Clin Periodontol*. 1977;4:250–262.

Lindhe J, Echeverria J. Consensus report of session II. In: *Proceedings of the 1st European Workshop on Periodontology*. London: Quintessence; 1993:212.

Moëne R, Décaillet F, Andersen E, Mombelli A. Subgingival plaque removal using a new air-polishing device. *J Periodontol*. 2010;81:79–88.

Mongardini C, Van Steenberghe D, Dekeyser C, Quirynen M. One stage full- versus partial mouth disinfection in the treatment of chronic adult or generalized early-onset periodontitis. 1. Long-term clinical observations. *J Periodontol*. 1999;70:632–645.

Moore J, Wilson M, Kieser JB. The distribution of bacterial lipopolysaccharide (endotoxin) in relation to periodontally involved root surfaces. *J Clin Periodontol*. 1986;13:748–751.

Nakib NM, Bissada NF, Simmelink JW, Goldstine SN. Endotoxin penetration into root cementum of periodontally healthy and diseased teeth. *J Periodontol*. 1982;53:368–378.

Nyman S, Westfelt E, Sarhed G, Karring T. Role of "diseased" root cementum in healing following treatment of periodontal disease. *J Clin Periodontol*. 1988;13:464–468.

Palmer RM, Floyd P. *A Clinical Guide to Periodontology*. 2nd ed. London: BDJ Books; 2006:28.

Pihlstrom BL, Hargreaves KM, Bouwsma OJ, Myers WR, Goodale MB, Doyle MJ. Pain after periodontal scaling and root planing. *J Am Dent Assoc*. 1999;130:801–807.

Quirynen M, Bollen CM, Vandekerckhove BN, Dekeyser C, Papaioannou W, Eyssen H. Full- vs partial-mouth disinfection in the treatment of periodontal infections: short-term clinical and microbiological observations. *J Dent Res*. 1995;74:1459–1467.

Quirynen M, Mongardini C, Pauwels M, Bollen CML, Van Eldere J, van Steenberghe D. One stage full- versus partial-mouth disinfection in the treatment of chronic adult or generalized early-onset periodontitis. 2. Long-term impact on microbial load. *J Periodontol*. 1999;70:646–656.

Quirynen M, Mongardini C, de Soete M, Pauwels M, Coucke W, van Eldere J, et al. The role of chlorhexidine in the one-stage full-mouth disinfection treatment of patients with advanced adult periodontitis. Long-term clinical and microbiological observations. *J Clin Periodontol*. 2000;28:578–589.

Salvi GE, Stahli A, Schmidt JC, Ramseier CA, Sculean A, Walter C. Adjunctive laser or antimicrobial photodynamic therapy to non-surgical mechanical instrumentation in patients with untreated periodontitis. A systematic review and meta-analysis. *J Clin Periodontol.* 2020;47(suppl 22):176–198.

Sanz M, Herrera D, Kebschull M, Chapple I, Jepsen S, Beglundh T, Sculean A, Tonetti M. Treatment of stage I-III periodontitis-The EFP S3 level clinical practice guideline. *J Clin Periodontol.* 2020;47(suppl 22):4–60.

Schmidlin PR, Beuchat M, Bussliger A, Lehmann B, Lutz F. Tooth substance loss resulting from mechanical, sonic and ultrasonic instrumentation assessed by liquid scintillation. *J Clin Periodontol.* 2001;28:1058–1066.

Sculean A, Schwarz F, Berakdar M, Romanos GE, Brecx M, Willershausen B, et al. Non-surgical periodontal treatment with a new ultrasonic device (Vector-ultrasonic system) or hand instruments. *J Clin Periodontol.* 2004;31:428–433.

Smart GJ, Wilson M, Kieser JB. The assessment of ultrasonic root surface debridement by determination of residual endotoxin levels. *J Clin Periodontol.* 1990;17:174–178.

Soo L, Leichter JW, Windle J, Monteith B, Williams SM, Seymour GJ, et al. A comparison of Er:YAG laser and mechanical debridement for the non-surgical treatment of chronic periodontitis: a randomized, prospective clinical study. *J Clin Periodontol.* 2012;39:537–545.

Suvan J, Leira Y, Moreno F, Graziani F, Derks J, Tomasi C. Subgingival instrumentation for treatment of periodontitis. A systematic review. *J Clin Periodontol.* 2020;47(suppl 22):155–175.

Tunkel J, Heinecke A, Flemmig TF. A systematic review of efficacy of machine-driven and manual subgingival debridement in the treatment of chronic periodontitis. *J Clin Periodontol.* 2002;13(suppl 3): 72–81.

Vandekerckhove BN, Bollen CM, Dekeyser C, Darius P, Quirynen M. Full- versus partial-mouth disinfection in the treatment of periodontal infections. Long-term clinical observations in a pilot study. *J Periodontol.* 1996;67:1251–1259.

Wennström JL, Tomasi C, Bertelle A, Dellasega E. Full-mouth ultrasonic debridement versus quadrant scaling and root planing as an initial approach in the treatment of chronic periodontitis. *J Clin Periodontol.* 2005;32:851–859.

Wennström JL, Dahlén G, Ramberg P. Subgingival debridement of periodontal pockets by air polishing in comparison with ultrasonic instrumentation during maintenance therapy. *J Clin Periodontol.* 2011;38:820–827.

West N, Chapple I, Claydon N, D'Aiuto F, Donos N, Ide M, Needleman I, Kebschull M. BSP implementation of European S3 - level evidence-based treatment guidelines for stage I-III periodontitis in UK clinical practice. *J Dent.* 2021;106:1–72:103562. https://doi.org/10.1016/j.jdent.2020.103562.

Zanatta GM, Bittencourt S, Nociti FH, Sallum EA, Sallum AW, Casati MZ. Periodontal debridement with povidone-iodine in periodontal treatment: short-term clinical and biochemical observations. *J Periodontol.* 2006;77:498–505.

5.3

ANTIBIOTICS IN THE MANAGEMENT OF PERIODONTAL DISEASES

ANDREW WALKER

CHAPTER OUTLINE

OVERVIEW OF THE CHAPTER

This chapter will explore the rationale for antibiotic use and indicate which periodontal conditions can be treated with antibiotics. It will examine the reasons for failure of root surface debridement (RSD) and assess the role of antibiotics as an alternative monotherapy to RSD. Local and systemic delivery of antibiotics will be compared, with reference to current evidence, and evaluation of such studies will be discussed. Current evidence to support or refute antibiotic use in daily practice will then be examined.

By the end of the chapter the reader should:

- Understand why RSD sometimes fails
- Recognise when it might be appropriate to use antibiotics in periodontal therapy
- Be able to evaluate studies which investigate antibiotic use in periodontal therapy.

The chapter covers the following topics:

- The rationale for antibiotic use
- Which periodontal conditions can be treated with antibiotics
- Reasons for the failure of RSD
- Antibiotics as an alternative monotherapy to RSD
- Comparison of local or systemic delivery of antibiotics
- Evaluating studies which use antibiotics as adjuncts to RSD
- The evidence for antibiotic use in periodontal therapy
- Recommendations on the use of antibiotics.

The Rationale for Antibiotic use

If it is believed that periodontal diseases are infections (which is in fact debatable – see Chapter 1.2), then we need to focus on controlling the infection in much the same way as we would control infection elsewhere in the body.

It is helpful to think of periodontitis as having parallels with an open wound on the forearm. Basic concepts of managing the forearm wound would involve debridement to remove foreign bodies and reduce bacterial load. If this does not succeed, we may employ chemicals in the form of antiseptics or antibiotics. Failure of these procedures to resolve the problem might result in the need for surgical excision to remove infected tissue. The wound can then be closed with healthy margins being opposed. If infection of the wound has become advanced, then more radical excision may need to be considered, which could include amputation of the limb. The parallels with periodontal management are clear:

1. wound debridement = root surface debridement
2. antiseptics or antibiotics = antiseptics or antibiotics

3. excision of wound margins = periodontal surgery
4. limb amputation = tooth extraction.

The sites which most commonly fail to respond to RSD are usually difficult to instrument, and this may be because the pocket depth is deep, there are multiple roots or there are infra-bony defects. This may result in an inability to reach and disrupt the biofilm in these areas. There may be a need for chemical agents, such as antibiotics, to act as an adjunct to the mechanical debridement at such sites. An alternative form of treatment would be periodontal surgery, which needs a higher level of training and skill, is more costly and more invasive. Therefore, if the effects of non-surgical periodontal therapy could be improved by the use of adjunctive antimicrobial therapies, it might be possible to achieve healthy tissues without the need for invasive surgical techniques.

Since bacteria are the initiating agents of periodontal diseases, systemically or locally administered antibiotics are considered as possible adjuncts for their control. However, studies on the efficacy of these agents show inconsistent results.

KEY POINT 1

Sites which most commonly fail to respond to root surface debridement are usually difficult to instrument.

KEY POINT 2

There may be a need for chemical agents such as antibiotics to act as an adjunct to mechanical debridement at non-responding sites.

KEY POINT 3

Because bacteria are the initiating agents of periodontal diseases, systemically or locally administered antibiotics are considered as possible adjuncts for their control. However, studies on the efficacy of these agents show inconsistent results.

Which Periodontal Conditions can be Treated with Antibiotics?

Several classification systems have been used over the years, and in 2017 a new worldwide classification system was introduced. Under the new classification (Tonetti & Sanz 2019, Dietrich et al. 2019), the first part of diagnosis involves *staging* the periodontitis by assessing the degree of bone loss. This allows the periodontitis to be classified as either initial (I), moderate (II), severe (III) or very severe (IV). The speed of progression is then estimated by comparing the bone loss against the age of the patient. The speed of progression is *graded* as slow (A), moderate (B), or rapid (C). For further information about the most recent classification, see Chapter 2.1.

Within the latest classification system, more acute conditions exist, such as necrotising periodontal diseases, abscesses of the periodontium and periodontitis associated with endodontic lesions. Although it may be tempting for the clinician to prescribe antibiotics immediately for these conditions, it is important to adhere to the principles for the management of infections in general. This focuses on removing the source of infection and establishing drainage when possible. Depending upon the clinical circumstances, this may be achieved through incision of the mucosa, debridement of the pocket or a pulpal access cavity. These actions along with mechanical debridement reduce the bacterial load and allow wound healing to occur in most instances. The presence of pyrexia, lymph node involvement and swelling in the fascial spaces may require the use of antibiotics, but this should be the exception rather than the norm.

KEY POINT 4

The presence of pyrexia, lymph node involvement and swelling in the fascial spaces may require the use of antibiotics, but this should be the exception rather than the norm.

Most periodontal treatment is focused on mild, moderate, or severe periodontitis (stages I–III), with a small but important percentage having very severe periodontitis (stage IV). Hospital and specialist practices may also encounter patients who have periodontitis as a manifestation of systemic disease. The use of antibiotics has been considered a possibility for the management of most types of periodontitis, apart from the most mild forms.

Reasons for the Failure of Root Surface Debridement

The conventional treatment of periodontal diseases involves cause-related therapy, directed at reducing the bacterial load. The objective is to cause a shift in the microflora of the gingival sulcus/pocket to one that is compatible with gingival health, allowing inflammatory resolution. Non-surgical periodontal therapy includes oral hygiene advice and professional debridement of the gum pocket (see Chapter 5.2). For most patients, this approach is effective, but the outcome varies depending upon the original pocket depth.

If the poor response is widespread then operator and patient-based factors should be considered. If sites have responded and others are refractory to treatment, then more local factors should be considered. Common causes for a poor response to RSD include:

1. Operator factors
   a. poor-quality RSD performed
   b. inexperienced operator
   c. not enough time allocated to instrument adequately all the sites
2. Patient factors
   a. poor oral hygiene
   b. smoking
   c. systemic diseases such as diabetes giving a poor response to treatment
3. Site factors
   a. very deep pockets, where the operator fails to instrument to the base
   b. intra-bony defects where the base is inaccessible without surgical access
   c. tooth and root morphology, such as furcation defects, grooves and hollows

4. Bacterial invasion of the tissues
   a. gingiva
   b. dentinal tubules.

If response has been poor, then further treatment options should be considered, including:

1. a second cycle of RSD
2. a second cycle of RSD with adjunctive antimicrobials
3. periodontal surgery
4. supportive periodontal care
5. extraction.

Periodontal therapy often results in pocket reduction, but it is common to find residual pockets of 4–5 mm post-treatment. At this stage, if the oral hygiene is good and there is no bleeding on probing, such pockets can be maintained with appropriate supportive periodontal care. It has been suggested that sites with pockets ≥6 mm have an increased risk of disease progression and an increased risk of tooth loss. As a consequence, this should be "viewed as incomplete periodontal treatment" (Matuliene et al. 2010) and further treatment should be provided.

Since bacteria have a causative role in periodontal disease aetiology, the use of antibiotics in therapy can be considered. Extensive research has investigated a wide range of drugs, at varying dosages, for different time periods, using different routes of administration, to patients with different forms of periodontal diseases. These have been evaluated both as adjuncts to non-surgical and surgical treatments and as monotherapies in the absence of RSD.

Antibiotics as an Alternative Monotherapy to RSD

There has been some research that shows antibiotics as a monotherapy may impact the bacteria and improve periodontal health equivalent to that achieved with RSD in the short term (López et al. 2006). This is a controversial issue, and whilst it does pose an interesting question, a high level of caution must be used when interpreting the results of this study and applying it to clinical practice. There are several flaws in the study by López et al., and for a more in-depth review of the paper the reader is directed to the online content.

Such an approach would flow against the drive for medical professionals to reduce the amount of antibiotics prescribed because of concerns surrounding hypersensitivity and development of resistant strains. Furthermore, using antibiotics as a monotherapy would be contrary to one of the paradigms of clinical periodontology: that RSD is the key intervention to treat periodontal diseases. Indeed, the European Federation of Periodontology S3 level clinical practice guideline (Sanz et.al. 2020), adopted by the British Society of Periodontology and Implant Dentistry (BSP) (West et al. 2021), recommends all periodontitis patients undergo oral hygiene instruction and professional debridement.

TABLE 5.3.1	Comparison of local and systemic antibiotic use	
	Systemic	**Local**
Sites treated	All sites including tongue, tonsillar tissues, etc.	Only treated pockets
Concentration	Spread all over body, lower at sites of interest	High in treated sites
Limitations	Relies on patient compliance, adverse side effects	Re-infection from non-treated sites, problems of GCF washing

GCF: gingival crevicular fluid.

COMPARISON OF LOCAL OR SYSTEMIC DELIVERY OF ANTIBIOTICS

The antibiotic agent needs to be in the right location, with a high enough concentration, for a long enough period of time, to be effective. There are different ways of delivering antimicrobial agents and, in periodontology, there is the choice of either systemic or local delivery. Systemic antibiotics are usually administered orally, and local antibiotics are placed directly into the periodontal pocket by means of a carrier. Comparisons of both delivery systems follow and are summarised in Table 5.3.1.

Systemic antibiotics have the advantage that all sites are treated, including areas such as the tongue and tonsillar crypts, which are areas thought to be implicated in the recolonisation of pockets. The disadvantages are more widespread adverse side effects, achieving high enough drug levels in periodontal pockets and the reliance on patient compliance.

Advantages of local delivery include assured compliance, minimal systemic exposure and drug levels which far exceed the mean inhibitory concentration for key periodontal pathogens. The time that therapeutic drug levels are maintained often depends on the delivery vehicle. Preparations such as gels are washed away from the pocket by gingival crevicular fluid, hence protocols usually recommend a second or third application. More solid vehicles, such as fibres or chips, are retained longer, but then have the problem of adequate and consistent drug release from the vehicle.

A wide range of systemic antibiotics have been evaluated in the management of chronic or aggressive periodontitis, and Table 5.3.2 lists some of the more widely used and investigated.

Local delivery systems include a range of different drugs and vehicles. Gel systems, applied by syringe, include 25% metronidazole and 2% minocycline. These are quickly and easily applied to pockets and can readily be used at multiple sites. However, their substantivity is less assured as they are

TABLE 5.3.2	Systemic antibiotics in the management of periodontal diseases	
Commonly used single therapies	**Combination therapies**	
Metronidazole	Amoxicillin and	
Tetracycline group	metronidazole	
Penicillin group		
Azithromycin		

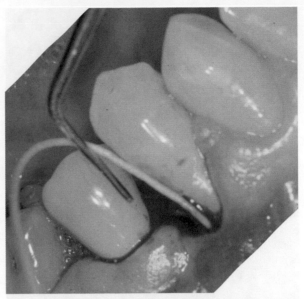

• **Figure 5.3.2** 25% tetracycline hydrochloride.

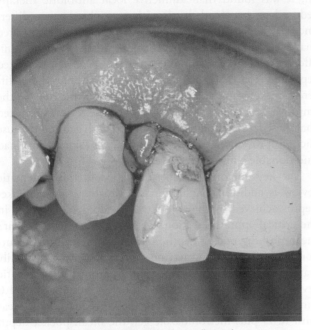

• **Figure 5.3.1** 2% minocycline gel.

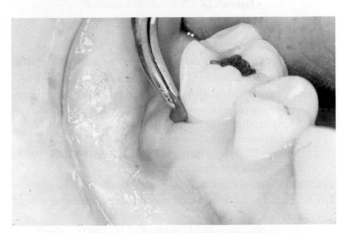

• **Figure 5.3.3** Chlorhexidine chip.

washed out of the pocket by crevicular fluid. Consequently, the protocols recommend that the dosage is repeated on several occasions. Chlorhexidine (2.5 mg) can be applied in a degradable gelatin chip, 25% tetracycline hydrochloride in a non-resorbable fibre and doxycycline hyclate in a gel/sol carrier. Examples of local delivery devices are shown in Figures 5.3.1–5.3.4.

KEY POINT 5

Locally applied systems for antibiotics are quickly and easily applied to pockets and can readily be used at multiple sites. However, their substantivity is less assured as they are washed out of the pocket by crevicular fluid.

Evaluating Studies which use Antibiotics as Adjuncts to RSD

As resistant strains of bacteria emerge, and new antibiotics are produced, it is impossible to provide specific protocols and regimens for clinical practice. Research into both local and systemic antibiotics is constantly published (more than 2000 papers on the subject), and this information is often distributed to the dental profession by manufacturers aiming to support a particular product. It is therefore important

for any professional to be able to critically appraise the literature so that they can provide the most clinically effective, and the most cost-effective, treatment for their patients.

The literature can be confusing, and similar studies undertaken by different research groups can often produce conflicting results. A few key skills in critical appraisal can equip the reader in analysing published papers. These are summarised below, but the reader is encouraged to use the online content for more in-depth guidance.

Carefully examine the research methods presented:

1. Is there a clear objective, asking a question that you are interested in?
   a. "Do antibiotics provide additional benefit when used as an adjunct to RSD?"
   b. "What degree of improvement do antibiotics give over RSD alone and is it clinically relevant?"
2. Are the outcomes clearly defined?
3. Is there a control group and is it appropriate? Was there adequate randomisation between the control and test groups?

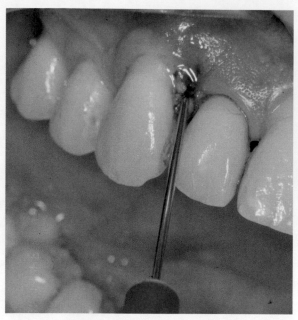

• **Figure 5.3.4** 25% metronidazole gel.

4. Were researchers blinded as to who was in the control and test groups?
5. Has a "power calculation" been performed to help determine appropriate sample size?
   a. Many studies have inadequate sample sizes
   b. Underpowered studies are misleading
   c. Systematic reviews and meta-analysis can to some extent compensate for small sample sizes.

Critical analysis of data:

1. Did the control group achieve the outcomes you would expect?
   a. Are results comparable to the Cobb (2002) review?
2. What is the magnitude of the difference between the test and control group?
   a. Described as a collective mean pocket depth reduction
   b. Subdivided into outcomes for shallow, moderate and deep pockets
3. Can I translate the outcomes to patients in my practice?
   a. The difference between treatment groups is usually described as the mean change in mm, yet we never calculate this for patients
   b. The percentage of sites that needed treatment initially and are then deemed healthy after treatment is a better measure of success:
      i. All sites >3 mm are treated so studies report the change in the number or % of such sites
      ii. Sites <6 mm are considered maintainable (Matuliene et al. 2010); the number or % of sites converting to this depth post-treatment would be another clinically relevant outcome.

> ### KEY POINT 6
> As resistant strains of bacteria emerge, and new antibiotics are produced, it is impossible to provide specific protocols and regimens for clinical practice.

The Evidence for Antibiotic use in Periodontal Therapy

Local Delivery Antibiotics

A systematic review (Matesanz-Pérez et al. 2013) reported on studies that tested one or more chemical antimicrobial agents as an adjunct to RSD alone or in comparison with placebo. Fifty-two studies were reported in 56 publications (some tested more than one antimicrobial agent). Overall, it was found that adjunctive local antibiotic therapy reduced pocket depth levels with a weighted mean difference (WMD) of 0.41 mm. However, the authors indicated that even when the differences were statistically significant, effects were modest in some studies. Data were reported separately for the different antimicrobials, but these differences were described as marginal and a fraction of the improvement achieved by RSD alone. The review suggested that these results should be interpreted with caution because such improvements, even if statistically significant, had questionable clinical relevance.

The key outcome variable described in this systematic review is additional reduction in "weighted mean pocket depth" achieved by the adjunctive therapy. As discussed in the critical appraisal section, we never measure a patient's mean probing pocket depth, and hence the improved outcome of 0.18–0.73 mm is not something we can readily translate to our patients. In one study from this systematic review (Griffiths et al. 2000), RSD alone resulted in a 1.0 mm mean pocket probing depth (PPD) reduction, whereas with RSD plus metronidazole gel, the mean pocket depth reduction was 1.5 mm. Because this means of reporting the data is not ideal, the study by Griffiths et al. (2000) and other more recent studies have tended to present the results using information that clinicians often use in practice. Table 5.3.3 shows the results as a percentage of the sites representing "successful treatment" or sites showing improvement by more than 2 mm.

A more recent systematic review of local antimicrobials (Herrera et al. 2020) reviewed 50 independent investigations and found that there was a range of study designs. The findings of this review were that in short-term studies of 6–9 months, local antimicrobials reduced pocket depth levels with a WMD of 0.37 mm. For longer-term studies (12–60 months) a statistically significant WMD in pocket depth reduction of 0.19 mm was found. Again, the data for individual antimicrobials were presented, as were changes in clinical attachment loss (CAL), and interestingly the data from the long-term studies did not show significant improvement in CAL for any of the antimicrobials.

Overall, the evidence suggests that most of the local adjuncts could confer an additional clinical benefit, and the European S3 level clinical practice guideline advises that they may be considered. However, it should be remembered that the results and conclusions drawn from a systematic review are only as good as the original studies. This was highlighted in the discussion of the 2020 review which also concluded that the high risk of bias and the heterogeneity of the studies makes it very difficult to define when and where such products would be of use. Another aspect the clinician must consider in relation to using a local antimicrobial is careful analysis of the cost of this gain in financial (Heasman et al. 2011) and environmental (Needleman and Wilson 2006) terms.

TABLE 5.3.3	"Clinically relevant measures of successful treatment" as alternatives to mean pocket reduction in studies examining the adjunctive effect of local delivery antibiotics

	RSD	RSD + gel	Difference
Mean reduction in PPD (mm)	1.0	1.5	0.5
% Improved to ≤3 mm	18.0	30.0	12.0
% Improved by ≥2 mm	32.0	47.0	15.0

Adapted from data presented in Griffiths et al. 2000. PPD: pocket probing depth; RSD: root surface debridement; RSD + gel: RSD with adjunctive metronidazole gel.

Systemic Delivery Antibiotics

Two systematic reviews, Herrera et al. (2002) and Haffajee et al. (2003), summarised the literature relating to the role of systemic antibiotics in the management of periodontal diseases defined by the 1999 classification. These reviews revealed that systemic antibiotics were consistently beneficial in providing an improvement in the clinical outcomes of gain in attachment and pocket depth reduction when used as adjuncts to RSD.

Chronic periodontitis (as defined by the 1999 classification): Systemic antibiotics used as an adjunct to RSD were found to offer additional benefits over RSD alone, especially in deep pockets.

Aggressive periodontitis (as defined by the 1999 classification): The limited information available showed that the adjunctive effect of some antimicrobials might be greater in aggressive forms of periodontitis. Figure 5.3.5 shows a patient with aggressive periodontitis who has been treated with systemic antibiotics as an adjunct to RSD.

These conclusions were based on mean change in PPD or mean gain in attachment. The mean gain in attachment was 0.3–0.4 mm at 6 months, but this was based on whole-mouth data and was diluted by the inclusion of healthy sites which would not be expected to change. These mean clinical values may have little clinical relevance, although Haffajee et al. (2003) put it into some clinical context when she described it as "equivalent to reversing 4–7 years of disease progression".

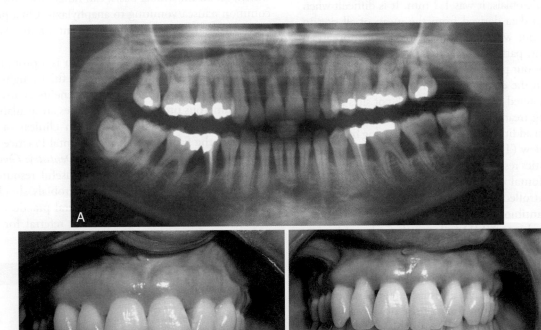

• **Figure 5.3.5** A patient diagnosed at the time with aggressive periodontitis treated with adjunctive systemic antibiotics. (A) Radiographic appearance on presentation. (B) Clinical appearance on presentation. (C) Clinical appearance after treatment.

TABLE 5.3.4	"Clinically relevant measures of successful treatment" as alternatives to mean pocket reduction in studies examining the adjunctive effect of systemic antibiotics.		
	RSD	RSD + adjunctive antimicrobials	Difference (mm)
Mean reduction in PPD (mm)	0.7	1.2	0.5
% Improved to ≤3 mm	37	55	18
% Improved by ≥2 mm	21	30	9

Clinically relevant data adapted from Guerrero et al. (2005) and Griffiths et al. (2011). PPD: pocket probing depth; RSD: root surface debridement; RSD + Adj: RSD plus adjunctive amoxicillin and metronidazole.

As illustrated previously with local delivery antibiotics, more clinically relevant methods of data presentation have been used. This is illustrated in Table 5.3.4, which shows results adapted from Guerrero et al. (2005) and Griffiths et al. (2011), which was a study comparing RSD alone with RSD plus adjunctive amoxicillin and metronidazole in patients with aggressive periodontal disease. The difference in the mean full-mouth PPD before and after RSD was 0.7 mm and, with adjunctive antimicrobials, it was 1.2 mm. It is difficult when using these mean data derived from the mean of all sites in all subjects to decide whether this has clinical relevance to an individual patient, particularly as these are not data that we usually record for our patients. Data presentation using information we use in the clinic showed that adjunctive systemic antimicrobials resulted in an additional 18% of sites converting from needing treatment to not needing treatment. They also resulted in an additional 9% of sites improving by ≥2 mm.

A further review (Teughels et al. 2020) again found that systemic antibiotics result in statistically significant improvements in periodontal parameters. This review identified 28 randomised controlled trials and found that the adjunctive use of systemic antibiotics in the active phase of periodontal treatment resulted in a WMD full-mouth pocket reduction of 0.45 mm and CAL gain of 0.39 mm at 6 months. It further found that these benefits were present for at least a year (PPD WMD 0.49 mm, CAL WMD 0.23). Specific data was reported for different antibiotic regimens, but the strongest evidence was found for the use of a combination of amoxicillin and metronidazole, and this was more pronounced in initially deep pockets. Interestingly, this review was unable to show any statistically significant difference in the benefit of using systemic antimicrobials for aggressive periodontitis over chronic periodontitis.

Similar to previous reviews, Teughels et al. (2020) concluded that it remained debatable whether the improvements found were clinically relevant, and it highlighted the lack of conclusive evidence for the long-term benefit of systemic antimicrobials. It was also noted that the vast majority of studies recruited patients with periodontitis stages III and IV. As such, it remains the case that systemic antibiotics may be considered for the management of periodontitis, but their use should be restricted to certain groups, such as those with severe and progressing forms of periodontitis. The S3 level clinical guideline further advises that systemic antibiotics should not be used routinely but may be considered for specific patient categories, such as generalised periodontitis stage III in young adults where a high rate of progression is documented.

Recommendations on the Use of Systemic Antibiotics in Periodontal Therapy

Despite the large number of research investigations in this area, it is still difficult to provide clear guidance on antibiotic use in periodontics because of small sample sizes and study heterogeneity. It seems clear that antibiotics confer therapeutic advantage, but questions still remain as to whether they should be part of routine use or restricted to individuals with "severe periodontal breakdown".

Further research needs to be undertaken to show efficacy in terms of patient-centred outcomes and cost-effectiveness. The timing of delivery of antibiotics is also important as shown by Griffiths et al. (2011), and this needs further investigation.

Side effects of antibiotic use should be considered, which, on an individual basis, can range from the relatively common nausea/vomiting to anaphylaxis. On a population basis, there are concerns over resistant strains (Feres et al. 2002, Needleman & Wilson 2006).

Appropriate antibiotic stewardship is a prominent issue for dental professionals, and so careful thought must be given to weighing up the risks and benefits of any prescription. Numerous professional guidelines are available to help with the decision-making process in clinical practice. In particular, the Faculty of General Dental Practice UK publication *Antimicrobial Prescribing in Dentistry: Good Practice Guidelines, 3rd Edition (2020)* is a useful resource. Alternative treatment options to antimicrobials should always be considered, and for those in general practice, that may include consideration as to whether referral for specialist opinion and/or treatment is warranted.

KEY POINT 7

Current recommendations are as follows:
- antibiotics should be considered in periodontal treatment planning
- antibiotics should not be used in all cases of periodontitis
  - if antibiotics may be required, consider seeking a specialist opinion
- antibiotics may be considered in the following circumstances:
  - severe periodontal disease (multiple deep sites with pus discharge)
  - patients who failed to respond to conventional periodontal therapy
  - young patients with severe disease

Multiple choice questions on the contents of this chapter are available online at Elsevier eBooks+.

References

Cobb CM. Clinical significance of non-surgical periodontal therapy: an evidence-based perspective of scaling and root planing. *J Clin Periodontol.* 2002;29(Suppl. 2):6–16.

Dietrich T, Ower P, Tank M, West NX, Walter C, Needleman I, Hughes FJ, Wadia R, Milward MR, Hodge PJ, Chapple ILC. Periodontal diagnosis in the context of the 2017 classification system of periodontal diseases and conditions – implementation in clinical practice. *Br Dent J.* 2019;226:16–22.

Faculty of General Dental Practice (UK). *GDP Antimicrobial Prescribing in Dentistry: Good Practice Guidelines.* 3rd ed. 2020.

Feres M, Haffajee AD, Allard K, Som S, Goodson JM, Socransky SS. Antibiotic resistance of subgingival species during and after antibiotic therapy. *J Clin Periodontol.* 2002;29:724–735.

Griffiths GS, Smart GJ, Bulman JS, Weiss G, Shrowder J, Newman HN. Comparison of clinical outcomes following treatment of chronic adult periodontitis with subgingival scaling or subgingival scaling plus metronidazole gel. *J Clin Periodontol.* 2000;27:910–917.

Griffiths GS, Ayob R, Guerrero A, Nibali L, Suvan J, Moles DR, Tonetti MS. Amoxicillin and metronidazole as an adjunctive treatment in generalized aggressive periodontitis at initial therapy or re-treatment: a randomized controlled clinical trial. *J Clin Periodontol.* 2011;38:43–49.

Guerrero A, Griffiths GS, Nibali L, Suvan J, Moles DR, Laurell L, Tonetti MS. Adjunctive benefits of systemic amoxicillin and metronidazole in non-surgical treatment of generalized aggressive periodontitis: a randomized placebo-controlled clinical trial. *J Clin Periodontol.* 2005;32:1096–1107.

Haffajee AD, Socransky SS, Gunsolley JC. Systemic anti-infective periodontal therapy. A systematic review. *Ann Periodontol.* 2003;8:115–181.

Heasman PA, Vernazza CR, Gaunt FL, Pennington MW. Cost-effectiveness of adjunctive antimicrobials in the treatment of periodontitis. *Periodontol 2000.* 2011;55:217–230.

Herrera D, Sanz M, Jepsen S, Needleman I, Roldán S. A systematic review on the effect of systemic antimicrobials as an adjunct to scaling and root planing in periodontitis patients. *J Clin Periodontol.* 2002;29(Suppl. 3):136–159.

Herrera D, Matesanz M, Conchita M, Oud V, Feres M, Teughels W. Adjunctive effect of locally delivered antimicrobials in periodontitis therapy: a systematic review and meta-analysis. *J Clin Periodontol.* 2020;47:239–256.

López NJ, Socransky SS, Da Silva I, Japlit MR, Haffajee AD. Effects of metronidazole plus amoxicillin as the only therapy on the microbiological and clinical parameters of untreated chronic periodontitis. *J Clin Periodontol.* 2006;33:648–660.

Matesanz-Pérez P, García-Gargallo M, Figuero E, Bascones-Martínez A, Sanz M, Herrera D. A systematic review on the effects of local antimicrobials as adjuncts to subgingival debridement, compared with subgingival debridement alone, in the treatment of chronic periodontitis. *J Clin Periodontol.* 2013;40:227–241.

Matuliene G, Studer R, Lang NP, Schmidlin K, Pjetursson BE, Salvi GE, et al. Significance of periodontal risk assessment in the recurrence of periodontitis and tooth loss. *J Clin Periodontol.* 2010;37:191–199.

Needleman I, Wilson M. Antimicrobial resistance in the subgingival microflora in patients with adult periodontitis. A comparison between The Netherlands and Spain. *J Clin Periodontol.* 2006;33:157–158.

Palmer, N. (Ed). Antimicrobial Prescribing in Dentistry: Good Practice Guidelines. 3rd Edition. London, UK: Faculty of General Dental Practice (UK) and Faculty of Dental Surgery; 2020.

Sanz M, Herrera D, Kebschull M, Chapple I, Jepsen S, Beglundh T, Sculean A, Tonetti MS. Treatment of stage I–III periodontitis—The EFP S3 level clinical practice guideline. *J Clin Periodontol.* 2020;47:4–60.

Teughels W, Feres M, Oud V, Martín C, Matesanz P, Herrera D. Adjunctive effect of systemic antimicrobials in periodontitis therapy: a systematic review and meta-analysis. *J Clin Periodontol.* 2020;47:257–281.

Tonetti MS, Sanz M. Implementation of the new classification of periodontal diseases: decision–making algorithms for clinical practice and education. *J Clin Periodontol.* 2019;46:398–405.

West N, Chapple I, Claydon N, D'Aiuto F, Donos N, Ide M, Needleman I, Kebschull M. BSP implementation of European S3 - level evidence-based treatment guidelines for stage I-III periodontitis in UK clinical practice. *J Dent.* 2021;106:1–72:103562. https://doi.org/10.1016/j.jdent.2020.103562.

5.4

Assessment of Treatment Outcomes and Supportive Periodontal Therapy

VALERIE CLEREHUGH

CHAPTER OUTLINE

Introduction

What is Supportive Periodontal Therapy?

Gingival Inflammation

Value of SPT

Assessment of Treatment Outcomes

When and How to Provide SPT

    SPT Plan

SPT Frequency

SPT Appointment

    Examination, Re-Evaluation, Re-Diagnosis

    Oral Hygiene Motivation and Re-Instruction

Risk Assessment

    Assessing Risk during SPT

OVERVIEW OF THE CHAPTER

This chapter explains the meaning of supportive periodontal therapy (SPT). The role of gingival inflammation in disease pathogenesis is explored. This leads into a discussion of the value of SPT in maintaining periodontal health and preventing tooth loss. Consideration is given to the assessment of treatment outcomes following SPT and when and how best to provide SPT, including the importance of plaque biofilm control and patient motivation in the context of the stepwise approach to periodontal therapy and the S3 clinical treatment guidelines. Various models of periodontal risk assessment during SPT are covered.

By the end of the chapter the reader should be able to:

- Explain what is meant by supportive periodontal therapy (SPT)
- Understand the role of SPT in managing patients with periodontal diseases
- Understand how SPT fits into the stepwise approach to periodontal therapy
- Outline the assessment of treatment outcomes following SPT
- Outline key aspects of SPT.

The chapter covers the following topics:

- Introduction
- What is SPT?
- Gingival inflammation
- Value of SPT
- Assessment of treatment outcomes
- When and how to provide SPT
- Risk assessment

Introduction

Periodontal therapy has traditionally been undertaken in three phases: initial, corrective and supportive, each with a number of stages. However, this approach has been superseded by a four-step *stepwise* approach to periodontal treatment which evolved following the 2017 World Workshop on Classification of Periodontal and Peri-implant Diseases and Conditions (Caton et al. 2018), and the development by the European Federation of Periodontology (EFP) of a set of stringent S3-level, evidence-based guidelines and clinical recommendations (CRs) for the management of stages I–III periodontitis (Sanz et al. 2020). The reader is directed to Chapter 4.3 and Appendix 3 for further details of the stepwise approach and an explanation of the development of the EFP S3 guidelines. The British Society of Periodontology and Implant Dentistry (BSP) adapted these EFP S3-level guidelines and produced UK Clinical Practice Guidelines for the Treatment of Periodontal Diseases illustrating the four-step sequence for the practitioner to follow for the treatment of periodontal diseases in the UK healthcare system, covering the spectrum from periodontal health to gingivitis and periodontitis (West et al. 2021; see Appendices 3 and 4), with SPT forming the basis of step 4.

What is Supportive Periodontal Therapy?

SPT (AAP 1998, Lang et al. 2008) embraces the philosophy that both the patient and dental professional are involved in maintaining the patient's periodontal health.

SPT is directed at supporting the patient in maintaining their periodontal health and preventing recurrence or progression of the disease. Although the dentist, hygienist or therapist is responsible for the provision of the professional periodontal treatments, the patient must be proactive if they are successfully to maintain periodontal stability. The maintenance of successful periodontal outcome is weighted heavily towards the contribution of the patient (Figures 5.4.1 and 5.4.2).

The main objective of SPT is to preserve the gingival and periodontal health achieved following the previous active phases of periodontal therapy. It is important to prevent or minimise the recurrence of disease progression in all patients treated for gingivitis, periodontitis and peri-implantitis and take account of their level of periodontal risk.

Other important goals are to:
- prevent or minimise any disease recurrence or progression
- prevent or reduce the incidence of tooth loss or implant loss by monitoring the dentition, prosthetic replacements and implants
- treat any diseases found during the examination
- ensure adequate control of supragingival plaque biofilm by the patient.

To achieve these goals, it is necessary to ensure:
- regular clinical assessments and recall periodontal maintenance visits tailored to each patient
- appropriate interceptive periodontal therapy
- continued psychological support, encouragement and motivation for the patient
- life long commitment by the patient
- life-long commitment by the dental professionals supporting the patient.

The biological basis of SPT takes into account several factors. These are shown in Box 5.4.1.

Gingival Inflammation

Although the microbial aetiology of periodontal diseases is well-documented, the role of gingival inflammation in disease pathogenesis has been increasingly recognised. In a classic longitudinal study of the natural history of periodontal diseases in 565 middle-class, dentally aware Norwegian males, it was reported that teeth with consistently inflamed gingiva showed greater clinical loss of attachment over 26-years observation (Schatzle et al. 2003, Lang et al. 2009). Sites with consistent bleeding (Gingival Index (GI) = 2) had 70% more clinical loss of attachment than sites that were consistently non-inflamed (GI = 0) (Figure 5.4.3).

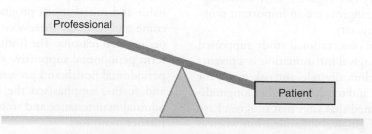

• **Figure 5.4.1** Balance of professional versus patient.

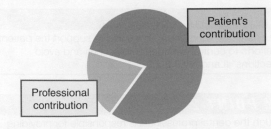

• **Figure 5.4.2** Patient's and professional's contribution to maintaining oral health.

• **BOX 5.4.1** Biological Basis of SPT

Plaque biofilm aetiology of periodontal diseases
Balance between microbial challenge, patient's host defences, conducive environment/plaque biofilm ecology
Individual patient risk assessment
Role of inflammation
Less clinical attachment loss (CAL) and tooth loss occur with regular SPT
Tooth loss is inversely proportional to SPT frequency
Recurrent periodontitis can be limited or prevented by optimal oral hygiene
SPT provides for monitoring following periodontal treatment or implant provision

---

Subgingival calculus formation increased the odds ratio of progressing from gingivitis to periodontitis (attachment loss) from 3.22 to 4.22 for the GI = 2 group compared to the GI = 0 group. Furthermore, there was significantly more cumulative tooth loss for those with the highest severity rating (GI severity group III) for teeth which consistently had bleeding on probing (GI = 2) in all sites and at all observations compared with GI severity group I, who never had bleeding on probing over the 26-year study period (Figure 5.4.4).

"Tooth age" was calculated in order to determine cumulative tooth survival data for the different levels of gingival inflammation – this was based on published national data on permanent tooth eruption dates and depended on the survey dates of when the tooth was last present and then subsequently lost (see Schatzle et al. [2004] for more information). Teeth with gingival tissues that always bled on probing (GI severity group III) had a 46 times higher likelihood to be lost than teeth always surrounded by healthy gingivae (GI severity group I). The data showed that well-maintained teeth with healthy gingivae were practically maintained for half a century (see Figure 5.4.4), which suggests that clinically healthy gingivae are an important prognostic indicator of tooth longevity.

This 26-year longitudinal observational study supported the widely held view that gingival inflammation is a precursor of periodontitis and a clinically relevant risk factor for periodontal attachment loss and tooth loss. Other longitudinal studies have also confirmed that sites that progress have persistently greater levels of gingival inflammation whereas

sites that do not progress have less gingival inflammation over time (Löe et al. 1986, Ismail et al. 1990, Clerehugh et al. 1995, Albandar et al. 1998, Schatzle et al. 2004, Tanner et al. 2007, Ramseier et al. 2017, Chapple et al. 2018).

For the first time, the 2017 World Workshop on classification gave clear definitions of periodontal health and gingivitis on an intact periodontium, on a reduced periodontium due to causes other than periodontitis and on a reduced periodontium due to periodontitis (Chapple et al. 2018).

KEY POINT 3

Gingival inflammation is a precursor of periodontitis and a clinically relevant risk factor for periodontal clinical attachment loss and tooth loss.

KEY POINT 4

Clinically healthy gingivae are a prognostic indicator of tooth longevity.

Overall these studies emphasise the importance of:
• the prevention and treatment of periodontal diseases
• maintaining periodontal health and avoiding recurrence of disease and inflammation
• the role of SPT.

Value of SPT

Many studies have been published since the 1970s that have demonstrated the value of SPT (including Suomi et al. 1971, Axelsson and Lindhe 1981, Becker et al. 1984a, b, Axelsson et al. 2004).

Compared to patients without SPT or with less SPT, patients receiving regular SPT have:
• reduced risk of tooth loss
• reduced risk of clinical attachment loss (CAL)
• decreased probing pocket depth (PPD).

Recurrence of periodontitis can be prevented, or limited, by optimal personal plaque control and through periodic professional SPT.

A systematic review (Chambrone et al. 2010) assessed factors influencing tooth loss during periodontal maintenance. Of 527 potentially eligible publications, 13 retrospective case series were scientifically robust enough and met the study criteria to include in the review. Most of the studies monitored patients for over 10 years. Of the 41,404 teeth present after active periodontal therapy, 3904 were lost during periodontal maintenance. Age, smoking habit and initial tooth prognosis affected tooth loss outcome and, overall, there were low rates of tooth loss for periodontal reasons. The findings demonstrated that long-term periodontal supportive therapy was able to maintain periodontal health and prevent tooth loss in most patients and further emphasised the importance of regular periodontal maintenance and smoking cessation in preventing further tooth loss.

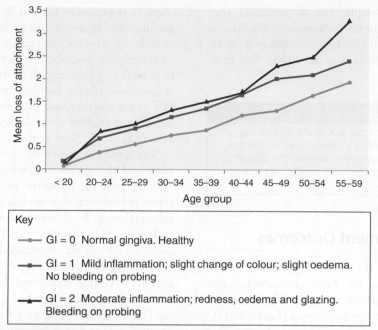

• **Figure 5.4.3** Effect of different gingivitis levels on attachment loss. From: Reprinted from *Journal of Clinical Periodontology,* 30(10):15, Niklaus P. Lang, Hans Boysen, Åge Ånerud et al. (2003), with permission from John Wiley & Sons.

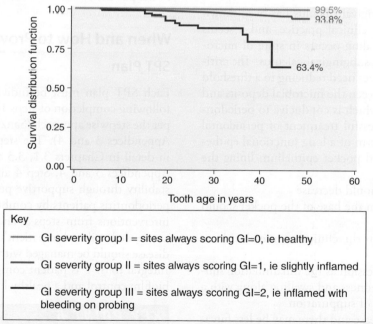

• **Figure 5.4.4** Effect of different gingivitis levels on tooth loss. Survival distribution function for different Gingival Index severity groups. After 50 years of tooth age, the cumulative survival for teeth with health gingivae is 99.5%. Teeth with always bleeding gingivae demonstrate a cumulative survival of 63.4% after 48 years of tooth age. From: Reprinted from *Journal of Clinical Periodontology,* 31(12):6, Hans Boysen, Åge Ånerud, Walter Bürgin, et al. (2004), with permission from John Wiley & Sons.

Based on the literature and biological plausibility, periodontitis patients with a low proportion of residual periodontal pockets and little inflammation have been deemed to be more likely to have periodontal stability and less tooth loss over time (Loos & Needleman 2020).

SPT needs to be undertaken in all patients who have been treated for periodontitis. However, it is fundamentally important to acknowledge that because of their inherent periodontal susceptibility, a periodontitis patient can never be deemed to be permanently "healed". Rather, albeit they can become periodontally "stable" (see Appendix 2), they will require ongoing periodontal maintenance for life, via SPT, to achieve tooth retention for life (Chapple et al. 2018, Kebschull & Chapple 2020, Sanz et al. 2020, West et al. 2021).

KEY POINT 5

Although a periodontitis patient can become periodontally stable after successful periodontal treatment, remember that "once a periodontitis patient, always a periodontitis patient", and ongoing SPT and periodontal maintenance are required for life.

Assessment of Treatment Outcomes

An evidence-based review of the clinical significance of non-surgical periodontal therapy has been conducted (Cobb 2002), and a systematic review on the effectiveness of mechanical non-surgical therapy performed (Suvan 2005).

At all stages of provision of periodontal therapy, it is important to recognise that the ability to remove all deposits is limited by the depth of the pocket, and this influences the amount of pocket reduction and attachment level gain ultimately achieved.

The removal of all subgingival calculus has been shown to be difficult to achieve in clinical practice, and it seems that clinically acceptable healing occurs in spite of microscopic aggregates of residual subgingival calculus. The critical mass of plaque biofilm does need reducing to a threshold where there is a balance between the microbial deposits and the patient's host response which is conducive to periodontal stability. Following successful treatment of periodontal pockets, healing takes the form of a long junctional epithelium, replacing the ulcerated pocket epithelium lining the pocket. Clinically:

- probing pocket depths should decrease
- bleeding on probing from the base of the pocket should reduce or resolve
- there should be a gain in the clinical connective tissue attachment
- there may be gingival recession as the inflammation subsides and normally less redness and swelling along with a reduction or elimination of suppuration
- tooth mobility may decrease and there may be less furcation involvement in some cases.

Radiographically, in due course, there may also be some bony infill at the base of angular defects where vertical bone loss had previously occurred.

After professional mechanical plaque removal (PMPR) and thorough subgingival instrumentation, junctional epithelium re-establishes quite quickly, within 2 weeks, but the granulation tissue is not yet mature and not replaced by collagen fibres. In fact, repair of connective tissue continues for 4 to 8 weeks after subgingival instrumentation and, therefore, although monitoring could be done at this stage, it is pertinent to wait 8 to 12 weeks to re-evaluate probing depths and measure the clinical attachment level in order to monitor the success of the treatment outcome. As subgingival microbial recolonisation can occur within 4 to 8 weeks of subgingival instrumentation in the absence of improved plaque biofilm control, an essential aspect of SPT is the maintenance of optimal oral hygiene and effective plaque biofilm control (Segelnick & Weinberg 2006, Sanz et al. 2020, West et al. 2021).

The position paper by Loos & Needleman (2020) addressed the question of which commonly applied periodontal probing measures recorded after completion of active periodontal therapy related to: stability of the clinical attachment level, tooth survival, need for re-treatment and oral health-related quality of life. From their extensive literature review, they concluded that: periodontitis patients with a low proportion of residual pockets are likely to have stability of clinical attachment levels and less tooth loss over time; probing pocket depths >6 mm and bleeding on probing (BOP) score >30% are a risk for tooth loss; there were no studies found that investigated the use of various periodontal probing measures on the need for re-treatment; and finally, there was a lack of evidence that periodontal probing measures after completion of active treatment were tangible to the patient.

When and How to Provide SPT

SPT Plan

Each SPT plan must be individually tailored for patients following completion of steps 1–3 of periodontal therapy as per the stepwise approach (Sanz et al. 2020, West et al. 2021; Appendices 3 and 4). The stepwise approach is described in detail in Chapters 3.1, 3.3 and 4.3 and is illustrated in Appendices 3 and 4. Step 4 aims to maintain periodontal stability through supportive periodontal care in all treated periodontitis patients by combining preventive/therapeutic interventions from steps 1 and 2. Regular recall intervals are needed, tailored to patient's individual needs. Recurrent disease should be managed with an updated treatment plan. Integral to SPT is patient compliance with optimal plaque biofilm control and a healthy lifestyle.

KEY POINT 6

Each SPT plan must be individually tailored for patients following completion of active periodontal therapy.

Following the development of the EFP S3-level treatment guidelines (Sanz et al. 2020) and the BSP implementation protocol (West et al. 2021), a number of CRs were produced for the UK healthcare system (see Chapter 4.3 for more information on this process). In respect to SPT in step 4 of the stairway, a total of 20 CRs were formulated (West et al. 2021). The following section describes those key CRs (reproduced from West et al. 2021) applicable to SPT.

TABLE 5.4.1	Frequency of SPT	
SPT frequency (months)	**Study**	
3–4	Most	
4–6	14 years (Lindhe and Nyman 1984)	
6–12, some tailored	15 years (Axelsson et al. 1991)	
	30 years (Axelsson et al. 2004)	
3, 6, 12, 18	5 years (Rosen et al. 1999)	

SPT Frequency

The frequency of SPT should be based on the patient's risk of disease progression. Studies ranging from 5 to 30 years (Table 5.4.1) have investigated different SPT intervals; the risk of insufficient SPT visits or excessively long intervals between visits may constitute under-treatment with the potential for disease recurrence and a lack of support to help the patient maintain adherence to oral hygiene procedures.

> ### KEY POINT 7
> The frequency of SPT should be based on the patient's risk of disease progression.

Although differences were not statistically significant, the 5-year study by Rosen et al. (1999) showed some rebound in the 18-month SPT group compared with those on more frequent SPT intervals.

> ### KEY POINT 8
> - Start with three monthly recalls
> - Maximum SPT interval should be 1 year

CR 4.1 (West et al. 2021) recommended that SPT visits should be scheduled at intervals of 3 to a maximum of 12 months and should be tailored to a patient's risk profile and periodontal conditions after active therapy. CR 4.2 recommended that adherence to SPT should be strongly promoted because it is crucial for long-term periodontal stability and potential further improvements in periodontal status.

SPT Appointment

It is likely that up to an hour will be required for the SPT appointment, but this will depend on individual patient requirements. Such treatment can be carried out by a dentist, hygienist or therapist. A typical SPT appointment is illustrated in Box 5.4.2. It is suggested by the EFP and BSP in CR 4.14 that routine PMPR be part of an SPT care plan in order to limit the rate of tooth loss and provide periodontal stability/improvement, as part of a supportive periodontal care programme, based on the systematic review and meta-analysis by Trombelli et al. (2020). However, the CRs

> ### • BOX 5.4.2 What Constitutes the SPT Appointment?
> Examination, re-evaluation, diagnosis
> Motivation, re-instruction (oral hygiene, smoking cessation/ modifiable risk-factor management)
> Treatment of re-infected sites, may need further appointment(s)
> - Non-surgical periodontal therapy
>   - Supragingival +/- subgingival PMPR with local analgesia as required
>   - Adjunctive local antimicrobials if indicated
> - Small surgicals
> Polishing, fluorides
> Determine future recall visit

suggested not to replace PMPR with alternative methods, e.g. Er: YAG laser treatment in SPT, nor to use adjunctive methods to PMPR (sub-antimicrobial dose doxycycline or photodynamic therapy) in SPT (Trombelli et al. 2020, West et al. 2021).

Examination, Re-Evaluation, Re-Diagnosis

During the SPT appointment the clinician should:
- update medical and dental history
- assess smoking status and other risk factor assessments including diabetes control if applicable
- assess oral hygiene/plaque score
- carry out a clinical examination and diagnosis
  - soft tissue evaluation
  - dental examination including fremitus and occlusal assessment
  - periodontal assessment – probing depths, BOP, plaque biofilm score, level of calculus, furcation involvement, suppuration, recession, mobility
  - radiographs if clinically justified
- reassess the patient's periodontal health status compared to baseline.

Oral Hygiene Motivation and Re-Instruction

Excellent plaque biofilm control is an essential feature of successful SPT in step 4 and throughout all steps of periodontal therapy, and patients need to be re-instructed and re-motivated if their plaque biofilm control is not optimal. CR 4.3 recommended repeated individually tailored instruction in mechanical oral hygiene, including interdental cleaning, in order to control inflammation (see also Figure 4.3.4 in Chapter 4.3). In respect of what additional strategies for motivation are useful, CR 4.9 recommended using step 1 of the stepwise approach.

> ### KEY POINT 9
> Excellent plaque biofilm control is an essential feature of successful SPT, and patients need to be re-instructed and re-motivated if their plaque biofilm control is not optimal.

Various methods of plaque biofilm control are available and should be tailored to each patient individually. A choice can be made between powered or manual brushes in conjunction with interdental cleaning aids, and where anatomically possible, interdental brushes are recommended in preference to floss (Slot et al. 2020), as reflected in the CRs of both the EFP and BSP (West et al. 2021). CR 4.10 stated that the basis of the management of gingival inflammation is self-performed mechanical removal of plaque biofilm, but adjunctive measures can be considered on an individual basis as part of a personalised plan (Figuero et al. 2020). The BSP were unable to make a clinical recommendation in respect of adjunctive use of antiseptics in dentifrices (CR 4.12) without further research but was able to suggest consideration of adjunctive use of mouthwashes containing chlorhexidine, essential oils and cetylpyridinium chloride in periodontitis patients undergoing SPT (CR 4.13). Based on the systematic review and meta-analysis by Figuero et al. (2020), it was stated by both EFP and BSP that it is not known if other adjunctive agents such as probiotics, prebiotics, anti-inflammatory agents and antioxidant micronutrients are effective in controlling gingival inflammation during SPT (West et al. 2021).

Patients need to understand the value of effective oral hygiene, but it is equally important to translate this understanding into action and behavioural change and for patients subsequently to adopt and maintain any oral hygiene changes (see Chapter 4.3 for more information and Figure 4.3.5 for the EFP/BSP CR on this).

> ### KEY POINT 10
> Patients need to understand the value of effective oral hygiene, but it is equally important to translate this understanding into action and behavioural change and for patients subsequently to adopt and maintain any oral hygiene changes.

The rationale and evidence base for oral hygiene measures and behavioural change are covered in Chapter 4.3.

Risk Assessment

Susceptibility to periodontitis varies from patient to patient and depends on several acquired and inherent risk factors (see Chapter 1.6). Risk assessment is different from diagnosis, because risk assessment predicts disease at some time in the future whereas diagnosis is an expression of current disease status (Kye et al. 2012).

Risk can be defined as "the probability that an event will occur in the future or the probability that an individual develops a given disease or experiences a change in health status during a specified interval of time" (Albandar 2002). *Risk factor* is a "characteristic, aspect of behaviour or environmental exposure associated with destructive periodontitis not necessarily causal" (Genco 1996). Local risk factors include subgingival calculus, furcations and restoration overhangs; systemic risk factors include smoking, poorly controlled diabetes, poor nutrition and stress.

Risk-factor control interventions have been recommended in periodontitis patients in SPT by the EFP and BSP (CR 4.17) to improve the maintenance of periodontal stability (Ramseier et al. 2020) – implementation of smoking cessation interventions was recommended (CR 4.18) and promotion of diabetes control interventions was suggested (CR 4.19); however, it was not known if physical exercise, dietary counselling or lifestyle modifications aimed at weight loss are relevant to SPT (CR 4.20) (Ramseier et al. 2020, West et al. 2021).

Assessing Risk during SPT

Numerous risk models have been introduced in which BOP is a key parameter for risk of future periodontal breakdown. These are largely based on the presence or absence of BOP and have shown the following.

Absence of bleeding on probing (Lang et al. 1986)
Low risk for disease progression

- Almost 100% predictable for periodontal health. Sites which do not exhibit BOP should not be instrumented during recall visits, the exception being in a smoker in whom the cigarette smoke may be associated with less bleeding.

Persistent bleeding on probing at successive recall visits (4/4)

- 30% of sites progress to develop CAL (but 70% do not!).
- Reinstrumentation of deep sites ≥5 mm may have a beneficial effect by altering the microbiota in the pocket to be less pathogenic.

> ### KEY POINT 11
> Absence of BOP is a better indicator of health than presence is of disease (Lang et al. 1990).

Different risk assessment models exist which share several common attributes. In general, they can evaluate future risk of disease based on current and past findings. Each finding provides a relative risk value and, taken collectively, they can assign a patient to a particular risk category indicating specific therapeutic approaches. Some models have been validated for new (untreated) patients, such as the Previser system (see Chapter 1.6), whereas others have been validated for SPT patients only. Examples of systems which are suitable for SPT patients include:

- Periodontal risk assessment (PRA) – six factors (Lang and Tonetti 2003):
  - % BOP, probing depth (PD) ≥5 mm, tooth loss, systemic and/or genetic conditions, ratio of radiographic bone loss to age, smoking
- Modified PRA – eight factors (Chandra 2007):
  - as above plus CAL-to-age ratio, diabetes, psychosocial factors; omitted radiographic bone loss-to-age ratio
- UniFe – five factors (Trombelli et al. 2009):
  - smoking, diabetes, PD ≥5 mm, BOP, bone loss/age
- DentoRisk – 20 factors (Lindskog et al. 2010):
  - various systemic and local predictors.

Table 5.4.2 and Figures 5.4.5A, B and C show the PRA model and how it can be used (Lang and Tonetti 2003).

A *low PRA* patient has all parameters in the low-risk categories, or maximum of one in the moderate risk category.

In the worked example, all parameters are in the low-risk category.

In Figure 5.4.5A, the patient: (1) has 5% sites with BOP; (2) has two sites with residual pockets of 5 mm or more; (3) has lost three teeth; (4) has a bone loss/age ratio of 0.25 derived from 10% bone loss at age 40 years (bone loss is calculated from the worst posterior site measured either on a periapical radiograph as % of root length, or from a bitewing, where 1 mm is considered to represent 10% bone loss); (5) has no systemic or genetic risk factors; and (6) is a non-smoker.

An online web tool is available to allow clinicians to calculate and complete the PRA template and also to access a link to a newly developed tool by Ramseier of the University of Bern for a personalised SPT interval (https://www.perio-tools.com/pra/en/index.php, accessed 09/08/21; see Figure 5.4.5A showing the previously mentioned low-risk example).

TABLE 5.4.2	Periodontal risk assessment (PRA) model
PRA parameter	**Risk of further breakdown**
1. Bleeding on probing % sites	<10% low risk; >25% high risk
2. Residual pockets of 5 mm or more	≤4 low risk; >8 high risk
3. Loss of teeth (from total of 28 teeth, excluding third molars)	≤4 low risk; >8 high risk
4. Loss of support related to age (% bone loss at worst site posteriorly/age)	<0.5 low risk; loss of higher % support than age = high risk
5. Systemic and genetic factors, e.g. diabetes	↑ Risk, if any of risk factors present
6. Environmental factors, e.g. smoking	Former smoker, low risk; occasional smoker (<10 cigarettes per day) and moderate smoker (10–19 cigarettes per day), moderate risk; ≥20 high risk

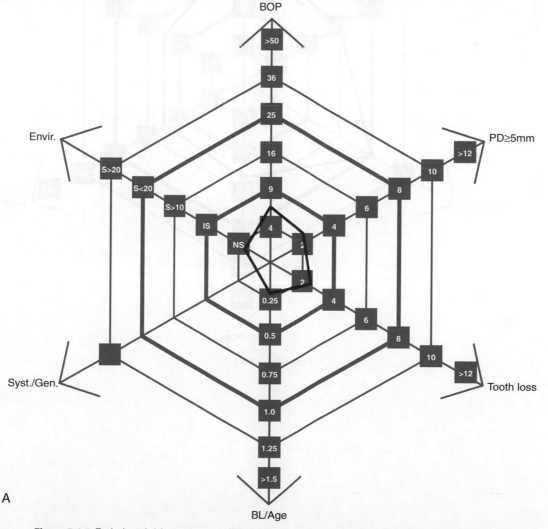

A

• **Figure 5.4.5** Periodontal risk assessment (PRA). (A) PRA low risk, worked example online tool for PRA available at https://www.perio-tools.com/pra/en/index.php, accessed 09/08/21. PRA low risk example in (A) shown.(B) PRA moderate risk, worked example.(C) PRA high risk, worked example. Source: Figures A–C are based on Functional Diagram Figure 1 from Lang and Tonetti (2003).

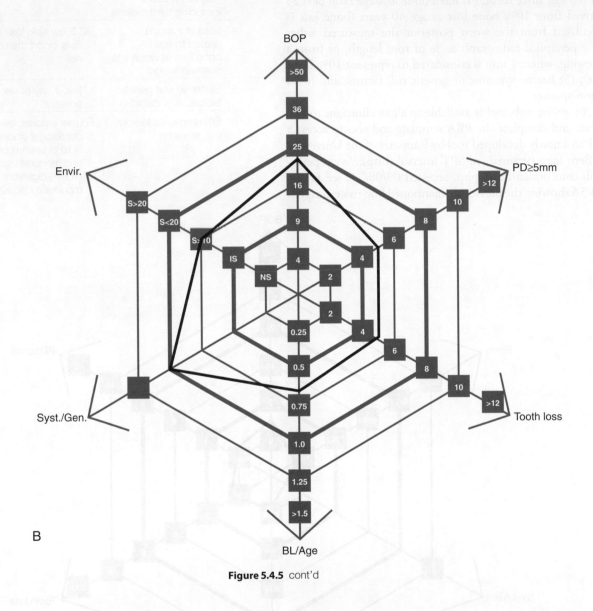

B

Figure 5.4.5 cont'd

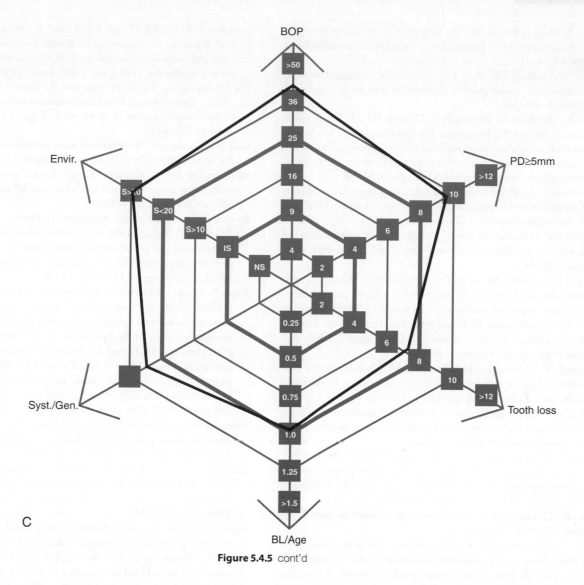

C

Figure 5.4.5 cont'd

A *moderate PRA* patient has at least two parameters in the moderate category, but at most one parameter in the high-risk category.

In the worked example, only one parameter (category 5) is high risk, and the rest are moderate risk.

In Figure 5.4.5B, the patient: (1) has 20% sites with BOP; (2) has five residual pockets of 5 mm or more; (3) lost five teeth; (4) has a bone loss/age ratio of 0.70 derived from 35% bone loss at age 50 years; (5) has type 1 diabetes mellitus; (6) is a smoker (10 cigarettes per day).

A *high PRA* patient has at least two parameters in the high-risk category.

In the worked example, four parameters are high risk (categories 1, 2, 5 and 6).

In Figure 5.4.5C, the patient: (1) has 40% of sites with BOP; (2) has nine residual pockets of 5 mm or more; (3) has lost seven teeth; (4) has a bone loss/age ratio of 1.0 (40% bone loss at 40 years of age); (5) is obese and has type 2 diabetes, treated by oral hypoglycaemic drugs and diet but is not compliant with the medication and does not adhere to dietary advice; (6) smokes 30 cigarettes per day.

Multiple choice questions on the contents of this chapter are available online at Elsevier eBooks+.

References

AAP. Position paper. Supportive periodontal therapy (SPT). *J Periodontol.* 1998;9:502–506.

Albandar JM. Global risk factors and risk indicators for periodontal diseases. *Periodontol 2000.* 2002;29:177–206.

Albandar JM, Kingman A, Brown J, Löe H. Gingival inflammation and subgingival calculus as determinants of disease progression in early–onset periodontitis. *J Clin Periodontol.* 1998;25:231–237.

Axelsson P, Lindhe J. The significance of maintenance care in the treatment of periodontal disease. *J Clin Periodontol.* 1981;8:281–294.

Axelsson P, Lindhe J, Nystrom B. On the prevention of caries and periodontal disease. Results of a 15 year longitudinal study in adults. *J Clin Periodontol.* 1991;18:182–189.

Axelsson P, Nystrom B, Lindhe J. The long term effect of plaque control program on tooth mortality, caries and periodontal disease in adults. Results after 30 years of maintenance. *J Clin Periodontol.* 2004;31:749–757.

Becker W, Berg L, Becker BE. The long term evaluation of periodontal maintenance in 95 patients. *Int J Periodontics Restorative Dent.* 1984a;4:54–71.

Becker W, Becker BE, Berg LE. Periodontal treatment without maintenance. A retrospective study in 44 patients. *J Periodontol.* 1984b;55:505–509.

Caton JG, Armitage G, Berglundh T, Chapple ILC, Jepsen S, Kornman KS, Mealey BL, Papapanou PN, Sanz M, Tonetti MS. A new classification scheme for periodontal and peri-implant diseases and conditions – Introduction and key changes from the 1999 classification. *J Clin Periodontol.* 2018;45(Suppl 20):S1–S8.

Chambrone L, Chambrone D, Lima LA, Chambrone LA. Predictors of tooth loss during periodontal maintenance: a systematic review of observational studies. *J Clin Periodontol.* 2010;37:675–684.

Chandra RV. Evaluation of a novel periodontal risk assessment model in patients presenting for dental care. *Oral Health Prev Dent.* 2007;5:39–48.

Chapple ILC, Mealey BL, et al. Periodontal health and gingival diseases and conditions on an intact and a reduced periodontium: Consensus report of workgroup 1 of the 2017 World Workshop on the Classification of Periodontal and Peri-implant Diseases and Conditions. *J Clin Periodontol.* 2018;45(Suppl 20):S68–S77. https://doi.org/10.1111/jcpe.12940.

Clerehugh V, Worthington HV, Lennon MA, Chandler R. Site progression of loss of attachment over 5 years in 14– to 19–year–old adolescents. *J Clin Periodontol.* 1995;22:15–21.

Cobb CM. Clinical significance of non-surgical periodontal therapy: an evidence-based perspective of scaling and root planing. *J Clin Periodontol.* 2002;29(Suppl. 2):6–16.

Figuero E, Roldán S, Serrano J, Escribano M, Martín C, Preshaw PM. Efficacy of adjunctive therapies in patients with gingival inflammation: a systematic review and meta-analysis. *J Clin Periodontol.* 2020;47:125–143. https://doi.org/10.1111/jcpe.13244.

Genco RJ. Current view of risk factors for periodontal diseases. *J Periodontol.* 1996;67:1041–1049.

Ismail AI, Morrison EC, Burt BA, Caffesse RG, Kavanagh MT. Natural history of periodontal disease in adults: findings from the Tecumseh Periodontal Disease Study, 1959–87. *J Dent Res.* 1990;69:430–435.

Kebschull M, Chapple I. Evidence-based, personalised and minimally invasive treatment for periodontitis patients - the new EFP S3-level clinical treatment guidelines. *Br Dent J.* 2020;229(7):443–449.

Kye W, Davidson R, Martin J, Engebretson S. Current status of periodontal risk assessment. *J Evid Base Dent Pract.* 2012;S1:2–11.

Lang NP, Tonetti MS. Periodontal risk assessment (PRA) for patients in supportive periodontal therapy (SPT). *Oral Health Prev Dent.* 2003;1:7–16.

Lang NP, Joss A, Orsanic T, Gusberti FA, Siegrist BE. Bleeding on probing – A predictor for the progression of periodontal disease? *J Clin Periodontol.* 1986;13:590–596.

Lang NP, Adler R, Joss A, Nyman S. Absence of bleeding on probing – an indicator of periodontal stability. *J Clin Periodontol.* 1990;17:714–721.

Lang NP, Bragger U, Salvi GE, Tonetti MS. Supportive periodontal therapy. In: Lang NP, Lindhe J, eds. *Clinical Periodontology and Implant Dentistry.* 5th ed. vol 2. Oxford: Wiley-Blackwell; 2008:1297–1321.

Lang NP, Schatzle MA, Löe H. Gingivitis as a risk factor in periodontal disease. *J Clin Periodontol.* 2009;36(Suppl. 10):3–8.

Lindhe J, Nyman S. Long-term maintenance of patients treated for advanced periodontal disease. *J Clin Periodontol.* 1984;11:504–514.

Lindskog S, Blomlof J, Persson I, Niklason A, Hedin A, Ericsson L, et al. Validation of an algorithm for chronic periodontitis risk assessment and prognostication: risk predictors, explanatory values, measures of quality, and clinical use. *J Periodontol.* 2010;81:584–593.

Löe H, Anerud A, Boysen H, Morrison E. Natural history of periodontal disease in man. Rapid, moderate and no loss of attachment in Sri Lankan laborers 14 to 46 years of age. *J Clin Periodontol.* 1986;13:431–445.

Loos BG, Needleman I. Endpoints of active periodontal therapy. *J Clin Periodontol.* 2020;47:61–71. https://doi.org/10.1111/jcpe.13253.

Ramseier CA, Ånerud A, Dulac M, et al. Natural history of periodontitis: disease progression and tooth loss over 40 years. *J Clin Periodontol.* 2017;44:1182–1191.

Ramseier CA, Woelber JP, Kitzmann J, Detzen L, Carra MC, Bouchard P. Impact of risk factor control interventions for smoking cessation and promotion of healthy lifestyles in patients with periodontitis: a systematic review. *J Clin Periodontol.* 2020;47:90–106. https://doi.org/10.1111/jcpe.13240.

Rosen B, Olavi G, Badersten A, Ronstrom A, Soderholm G, Egelberg J. Effect of different frequencies of preventive maintenance treatment on periodontal conditions. Five-year observations in general dentistry patients. *J Clin Periodontol.* 1999;26:225–233.

Sanz M, Herrera D, Kebschull M, Chapple I, Jepsen S, Beglundh T, Sculean A, Tonetti MS; On behalf of the EFP Workshop Participants and Methodological Consultants. Treatment of stage I–III periodontitis—The EFP S3 level clinical practice guideline. *J Clin Periodontol.* 2020;47:4–60. https://doi.org/10.1111/jcpe.13290.

Schatzle M, Löe H, Burgin W, Anerud A, Boysen H, Lang NP. Clinical course of chronic periodontitis. I. Role of gingivitis. *J Clin Periodontol.* 2003;30:887–901. Erratum in J Clin Periodontol 2004, 31, 813.

Schatzle M, Löe H, Lang NP, Burgin W, Boysen H, Anerud A. The clinical course of chronic periodontitis. IV. Gingival inflammation as a risk factor in tooth mortality. *J Clin Periodontol.* 2004;31:1122–1127.

Segelnick SL, Weinberg MA. Reevaluation of initial therapy: when is the appropriate time? *J Periodontol.* 2006;77:1598–1601.

Slot DE, Valkenburg C, Van der Weijden GA. Mechanical plaque removal of periodontal maintenance patients: a systematic review and network meta-analysis. *J Clin Periodontol.* 2020;47:107–124. https://doi. org/10.1111/jcpe.13275.

Suomi JD, Greene JC, Vermillion JR, Doyle J, Chang JJ, Leatherwood EC. The effect of controlled oral hygiene procedures on the progression of periodontal diseases in adults: results after third and final year. *J Periodontol.* 1971;42:152–160.

Suvan JE. Effectiveness of mechanical non-surgical periodontal therapy. *Periodontol 2000.* 2005;37:48–71.

Tanner ACR, Kent Jr R, Kanasi E, et al. Clinical characteristics and microbiota of progressing slight chronic periodontitis in adults. *J Clin Periodontol.* 2007;34:917–930.

Trombelli L, Farina R, Ferrari S, Pasetti P, Calura G. Comparison between two methods for periodontal risk assessment. *Minerva Stomatology.* 2009;58:277–287.

Trombelli L, Farina R, Pollard A, et al. Efficacy of alternative or additional methods to professional mechanical plaque removal during supportive periodontal therapy: a systematic review and meta-analysis. *J Clin Periodontol.* 2020;47:144–154. https://doi. org/10.1111/jcpe.13269.

West N, Chapple I, Claydon N, D'Aiuto F, Donos N, Ide M, Needleman I, Kebschull M. BSP implementation of European S3-level evidence-based treatment guidelines for stage I-III periodontitis in UK clinical practice. *J Dent.* 2021;106:1–72. 103562 https://doi.org/10.1016/j.jdent.2020.103562.

Surgical Periodontal Therapy

6.1

Rationale for Periodontal Surgery

JOSÉ ZURDO

CHAPTER OUTLINE

OVERVIEW OF THE CHAPTER

This chapter explains the basis to considering periodontal surgery as an additional therapeutic measure in the management of periodontitis. It outlines the most common surgical approaches, describing the specific objectives, techniques and expected outcomes.

By the end of the chapter the reader should:

- Understand the principles of periodontal surgery
- Be able to describe the objectives of the most common surgical approaches
- Recognise the potential benefits and risks associated with periodontal surgery
- Appreciate the importance of case selection.

The chapter covers the following topics:

- Introduction
- When is periodontal surgery appropriate?
- Surgical approaches
- Surgical treatment of furcation-involved, multi-rooted teeth
- Regenerative techniques
- Summary

Introduction

The ultimate goal of all forms of periodontal therapy is commonly considered to be the prevention of tooth loss (true end point). For the clinician, surrogate end points of success may be defined as no bleeding on probing (BoP) and probing pocket depths (PPD) of ≤4 mm.

Following periodontal therapy, an increased resistance of the gingival tissues to probing and the absence of BoP are signs of resolution of the inflammatory lesion and useful indicators that the risk of further attachment and tooth loss is minimised.

There is evidence that non-surgical therapy, with a combination of root instrumentation and optimal supragingival plaque-control measures, is an effective treatment modality in reducing PPD and BoP in the majority of the cases and sites (Figure 6.1.1). Nevertheless, some patients and/or sites can show persistent disease that is difficult to control and may be considered for more complex corrective treatment (Heitz-Mayfield et al. 2002). Because periodontitis is a plaque-induced disorder, surgical therapy should be considered on the basis of its potential to facilitate the removal of subgingival deposits and to enhance the long-term preservation of the periodontal tissues.

When is Periodontal Surgery Appropriate?

Control of Disease

Periodontal surgery is elective; therefore a careful assessment should be made to identify the potential benefits and risks involved.

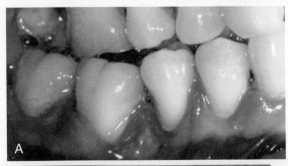
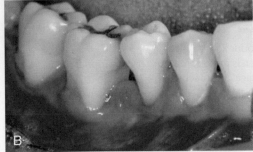

• **Figure 6.1.1** Gingival tissues (A) before and (B) after a course of non-surgical treatment.

There are standardised surgical protocols with supportive research evidence about their potential advantages, but a special effort should be made to consider all the risk factors on a case-by-case basis, keeping in mind that the main objective is to provide a significant clinical improvement with tangible benefits for the patient. In terms of overall treatment planning and the scheduling of periodontal surgery, the European Federation of Periodontology (EFP) S3-level clinical treatment guideline (Kebschull & Chapple 2020, Sanz et al. 2020) should be followed; details of this guideline, and the British Society of Periodontology and Implant Dentistry (BSP) implementation of this guideline (West et al. 2021), can be found in Chapter 4.3 and in Appendices 3 and 4. Thus it can be seen that usually periodontal surgery should only be considered during step 3 of the stepwise approach – that is, when interventions to control poorly or non-responding sites need to be employed and after adequate execution of steps 1 and 2. The guideline suggests that residual 4–5 mm pockets should receive repeat subgingival instrumentation whereas pockets of 6 mm or greater may benefit from surgical procedures (Sanz-Sanchez et al. 2020).

Surgical management requires adequate planning and specific skills in tissue handling that are critical to the success of the treatment; therefore, the operator should anticipate the level of difficulty and evaluate their own skills to undertake cases within their own limits of competence. The EFP S3-level guideline recommends, based on expert opinion rather than evidence, that surgical periodontal treatment should only be carried out by specialists or dentists with appropriate training (consensus-based clinical recommendation 3.4).

General Objectives

The main objective of periodontal surgery is to improve the prognosis of the tooth by one or more of the following means:

- Creating accessibility for effective root surface debridement (Figure 6.1.2)
- Improving the gingival or tooth morphology to facilitate the patient's self-care
- Regenerating lost periodontal attachment.

Traditionally, persistent increased PPD following initial therapy has been the main parameter used to assess the indication for periodontal surgery and the classic main objective was "pocket elimination".

Evidence suggests that pocket depth does not necessarily correlate with active disease and that clinical signs of inflammation (BoP) should be considered. Although the presence of inflammation has a poor positive predictive value for disease progression (Joss et al. 1994), the lack of it may be a more reliable indication of disease control/stability. The emphasis is now less on pocket elimination and more on control of inflammation. Thus deeper sites of pocketing with persistent

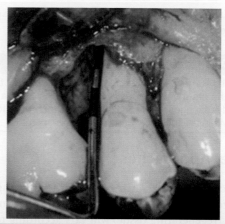

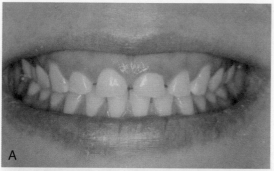

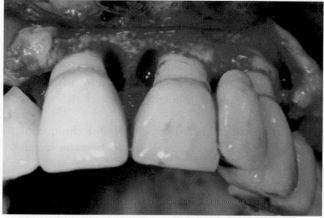

• **Figure 6.1.2** Examples of intra-osseous defects. These types of defects often limit access for root surface debridement.

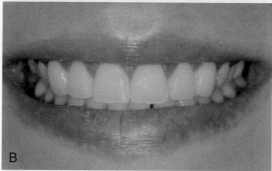

• **Figure 6.1.3** (A) An example of a "gummy smile" with short clinical crowns and diastemas. (B) This patient received crown-lengthening surgery and cosmetic rehabilitation with porcelain veneers.

inflammation (BoP) may be candidates for additional treatment (Tomasi et al. 2006).

KEY POINT 1

Periodontal surgery is only appropriate when it is used as part of a well-formulated treatment plan and the objectives are clearly defined and reasonable.

Periodontal Plastic Surgery

Additional objectives of periodontal surgery unrelated to the treatment of periodontal diseases are:

• Correction of gingiva–alveolar mucosal problems (Figure 6.1.3)
• Preparation of adequate periodontal architecture prior to restorative treatment
• Aesthetic improvement (Figure 6.1.4).

Case Selection for All Forms of Periodontal Surgery

The selection of patients for surgical periodontal therapy is a delicate decision-making process in which subject, tooth

and site-specific factors have to be considered, and patients may need to be referred to a specialist for this.

Subject Factors

• Compliance: a patient with poor plaque control and who has shown a poor response to initial therapy is not a good candidate for surgical treatment. Periodontal surgery without appropriate plaque control and maintenance care may result in a sub-optimal treatment outcome.
• Patient coping skills and operator skills: periodontal surgery is technically demanding for the operator and requires high levels of cooperation from the patient.
• Wound-healing potential: general factors such as poorly controlled diabetes, smoking or stress may influence the response to the treatment.

Tooth Factors

• Anatomic factors such as furcation anatomy and location, malposition or root proximity to adjacent teeth, position of the tooth in the dental arch, tooth mobility and occlusal factors may have a significant impact in the response to treatment.
• Restorative, cosmetic and endodontic considerations will influence the treatment approach and outcome.

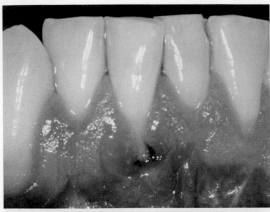

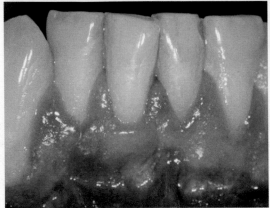

• **Figure 6.1.4** Surgical correction of gingival recession at LR1 with a laterally repositioned flap.

• Poor-quality, non-surgical root debridement is not an indication for surgical debridement; it is an indication for improved instrumentation.

KEY POINT 2

Periodontal surgery should not be used to compensate for inadequate non-surgical debridement.

Site Factors

• Adverse root morphology, pocket depth, bone and soft tissue anatomy will also influence the healing potential and the technique of choice.

Medical Contraindications

There are some conditions that may require further investigation or advice from the patient's physician prior to surgery being undertaken. These conditions include:

• Bleeding predisposition
  • Blood disorders (e.g. haemophilia)
  • Medication with anticoagulant treatment (e.g. warfarin resulting in a high INR)
• Poorly controlled diabetes
• Uncontrolled hypertension
• Immunocompromised patients
• Blood disorders (e.g. leukaemia)

• Medication with immunosuppressive drugs (e.g. cyclosporine A).

KEY POINT 3

Periodontal surgery should be regarded as a potential tool to improve the prognosis of specific teeth with lesions that are realistically manageable and as long as the technique to be used is within the technical capability of the operator.

Surgical Approaches

The choice of a conservative approach (preserving tissue), a resective approach (removing tissues) or reconstructive approach (regenerating tissue) will vary according to various factors. The following factors should be considered:

• The anatomy of the residual pocket (e.g. supra-bony or infra-bony lesion, amount of keratinised gingiva)
• The anatomy of the tooth (e.g. single-rooted or multi-rooted tooth with or without furcation involvement)
• The position of the tooth in the dental arch (e.g. cosmetic area)
• The complexity and predictability of the technique in different case scenarios (e.g. patient and operator factors).

Historically, periodontal surgery has comprised several techniques and multiple variations within each technique, giving a confusing picture of the appropriate surgical approach in individual cases. Evidence suggests that the choice of technique is not a determinant in successful treatment outcomes.

Pocket Production Procedures

• Open flap debridement
  • Papillae preservation technique, simplified papilla preservation technique
• Modified Widman flap

Pocket Elimination Procedures

• Soft tissue
  • Gingivectomy
  • Apically repositioned flap
• Hard tissue
  • Osseous surgery
  • Osteoplasty
  • Ostectomy
• Resective procedures of furcation-involved teeth
  • Furcation plasty
  • Root separation and resection

Regenerative Procedures

• Guided tissue regeneration (GTR)
• Root surface modification
• Other grafting biomaterials

Open Flap Debridement (OFD)
Objectives

The main goal of the "replaced flap", "access flap" or "open flap debridement" is to obtain improved visibility and accessibility for subgingival instrumentation of both soft and hard root surface deposits which have not been removed by non-surgical means.

Technique

The technique for this procedure is as follows:

- Intrasulcular incisions and full-thickness mucoperiosteal flaps (buccal and lingual/palatal) preserving the interdental soft tissue ("papilla preservation") in the flaps (Cortellini et al. 1995)
- Removal of granulation tissue
- Thorough root surface debridement
- Replacement of the flap margins to their original position and held with sutures.

Note: The flap should be of sufficient size to expose the area that requires instrumentation.

Vertical relieving incisions can facilitate the access and reduce the tension of the flap, but such incisions should be used with caution as they can reduce blood supply and stability of the flap.

Complete soft tissue coverage of the alveolar bone should be achieved at the termination of the surgery.

Outcomes

Although pocket reduction is not the intention of this technique, some pocket reduction may result from postoperative gingival recession. This will depend on soft tissue biotype (thick or thin) and the morphology of any underlying bone lesions (supra- or infra-bony). Gingival recession can be minimised by using microsurgical techniques and a minimally invasive surgical approach.

> **KEY POINT 4**
>
> OFD is the most reasonable surgical approach when the objective is to carry out effective root surface debridement in areas with difficult access.

Modified Widman Flap (MWF)

Objective

The modified Widman flap was historically designed as an access flap with removal of the inflamed pocket epithelium (Ramfjord & Nissle 1974). This technique aims to excise a marginal tissue cuff to facilitate direct postoperative pocket depth reduction (Figure 6.1.5).

Technique

The technique for this procedure is as follows:

- Initial scalloped inverse bevel incision 1 mm from the gingival margin and parallel to the long axis of the tooth
- Muco-periosteal flaps *within* the attached gingiva
- Second intrasulcular incision to the bone crest to separate the tissue collar from the root surface
- Removal of the soft tissue collar
- As described with OFD, removal of granulation tissue, mechanical instrumentation of the root surface and replacement of the flap.

Outcomes

MWF may result in greater pocket reduction than OFD because of the greater potential for gingival recession postoperatively. It is technically more demanding than OFD.

Gingivectomy

Objective

This procedure involves the excision of the soft tissue wall of the periodontal pocket aiming for pocket elimination (Goldman 1951). Currently, it is commonly used for the surgical management of gingival overgrowth (hyperplasia) characterised by enlargement of the gingival tissues without apical migration of the junctional epithelial attachment ("false pocketing") (Figure 6.1.6).

Control of the causative factors should be completed before surgical treatment is considered.

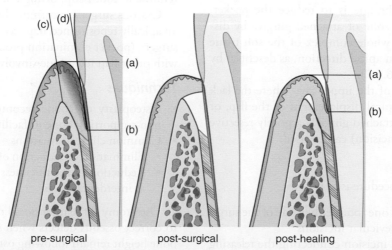

• **Figure 6.1.5** Stages in a modified Widman flap procedure. Lines: (a) gingival margin; (b) bottom of pocket; (c) scalloped inversed bevel incision; (d) intrasulcular incision.

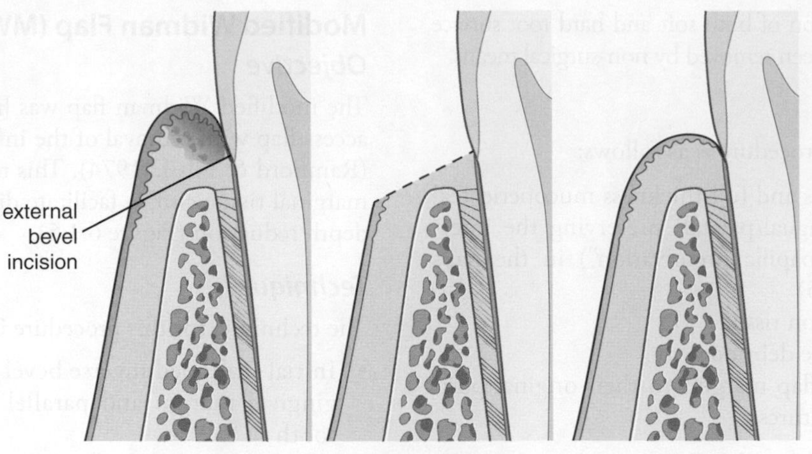

external
bevel
incision

pre-surgical   post-surgical   post-healing

• **Figure 6.1.6** Stages in a gingivectomy.

Technique

The technique for this procedure is as follows:

- Identification of the bottom of the pocket with the probe
- Marking the outer aspect of the gingiva creating a bleeding point
- First scalloped external bevel incision (45 degrees to the long axis of the roots) apical to the bleeding points to terminate at a level slightly apical to the "bottom" of the pocket
- Removal of the detached gingiva
- Gingivoplasty to create a better aesthetic contour.

Outcomes

The exposed tissue will heal by secondary intention. Periodontal dressing should be used to cover the wounded area and reduce postoperative discomfort and bleeding. If there is limited attached gingiva, a modified Widman flap approach may be more appropriate.

Apically Repositioned Flap (ARF)

Objective

The objective of this technique is to reduce the pocket, maintaining an adequate zone of attached gingiva by displacing the flap with the whole complex of the soft tissue (gingiva and mucosa) in an apical direction, as described by Friedman (1962) (Figure 6.1.7).

In the palatal surfaces of the upper jaw, where the lack of mucosa impedes any apical displacement of the flap, or where there is sufficient attached gingiva, a purely resective technique (inverse bevel incision) can be used.

Technique

The technique for this procedure is as follows:

- Create horizontal relief one tooth either side of the surgical field by means of crevicular incisions
- Scalloped inverse bevel incision connecting the releasing incisions

- Mucoperiosteal flap and crevicular incision removing a collar of gingival tissue
- Exposure of the bone margins and possible bone reshaping, avoiding removal of tooth-supporting bone
- Repositioning of the flaps at the level of alveolar bone crest, securing them in this position with adequate suturing.

Outcomes

Pocket reduction should result where the soft tissues have been apically displaced, although there may be residual pocketing in areas of greater bone loss.

Osseous Surgery

Objective

The most significant factor in the final position of the gingival margin following any periodontal surgical technique is the anatomy of the underlying bone. Therefore, the objective of bone surgery is to establish a "physiological" anatomy of the alveolar bone but at a more apical level. However, the removal of tooth-supporting bone should be avoided.

Osseous surgery is commonly used in conjunction with an apically repositioned flap (see Figure 6.1.7) and resective surgery (pocket elimination procedures), but it can be used with other flap techniques involving pocket reduction.

Techniques

- Osteoplasty or "bone recontouring" is the removal of non-supporting bone to facilitate flap adaptation
- Common clinical situations
  - Elimination or reduction of shallow intra-bony defects
  - Reduction of the thickness of the buccal/lingual bone at interdental areas

Ostectomy is the intentional removal of supporting bone to correct osseous defects when significant discrepancies in bone height remain following osteoplasty around teeth with sufficient periodontal support.

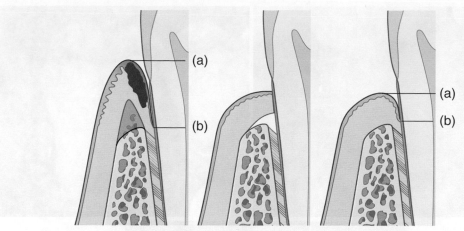

• **Figure 6.1.7** Stages during an apically repositioned flap procedure. Lines: (a) gingival margin; (b) bottom of pocket.

Common clinical situations in which osseous surgery is indicated:

- Elimination of small peaks of bone that often remain in the line angles
- Correction of reversed osseous architecture.

> ### KEY POINT 5
> Resective surgical therapies are destructive to the tissues and should be undertaken with restraint. The most common clinical indications involve the management of molars with furcation lesions and cosmetic or restorative crown lengthening.

Surgical Treatment of Furcation-Involved, Multi-Rooted Teeth

Molars with periodontal breakdown affecting the furcation area tend to respond less favourably to non-surgical periodontal therapy and, although earlier evidence suggested that they have reduced prognosis (Hirschfeld & Wasserman 1978), more recent studies suggest that, properly managed and maintained, furcation-involved molars may survive for long periods (Huynh-Ba et al. 2009). The EFP S3-level treatment guideline recommends the retention and treatment of teeth with class II and III furcation involvement and that furcation involvement is not a reason for extraction (clinical recommendation 3.10, based on Jepsen et al. [2020] and Dommisch et al. [2020]). However, if non-surgical treatment of furcation lesions has not been successful, various surgical options may be considered.

Surgical Treatment Options

These are as follows:

- Resective surgery:
  - Furcation plasty
  - Root separation or root resection
- Regenerative surgery.

Furcation Plasty

Significant variations in the morphology of multi-rooted teeth explain the difficulties in diagnosing, treating and managing furcation areas and in predicting their prognosis.

Objective

The periodontal pocket in a furcation lesion is influenced by the anatomy of the soft tissue (thick or thin), the bone (horizontal or angular loss) and the inter-radicular anatomy of the tooth. Odontoplasty (reshaping the tooth), osteoplasty (reshaping bone) or gingivoplasty (reshaping gingiva) may be used to enhance the probability of pocket and furcation closure following open debridement (Figure 6.1.8).

Technique

The technique for this procedure is as follows:

- OFD to access the inter-radicular area
- Odontoplasty to reduce the horizontal component of the defect and widen the furcation entrance
- Osteoplasty to reduce the vertical component of the defect (e.g. eliminating the intra-bony lesion) and the horizontal component (e.g. decreasing the thickness of the bone)
- Positioning the flap at the level of the alveolar bone crest.

Outcomes

Improved access for self-care and professional supportive care should result. Aggressive odontoplasty should be avoided on vital teeth due to the risk of hypersensitivity.

Root Resection or Amputation
Objective

Complete elimination of the furcation defect is frequently only possible if the roots are sectioned. Root separation involves keeping all the roots, and root resection involves the removal of one or more of the roots (Figure 6.1.9).

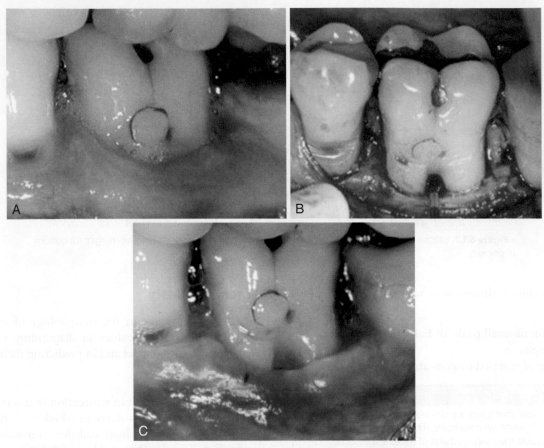

• **Figures 6.1.8** Result after periodontal flap surgery with osteoplasty and odontoplasty to reduce the vertical and horizontal components of the pocket.

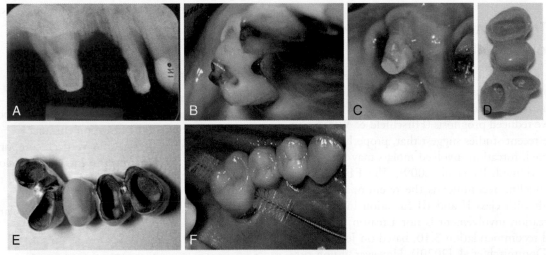

• **Figures 6.1.9** Disto-buccal (DB) root resection and mesio-distal tunnelling case. The patient presented with a class 3 furcation involvement. The DB root was sectioned and removed and the mesio-distal furcation entrance exposed to facilitate oral hygiene. A four-unit bridge has stabilised the remaining roots.

This treatment requires a multidisciplinary approach (endodontic and restorative treatment) and aims to reserve the tooth or part of it when no other alternative is effective and the tooth has a high strategic value.

Methodical treatment planning is critical in the success of this therapy. Endodontic treatment should be done before surgery; occasionally, the decision to resect a root is made during surgery, in which case, the endodontic treatment is carried out as soon as possible after surgery.

Technique

The technique for this procedure is as follows:

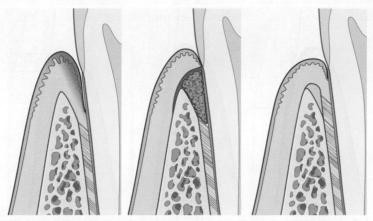

• **Figure 6.1.10** Use of a barrier membrane. The membrane (in blue) acts as a barrier to the down growth of epithelial cells, the "sprinter" cells in wound healing. It also helps protect and stabilise the blood clot within the defect area.

- Mucoperiosteal flap to expose the furcation area
- Root sectioning with straight line cut and preparation of the roots avoiding undercuts or ledges
- Careful removal of the root selected for extraction without damaging the adjacent roots
- Repositioning of the flaps at the level of the bone crest.

Outcomes

The remaining root(s) should have adequate bone support. Failures are usually related to non-periodontal complications, so care should be taken to ensure sound endodontic therapy and a balanced occlusion (Carnevale et al. 1998).

Regenerative Techniques

Objective

The ultimate and realistic goal of periodontal therapy is to stop the progression of the disease.

Although conventional non-surgical and surgical techniques can lead to predictable pocket reduction and decrease risk of disease progression, they are characterised by repair, often associated with recession and formation of long-junctional epithelium (the majority of the repaired soft tissue in contact with the treated root surface being epithelium).

A more idealistic goal is to restore completely the structure and function of the lost periodontal tissues (root cementum, periodontal ligament, alveolar bone and connective tissue attachment).

Although there is histological evidence demonstrating that partial periodontal regeneration is possible, complete periodontal restoration is an elusive goal (Needleman et al. 2002). Regeneration can only be attempted in vertical bone defects. The EFP S3-level guideline recommends treating teeth with residual deep pockets associated with intra-bony defects of 3 mm or more with periodontal regenerative surgery (clinical recommendation 3.7, based on Nibali et al. 2020).

Techniques

Guided Tissue Regeneration (Gtr)

Following open debridement of a periodontal lesion, barrier membranes can prevent the epithelium and connective tissue from contacting the root surface during the periodontal wound healing, allowing the undifferentiated cells from the periodontal ligament and bone to populate the area and promote new attachment formation (Figure 6.1.10). Cortellini et al. (2017) compared GTR with access flap (OFD) alone in 45 patients over a 20-year follow-up period and found that regeneration provided better long-term benefits than OFD alone.

Biological Root Modifiers

Biologic root modifiers, such as enamel matrix proteins (EMPs) obtained from porcine tooth follicles, have been shown to induce proliferation of periodontal ligament cells, gingival fibroblasts and osteoblasts; increase the rate of periodontal ligament cell attachment; and inhibit epithelial down growth when applied to a treated root surface following open debridement (Figure 6.1.11). The biological effects also include upregulation of markers of bone formation (Bosshardt 2008).

The clinical cases in Figures 6.1.12 and 6.1.13 illustrate the regenerative capacity of these biological root surface modifiers.

Grafting and Combined Therapies

A huge number of materials, techniques and combined therapies claim to promote periodontal regeneration, which makes it very difficult for the clinician to choose the most appropriate therapy (Figures 6.1.14 and 6.1.15).

Only a few techniques, namely GTR and EMPs (the most documented), are supported by sound scientific evidence.

> **KEY POINT 6**
>
> Regenerative therapy is demanding and in general has low cost-effectiveness. Case selection is important.

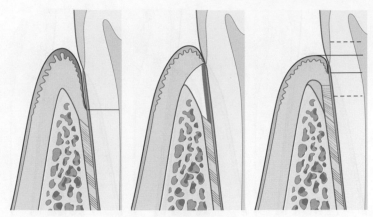

• **Figure 6.1.11** Use of enamel matrix protein (EMP). The blue zone on the root surface represents the EMP.

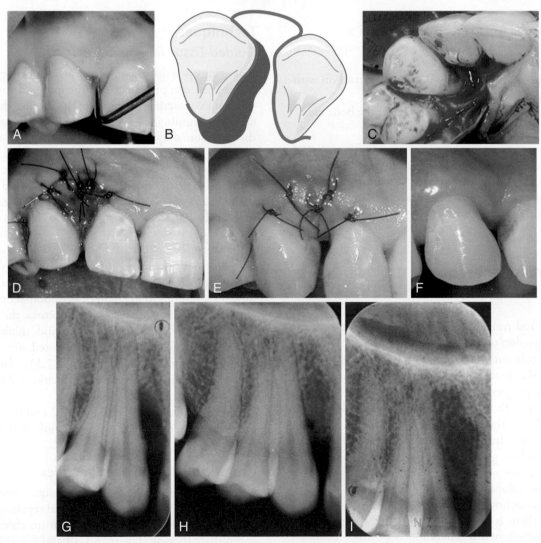

• **Figure 6.1.12** A case treated with EMP (alone). The blue line in the diagram represents the incision line and borders of the flap (intrasulcular incisions on both teeth connected by a semilunar incision). At the root surface of UR3 there was 13+ mm of attachment loss on the mesial surface and UR1 palatally. The flap involved a papilla preservation technique, as there was enough space to bring the whole tissue to the palatal side. EMP was used according to manufacturer's instructions. The three radiographs show the situation before surgery, at 6 months follow-up and 1 year. Note the bone fill at 1 year.

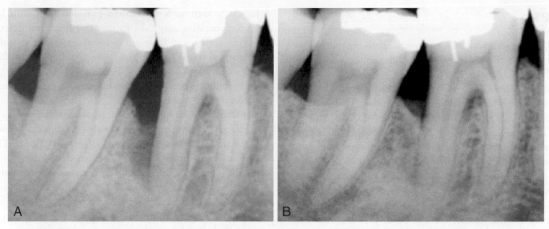

• **Figure 6.1.13** Another case (intra-bony defect involving only the distal aspect of a vital LR6) where root surface modifiers were used. (A) The preoperative radiograph and (B) the 1-year postoperative control radiograph.

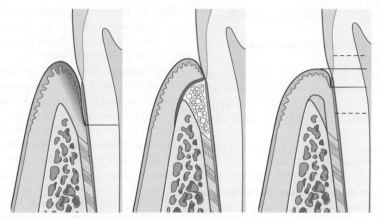

• **Figure 6.1.14** Combined regenerative approach using a barrier membrane and a bone "filler", intended to keep space for the blood clot and prevent membrane collapse into the defect.

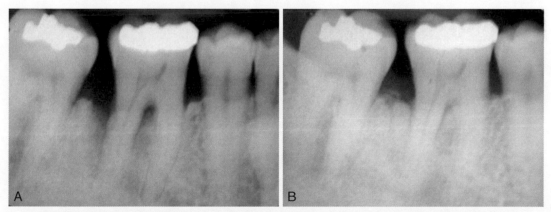

• **Figure 6.1.15** Intra-bony defect at LR6 distally with involvement of the furcation, treated with GTR combined with a xenographic bone substitute. Preoperative radiograph and healing control after 6 months.

Summary

The aim of non-surgical periodontal therapy (NST) is to control the cause-related factors, allow resolution of the inflammation and establish a clinical condition that can be easily maintained by the patient. Periodontal surgery should only be considered when non-surgical therapy has failed to produce adequate healing because of identifiable local factors and in spite of a high standard of care.

Multiple choice questions on the contents of this chapter are available online at Elsevier eBooks+.

References

Bosshardt DD. Biological mediators and periodontal regeneration: a review of enamel matrix proteins at the cellular and molecular levels. *J Clin Periodontol.* 2008;35:87–105.

Carnevale GG, Pontoriero RR, di Febo GG. Long-term effects of root-resective therapy in furcation-involved molars. A 10-year longitudinal study. *J Clin Periodontol.* 1998;25:209–214.

Cortellini PP, Prato GPG, Tonetti MSM. The modified papilla preservation technique. A new surgical approach for interproximal regenerative procedures. *J Periodontol.* 1995;66:261–266.

Cortellini PP, Buti J, Pini Prato G, Tonetti MS. Periodontal regeneration compared with access flap surgery in human intra-bony defects 20-year follow-up of a randomised clinical trial: tooth retention, periodontitis recurrence and costs. *J Clin Periodontol.* 2017;44:58–66.

Dommisch H, Walter C, Dannewitz B, Eickholz P. Resective surgery for the treatment of furcation involvement - a systematic review. *J Clin Periodontol.* 2020;47(suppl 22):375–391.

Goldman HMH. Gingivectomy. *Oral Surg Oral Med Oral Pathol.* 1951;4:1136–1157.

Friedman N. Mucogingival surgery. The apically repositioned flap. *J Periodontol.* 1962;33:328–340.

Heitz-Mayfield LJA, Trombelli F, Needleman I, Moles D. A systematic review of the effect of surgical debridement vs non-surgical debridement for the treatment of chronic periodontitis. *J Clin Periodontol.* 2002;29(suppl 3):92–102;discussion 160–162.

Hirschfeld L, Wasserman B. A long-term survey of tooth loss in 600 treated periodontal patients. *J Periodontol.* 1978;49:1–13.

Huynh-Ba G, Kuonen P, Hofer D, Schmid J, Lang NP, Salvi GE. The effect of periodontal therapy on the survival rate and incidence of complications of multirooted teeth with furcation involvement after an observation period of at least 5 years: a systematic review. *J Clin Periodontol.* 2009;36:164–176.

Jepsen S, Gennai S, Hirschfeld J, Kalemaj Z, Buti J, Graziani F. Regenerative surgical treatment of furcation defects: a systematic review and Bayesian network meta-analysis of randomized clinical trials. *J Clin Periodontol.* 2020;47(suppl 22):352–374.

Joss A, Adler R, Lang NP. Bleeding on probing. A parameter for monitoring periodontal conditions in clinical practice. *J Clin Periodontol.* 1994;21:402–408.

Kebschull M, Chapple I. Evidence-based, personalised and minimally invasive treatment for periodontitis patients - the new EFP S3-level clinical treatment guidelines. *Br Dent J.* 2020;229(7):443–449.

Needleman I, Tucker R, Giedrys-Leeper E, Worthington H. A systematic review of guided tissue regeneration for periodontal infrabony defects. *J Periodontal Res.* 2002;37:380–388.

Nibali L, Koidou VP, Nieri M, Barbato L, Pagliaro U, Cairo F. Regenerative surgery versus access flap for the treatment of intrabony periodontal defects. A systematic review and meta- analysis. *J Clin Periodontol.* 2020;47(suppl 22):320–351.

Ramfjord SP, Nissle RR. The modified Widman flap. *J Periodontol.* 1974;45:601–607.

Sanz M, Herrera D, Kebschull M, Chapple I, Jepsen S, Beglundh T, Sculean A, Tonetti M. Treatment of stage I-III periodontitis-The EFP S3 level clinical practice guideline. *J Clin Periodontol.* 2020;47(suppl 22):4–60.

Sanz-Sanchez I, Montero E, Citterio F, Romano F, Molina A, Aimetti M. Efficacy of access flap procedures compared to subgingival debridement in the treatment of periodontitis. A systematic review and meta-analysis. *J Clin Periodontol.* 2020;47(suppl 22):90–106.

Tomasi C, Bertelle A, Dellasega E, Wennström J. Full-mouth ultrasonic debridement and risk of disease recurrence: a 1-year follow-up. *J Clin Periodontol.* 2006;33:626–631.

West N, Chapple I, Claydon N, D'Aiuto F, Donos N, Ide M, Needleman I, Kebschull M. BSP implementation of European S3-level evidence-based treatment guidelines for stage I-III periodontitis in UK clinical practice. *J Dent.* 2021;106:1–72:103562. https://doi.org/10.1016/j.jdent.2020.103562.

Interaction with Other Dental Disciplines

7.1

The Periodontal–Restorative Interface

EWEN MCCOLL

CHAPTER OUTLINE

OVERVIEW OF THE CHAPTER

This chapter examines the relationship and interactions between the periodontium and a range of aspects of restorative dentistry.

By the end of the chapter the reader should:

- Understand the importance of a healthy periodontium and meticulous oral hygiene in restorative dentistry
- Be able to describe the key phases of restorative treatment planning
- Recognise the practical and aesthetic challenges of restorative dentistry in treated periodontal patients
- Understand the importance of a structured periodontal maintenance regimen in successful restorative dentistry.

The chapter covers the following topics:

- General restorative considerations
- Crown and bridge construction
- Supracrestal tissue attachment
- Partial dentures
- Occlusion
- Mobility
- Implant dentistry
- Pulpal tissues
- Summary and conclusions.

General Restorative Considerations

Periodontal health is the foundation for successful restorative dentistry whether the treatment involves a single occlusal amalgam restoration or full-mouth rehabilitation. Often, in the rush to proceed to the corrective phase of treatment, insufficient attention is paid to the control of active disease. This may be due to lack of clinical awareness, lack of clinical time, patient impatience, or financial imperatives. However, if the cause-related phase of disease management is ignored, this may risk treatment failure and the potential for litigation. Thus the importance of a structured and phased

treatment-planning approach in restorative dentistry cannot be over-emphasised. These phases are often categorised as:

1. Emergency treatment
2. Cause-related therapy
3. Re-evaluation
4. Corrective therapy
5. Maintenance/supportive therapy.

KEY POINT 1

Periodontal health is the foundation stone for successful restorative dentistry.

One of the most important elements of cause-related therapy is the control of gingivitis and periodontitis.

The most important aspect of regaining and retaining periodontal health is improving levels of self-performed oral hygiene. Behavioural change can take time, whether improving oral hygiene or altering lifestyle habits. It is crucial that patients, with guidance from their clinician, establish these changes prior to embarking on complex restorative treatment plans. This concept is now referred to as "patient engagement".

Patient Engagement

The British Society of Periodontology and Implant Dentistry have defined patients as being engaging or non-engaging depending on their compliance or ability to comply with recommended oral hygiene regimens (https://www.bsperio.org.uk/assets/downloads/Delivering_phased_Care_Final_6th_May_2021_1.pdf).

Engaging Patient

The average engaging patient demonstrates a favourable response to self-care advice and sufficient improvement in oral hygiene as indicated by a 50% or greater improvement in plaque (disclosing is required) and marginal bleeding scores OR:
- Indicative bleeding levels <30%
- Indicative plaque levels <20%
- AND a stated preference to achieving periodontal health.

Non-Engaging Patient

The non-engaging patient demonstrates an unfavourable response to self-care advice and insufficient improvement in oral hygiene as indicated by less than a 50% improvement in plaque and marginal bleeding scores OR:
- Indicative bleeding levels >30%
- Indicative plaque levels >20%
- OR a stated preference to a palliative approach to periodontal care.

Most restorative treatment will occur in the corrective phase of treatment, and it is essential that, prior to this, patient engagement and periodontal stability has been achieved.

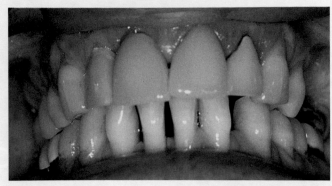

• **Figure 7.1.1** "Black triangle" effect at lower anteriors.

The periodontal tissues should be sufficiently healthy to facilitate soft tissue management, allowing better moisture control during restorative procedures. This will help with long-term restoration marginal stability.

Crown and Bridge Construction

While the control of active disease (gingivitis, periodontitis and caries) is the key to successful restorative dentistry, the importance and relevance of the periodontal condition in more advanced restorative dentistry will be discussed here.

Fixed prosthodontics can be a challenge at the best of times, but it can become even more demanding in the treated periodontal patient. In a successfully treated periodontal patient, gingival recession may be an unavoidable result of the reduction in inflammation and loss of clinical attachment. Apart from the obvious aesthetic concerns that patients may have, the appearance of triangular spaces between the teeth (the "black triangle" effect) may mean crowns need to have longer contact points to mask this effect (Figure 7.1.1).

However, these long contact points may make oral hygiene measures more challenging interdentally, and close liaison with the laboratory will be necessary to ensure that patients are able to carry out effective oral hygiene measures.

The production of high-quality temporary crowns is essential to allow optimal oral hygiene practices and avoid inflammation of the marginal periodontal tissues. The resolution of any inflammation that is present at the provisional stage may result in some recession when the final restorations are cemented, as this may lead in turn to exposure of restorative margins.

From an operative dentistry perspective, it is also important to remember that in teeth with conical roots where recession has occurred, the circumference of the root decreases the more apically you prepare, and this may mean there is an increased risk of pulpal exposure if margins are cut too heavily. Where recession has occurred around furcations, the anatomy of the exposed cement–enamel junction may also increase the difficulties of marginal preparation around the curvature of this margin, so careful pretreatment planning is of paramount importance.

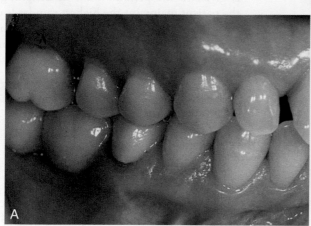
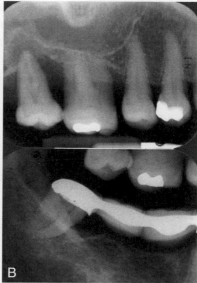

• **Figure 7.1.2** Poor pontic design making patient oral hygiene more difficult.

Bridges should be designed to ensure that gingival papillae are not traumatised, and pontic design should allow adequate oral hygiene to be performed by the patient (Figure 7.1.2).

> ### KEY POINT 4
> Abutment preparations may be more complex where periodontal attachment loss has occurred.

Pontic design in bridgework (Figure 7.1.3) can be categorised as follows:
1. Hygienic
2. Ridge lap/saddle
3. Modified ridge lap
4. Ovate pontic.

Although the hygienic pontic does not contact the edentulous ridge and is in effect self-cleansing, it will not provide adequate aesthetics and, for many patients, is unacceptable. The ridge lap/saddle design can limit oral hygiene measures, and the modified ridge lap or ovate pontic tend to be favoured to allow for adequate aesthetics and oral hygiene measures. The crucial element of pontic design is that the patient can use interdental aids to access abutments and associated margins so that the risk of bacterial recolonisation and disease recurrence is kept to a minimum. At the fit appointment, it is essential to ensure that the patient can still reach all areas of potential bacterial accumulation for oral hygiene to prevent the recurrence of inflammation. Close liaison with the laboratory is necessary to minimise this risk. At the cementation stage of crown and bridge work, it is important to ensure that excess cement is not left as a long-term irritant to the periodontal tissues.

> ### KEY POINT 5
> **Pontic design**
> Ensure pontic design does not compromise patient's ability to carry out oral hygiene measures.

Supracrestal Tissue Attachment

Although margins of crowns and bridges need to be slightly subgingival in aesthetic zones, i.e. where the gingival margins are visible when a patient smiles, it is crucial that these do not impinge on the supracrestal tissue attachment. Gargiulo et al. (1961) established the concept of biological width (now referred to as supracrestal tissue attachment) by looking at the dento-gingival complex in cadavers. They established that the supracrestal tissue attachment (Figure 7.1.4) in humans is approximately 2 mm, extending from the base of the gingival sulcus to the alveolar crest. This was found to comprise an epithelial attachment of about 1 mm and a connective tissue component of about 1 mm. Although this study established these dimensions, it is difficult to measure this clinically when preparing crown margins, so a figure of 3 mm is used, taking into account possible measurement error (Figure 7.1.5). Subgingival margins of crowns or restorations can impinge on the supracrestal tissue attachment causing inflammatory change and the risk of alveolar bone resorption. Impinging on the supracrestal tissue attachment can result in recession in patients with a thin gingival tissue biotype and inflammation and periodontal pocketing where there is a thick gingival biotype.

> ### KEY POINT 6
> **Supracrestal tissue attachment**
> - Approximately 2 mm, consisting of epithelial (junctional) and connective tissue attachment
> - Impinging on the supracrestal tissue attachment may lead to inflammation (in thick biotypes) or recession (in thin biotypes)

The concept of supracrestal tissue attachment is important when planning for the location of crown margins. In wear cases, or where the crown margins are likely to impinge upon the supracrestal tissue attachment, crown lengthening surgery may be necessary. The basic principle is that, in order to avoid impinging on the supracrestal tissue attachment, 3 mm of space is needed between the restoration margin and the alveolar bone.

Partial Dentures

With any prosthesis, whether fixed or removable, it is important to ensure that the prosthesis does not have any negative impact on the periodontal tissues.

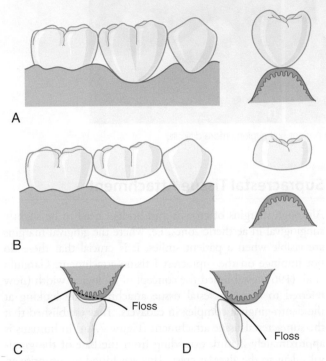

• **Figure 7.1.3** (A) Bullet pontic: makes point contact with tip of ridge; (B) hygienic pontic: easy to clean molars only; (C) saddle pontic: difficult to clean; (D) ridge lap: minimal contact with buccal aspect of ridge.

Poorly designed dentures in poorly maintained patients may lead to increased mobility of abutment teeth and breakdown of the periodontium. However, if consideration is given to the periodontium in designing dentures, and the patient maintains the highest standards of oral hygiene, then this can be avoided. The classic "gum stripper" style of denture can be damaging to the periodontal tissues and should be avoided.

Where an acrylic denture is indicated, the "Every" design of denture, first described by Every in 1949, incorporates features in an acrylic denture conducive to maintaining periodontal health. Key to this design is that coverage of the gingival margin is kept to a minimum to prevent gingival damage, and lateral interdental forces are kept to a minimum (Figure 7.1.6).

Bates & Addy (1978) established that removable partial dentures performed best when given to patients with good oral hygiene, where tissue coverage was kept to a minimum and the dentures were kept out at night.

Similar principles apply to chrome cobalt dentures where the design should be such that gingival coverage is kept to a minimum, clasps are passive and rest seats are designed so that forces are axial rather than lateral in order to reduce the likelihood of tooth mobility.

Where the clinician is faced with a Kennedy class 1 situation with bilateral free end saddles, the risk of overloading the last standing tooth is increased and denture design

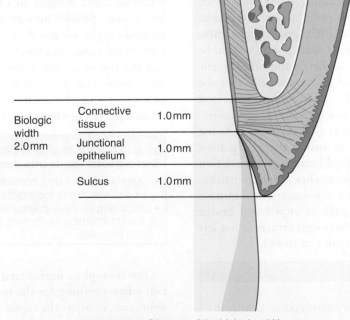

Biologic width 2.0mm	Connective tissue	1.0mm
	Junctional epithelium	1.0mm
	Sulcus	1.0mm

• **Figure 7.1.4** Diagram of the biologic width.

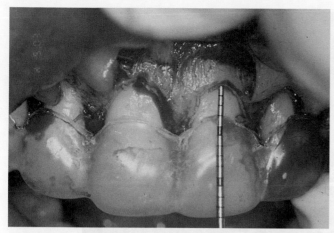

• **Figure 7.1.5** 3 mm of clearance between predicted crown margin and alveolar bone.

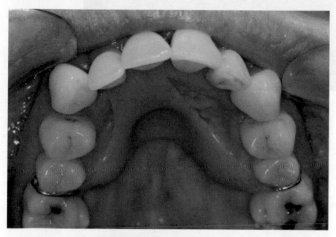

• **Figure 7.1.6** Every style denture.

becomes more challenging. This emphasises the importance of retaining molar teeth wherever possible to allow some posterior support. In many cases, the shortened dental arch, as suggested by Kayser (1989), may be preferable to overloading the remaining teeth.

Occlusion

It was initially suggested by Glickman (1965) that angular bony defects and increasing tooth mobility were caused by trauma from occlusion. However, further studies by Waerhaug & Randers-Hansen (1966) established the presence of such bone defects in teeth unaffected by trauma from occlusion. A study by Ericsson & Lindhe (1977) established that occlusal overload does not cause periodontal breakdown. Periodontitis was caused in dogs by allowing the animals to accumulate plaque and calculus around the teeth. When almost 50% of bone loss occurred, the animals were brought back to periodontal health by undergoing a meticulous oral hygiene regimen including scaling, root planing and pocket elimination. Certain teeth were then exposed to jiggling forces and, although the teeth became mobile, there was no increase in attachment loss or development of periodontitis.

Further animal studies by Lindhe & Ericson (1982) suggested that, in the presence of uncontrolled periodontitis, greater attachment loss could occur in the presence of occlusal trauma. This suggested that occlusal trauma may exacerbate periodontitis. However, this effect has only been shown in some animal studies, and the evidence for this so-called co-destructive effect is weak. Such effects have not been shown in human studies, and there is a lack of evidence from such human studies to implicate occlusal trauma in the progression of attachment loss in periodontitis. Whereas some clinicians advocate occlusal intervention to reduce occlusal trauma in periodontitis patients, a recent Cochrane systematic review showed that there was insufficient evidence to justify such treatment in periodontitis cases (Weston et al. 2008). The World Workshop on the Classification of Periodontal and Peri-implant Diseases and Conditions (2018) has stated that there is no evidence that traumatic occlusal forces cause periodontal attachment loss in humans.

Mobility

From a clinical relevance perspective, where treatment has been completed and attachment loss has occurred, occlusal overload may contribute to the mobility of teeth. It should be remembered that mobility is not just the result of occlusal loading of teeth but that the level of bone support and the inflammatory status of the soft tissues are also contributory factors. In patients for whom the mobility is a problem, occlusal analysis to eliminate premature contacts may help to reduce the extent of tooth mobility. Splinting such problematic teeth where the mobility is causing the patient discomfort may also be an option. In these patients, occlusal analysis to eliminate premature contacts may address this problem.

Numerous types of splint design have been suggested over the years. Direct types involve splinting the teeth directly with composite material. In addition, orthodontic wire can be used to run between the teeth which allows some flexion on occlusion. Additionally, composite fibre mesh has become available which may also be used for direct splinting (Figure 7.1.7).

Indirect methods of splinting may involve the use of orthodontic wire with composite. The bending of the wire in the laboratory may allow a more accurate fit, although difficulties may be encountered when taking impressions of very mobile teeth which may also affect the accuracy of any laboratory work. Another method of indirect splinting is to use an adhesive bridge-style, nickel-chromium backing. However, there may be aesthetic issues as, normally, in mobile periodontally involved teeth there is spacing and the metal will show. The same can be said for orthodontic wire

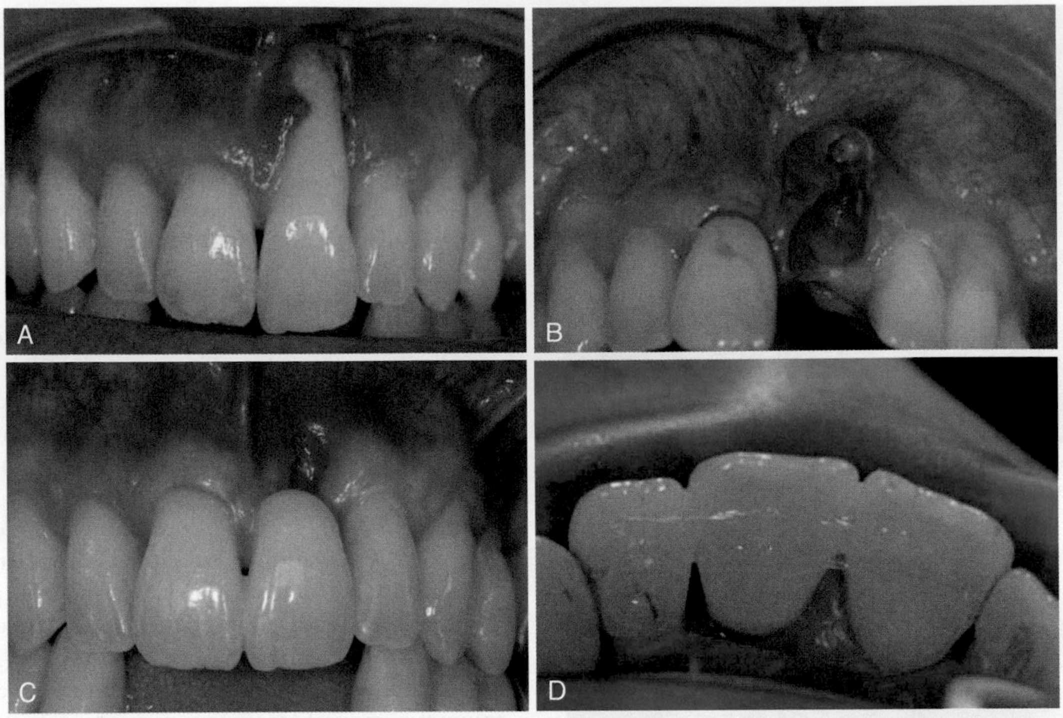

• **Figure 7.1.7** Use of composite mesh in immediate adhesive bridge. Photos courtesy of Dr Neil Macbeth.

palatally. This means the most practical and aesthetic solution is often directly applied composite.

The key component of splint design is that it does not impede the patient's oral hygiene measures and careful monitoring and maintenance are essential.

The splint should be designed in such a manner that interdental brushes can still easily access interdental spaces so that oral hygiene is not compromised in any way.

When hopeless periodontally involved teeth are extracted in the short term, they can be splinted back in place to provide the patient with an aesthetic fixed tooth replacement (Figure 7.1.7). This will allow healing to take place prior to construction of a definitive restoration.

> ### KEY POINT 9
> Splints may be indicated where mobility is causing patient discomfort.

Periodontitis and Implant Dentistry

As periodontitis may result in the loss of teeth, patients with a history of periodontitis will sometimes seek implant treatment to replace these missing teeth.

However, many patients do not realise that implants may themselves be exposed to disease processes similar to gingivitis and periodontitis (peri-implant mucositis and peri-implantitis), particularly in those patients who have a history of periodontitis. This is not surprising given that the microflora around implants is similar to that around teeth, and many of the host factors involved in periodontitis remain the same.

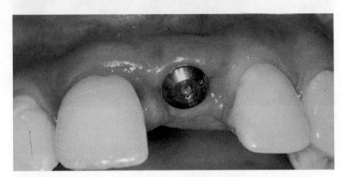

• **Figure 7.1.8** Implant placement in a treated periodontal patient with meticulous oral hygiene.

> ### KEY POINT 10
> Implants may suffer peri-implant mucositis or peri-implantitis. Supportive care, maintenance and monitoring are essential for implants, especially in patients with a history of periodontitis.

Risk indicators for peri-implant disease are essentially the same as those for periodontitis. In implant cases that are managed in a general practice, a strict periodontal and peri-implant maintenance and monitoring regimen is essential (Figure 7.1.8).

Periodontally susceptible patients should be warned that they may be at higher risk of implant complications and also that implant treatment should not be carried out unless there is no uncontrolled disease present and an optimal level of plaque control is maintained (Lindhe & Meyle 2008). The management of implants and their complications is discussed in detail in Chapter 7.3.

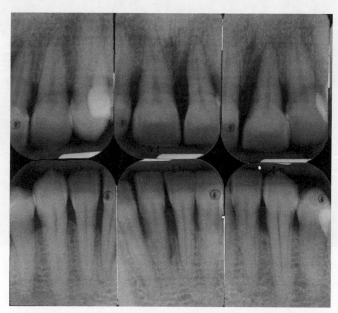

• **Figure 7.1.9** Radiographic appearance of an endo-periodontal lesion at tooth 21.

Endodontic/Periodontal Relationships

The close relationship between the pulpal complex and the periodontium via the apical foramina and lateral canals means that infection in one may result in infection in the other. These lesions have been classified by the World Workshop on the Classification of Periodontal and Peri-implant Diseases and Conditions (2018) as endo-periodontal lesions (Herrera et al. 2018). Where periodontal infection has led to pulpal necrosis, this is classed as a primary periodontal lesion. Where pulp necrosis has occurred and the infection drains through the periodontal ligament, this often presents as an isolated narrow pocket (often in the absence of periodontal lesions elsewhere), and the lesion is classed as primarily endodontic in origin. Where both a periodontal infection and endodontic infection are present together, this is classed as a true combined lesion and such lesions can be difficult to diagnose (Figure 7.1.9).

In all cases, pulp vitality should be established, and if the pulp is found to be non-vital then endodontic treatment should be carried out first. No periodontal treatment should be carried out until the endodontic lesion has had an opportunity to resolve. In those cases where the lesion is of primary endodontic origin, the periodontal component of the lesion may resolve completely.

Where the lesion is suspected to be primarily periodontal in origin, providing the tooth has a reasonable prognosis, endodontic treatment should still be carried out first and again periodontal treatment delayed until the endodontic infection has been resolved. Careful assessment of prognostic indicators such as bone volume, furcation involvement, probing depth and mobility should be assessed before embarking on complex treatment of this sort.

KEY POINT 11

When managing a tooth with a suspected endo-periodontal lesion, always test pulp vitality of suspect tooth and, if vitality is lost, always carry out endodontic treatment first, followed by periodontal therapy if required.

Summary

The key element in the provision of restorative treatment for periodontally susceptible patients is control of active disease prior to definitive restorative treatment and maintenance of a healthy periodontium. It is important to ensure that there are regular periodontal reviews and that self-performed plaque control is maintained at an optimal level.

Multiple choice questions on the contents of this chapter are available online at Elsevier eBooks+.

References

Bates JF, Addy M. Partial dentures and plaque accumulation. *J Dent.* 1978;6:285–293.

Ericcson I, Lindhe J. Lack of effect of trauma from occlusion on the recurrence of experimental periodontitis. *J Clin Periodontol.* 1977;9.497–503.

Gargiulo AW, Wentz FM, Orban B. Dimensions and relations of the dentogingival junction in humans. *J Periodontol.* 1961;39:261–267.

Glickman I. Clinical significance of trauma from occlusion. *J Am Dent Assoc.* 1965;70:607–618.

Herrera D, Retamal-Valdes B, Alonso B, Feres M. Acute periodontal lesion (periodontal abscesses and necrotizing periodontal diseases) and endo-periodontal lesions. *J Periodontol.* 2018;89(Suppl 1):S85–S102.

Kayser AF. Shortened dental arch a therapeutic concept in reduced dentitions and certain high risk groups. *Int J Periodontics Restorative Dent.* 1989;9:426–449.

Lindhe J, Ericcson I. The effect of elimination of jiggling forces on periodontally exposed teeth in the dog. *J Periodontol.* 1982;53:562–567.

Lindhe J, Meyle J. Peri implant diseases: Consensus report of the sixth European Workshop on periodontology. *J Clin Periodontol.* 2008;35(Suppl. 8):282–285.

Papaspyridakos P, Chen CJ, Singh M, Galluci GO. Success criteria in implant dentistry: a systematic review. *J Dent Res.* 2012;91:242–248.

Proceedings of the World Workshop on the Classification of Periodontal and Peri-implant Diseases and Conditions. *J Clin Periodontol.* 2018;45(Suppl 20):S1–S291.

Waerhaug J, Randers-Hansen E. The infrabony pocket and its relationship to trauma from occlusion and subgingival plaque. *J Periodontol.* 1966;50:355–365.

Weston P, Yaziz YA, Moles DR, Needleman I. Occlusal interventions for periodontitis in adults. *Cochrane Database Syst Rev.* 2008: CD004968.

7.2

The Periodontal–Orthodontic Interface

IAN DUNN

CHAPTER OUTLINE

OVERVIEW OF THE CHAPTER

This chapter describes the interactions between periodontal and orthodontic treatment. It explains the need for a stable and healthy periodontium before, during and after orthodontic treatment and how orthodontically moving teeth can reposition them such that they and the associated gingivae are easier to maintain.

By the end of the chapter the reader should:

- Understand how orthodontics can benefit a periodontal patient (a patient who has suffered from periodontal attachment loss)
- Understand how periodontitis affects orthodontic treatment planning
- Know how to prepare a periodontal patient for orthodontic treatment
- Understand how periodontics can help orthodontics.

The chapter covers the following topics:

- Introduction
- The role of the orthodontics in periodontal therapy
- The role of periodontics in orthodontic therapy
- Preparing periodontal patients for orthodontic treatment.

Introduction

Adult orthodontic treatment is a growing area of orthodontic practice because of the increased desire by patients to improve the appearance of their teeth. As already discussed in previous chapters, periodontal diseases can have devastating effects on both the appearance and function of a dentition. As such, for many periodontal patients, as long as their periodontium has been stabilised, orthodontic therapy can be beneficial in improving the appearance and function of a periodontally compromised dentition. This chapter will look at the ways in which orthodontic treatment can complement periodontal therapy; the potential issues that may arise; how the reduced periodontium affects orthodontic treatment planning; how to prepare a patient for, and maintain a patient during, orthodontic treatment; and look at how periodontics can assist orthodontics.

The Role of Orthodontics in Periodontal Therapy

In the following section, a series of clinical problems and how orthodontic treatment may solve them will be described. It should be stressed that, in all cases, the patient should be displaying optimal oral hygiene before any orthodontic treatment commences and that, although the periodontal support for the teeth may be reduced, there should be no evidence of ongoing periodontal breakdown, such as bleeding on probing or pus from periodontal pockets.

1. Crowded Teeth, Anterior Splaying or Over Eruption

Periodontal patients may suffer from the same malocclusions as non-periodontal patients, i.e. crowding, over-jets and cross-bites. In addition, because of the reduced periodontal support and inflammatory status of the tissues, teeth can also drift or splay and over-erupt.

Orthodontic Treatment

Correction of tooth position through routine orthodontics is achievable in periodontal patients (Figure 7.2.1). Teeth can be aligned, de-rotated, extruded or intruded to improve the appearance. Intrusion, in particular, is not without its risks, as this often leads to some apical resorption of the intruded tooth without any additional gain in periodontal support effectively leading to reduced periodontal support. A study by Melsen et al. (1989) showed that when intruding teeth, apical resorption could be as much as 3 mm (Figure 7.2.2). Whereas the primary goal in these cases is improved aesthetics, improved alignment may make cleaning and periodontal maintenance easier.

> **KEY POINT 1**
>
> Intruding teeth may lead to up to 3 mm of apical resorption.

2. Infra-Bony Defects

Although the majority of patients exhibit horizontal bone loss, it is not unusual for vertical bone defects to occur, resulting in infra-bony defects. As discussed in previous chapters, it is possible to regenerate this type of defect using biomaterials and surgical techniques. However, patients planning to undergo orthodontics with infra-bony defects may benefit from having any surgical periodontal treatment well in advance of any orthodontic intervention(s),

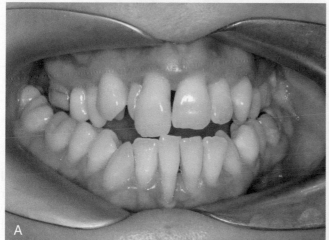

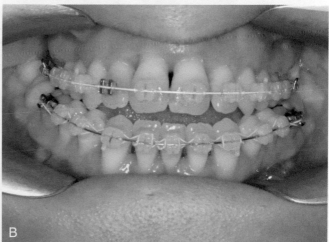

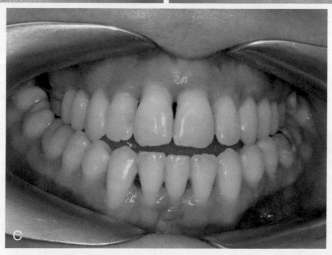

• **Figure 7.2.1** A 30-year-old patient who presented with an aggressive form of periodontitis that was successfully treated. (A) clinical appearance on presentation. (B) Fixed orthodontic appliances in place. (C) Final post-orthodontic result.

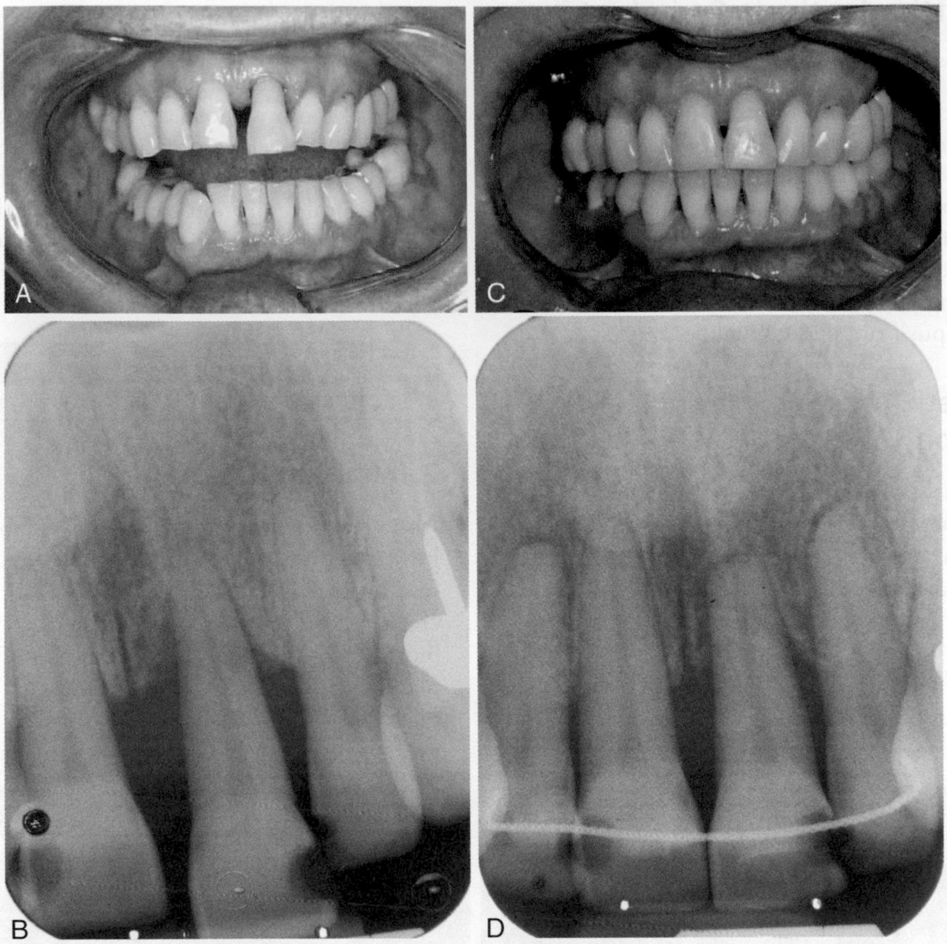

• **Figure 7.2.2** Apical resorption in a periodontally susceptible, orthodontically treated patient. (A) The patient before orthodontic treatment; (B) the UL1 before orthodontic treatment; (C) the patient after orthodontic treatment; (D) the UL1 after orthodontic treatment.

highlighting the need for multidisciplinary treatment planning for these complex cases.

Orthodontic Treatment

In one cohort study (Corrente et al. 2003), 10 patients were treated initially non-surgically and then surgically at the infra-bony defect sites followed by constant, light force orthodontic treatment started within 2 weeks. This resulted in significant gains in all the usual parameters when moving the teeth into the defect sites. It should be noted that, as a cohort study, there was no control group to allow for assessment of the additional effect of the orthodontic treatment.

> #### KEY POINT 2
> Patients planning to undergo orthodontics with infra-bony defects may benefit from having any surgical periodontal treatment well in advance of any orthodontic intervention(s).

3. Gingival Asymmetry

Some patients have asymmetrical teeth or gingival anatomy. While gingival anatomy can be altered surgically using techniques such as crown lengthening, this usually results in the need to restore the exposed crown or root structure, possibly with veneers. However, the need for restorative intervention for aesthetic gain must be balanced against the desirability of retaining tooth structure.

Orthodontic Treatment

Patients undergoing orthodontic treatment to correct malpositioned teeth or for pre-restorative purposes should have their gingival margin positions assessed. Combinations of intrusive and extrusive tooth movements can lead to a more favourable gingival margin symmetry. It should be noted that teeth requiring extrusion, where the gingival margin is already in the correct position, may also require pericision to prevent the alveolar and gingival architecture from being brought down with the extruded tooth. Pericision or fibreotomy involves anaesthetising the soft tissues and, with a blade held in the long axis of the tooth concerned, cutting through the gingival epithelium and connective tissue attachment down to the crest of the alveolar bone with the aim of severing the soft tissue attachment. This eliminates the "pull" on the root from these tissues and makes it easier to move the tooth vertically out of the bone.

4. Loss of Interdental Papillae

Patients undergoing periodontal treatment will often experience gingival recession and loss of the interdental papillae as a result of the bone loss and resolution of the inflammation within the periodontal tissues. The loss of interdental papillae is often, unkindly, referred to as "black triangle disease" because of the resulting interdental spacing. Surgical attempts at regenerating lost interdental papillae have generally been unsuccessful around teeth and most techniques involve masking the spaces with either fixed or removable prostheses such as porcelain veneers with longer contact points or removable silicone gingival veneers.

Orthodontic Treatment

In cases where there is minimal labial recession but loss of interdental tissue, it may be possible to improve the appearance with orthodontics. This involves interproximal "stripping", another term for reduction of the interproximal enamel, to create small spaces between the teeth, allowing the orthodontist to move the teeth together. This in turn lengthens the contact points and reduces the interdental papilla space. The technique is particularly useful in patients with triangular-shaped incisors, where the contact point between adjacent teeth is often small and towards the incisal edge. In these cases, when the reduction and space closure is complete, a more rectangular tooth shape is achieved, and the interdental space is reduced. Tarnow et al. (1992) investigated the distance between the contact point and the alveolar crest and found that if this distance was 5 mm or less, then an interdental papilla was present nearly 100% of the time. When this distance was only 1 mm more, i.e. 6 mm, there was only a papilla approximately 56% of the time. Although orthodontics cannot predictably produce a contact point to bone distance and hence a papilla, reducing the size of the "black triangles" usually leads to a significant aesthetic improvement.

The Role of Periodontics in Orthodontic Therapy

Orthodontic treatment involves applying a force to a tooth that in turn induces osteoclastic and osteoblastic activity, allowing the tooth to be moved within the alveolar bone. As the tooth is moved, bone resorption takes place in the direction of the movement and bone deposition occurs on the opposite side. Patients who are susceptible to periodontitis have dentitions with reduced bone levels around some, or sometimes all, of their teeth. They require regular professional maintenance (supportive periodontal care) by the dental team and self-performed plaque removal. As such, these factors may influence the orthodontic management. Periodontal problems which influence orthodontic treatment will now be considered.

1. Oral Hygiene

Oral hygiene and supportive periodontal care can become more difficult when orthodontic appliances are present.

Influence on Treatment

Wherever possible, orthodontists should avoid using bands on molar teeth, as Boyd & Baumrind (1992) have shown an increase in plaque retention around such bands. Anything that encourages plaque accumulation can be detrimental to periodontal health. Patients should also be taught how to clean around any appliance so that plaque accumulation is minimised.

2. Tooth Crowding

Many dentitions suffer from crowding, which can be aesthetically displeasing and can also create difficulties in oral hygiene for patients. A common solution for crowding is extraction, and this is usually done through loss of a number of premolars in certain combinations depending on the desired tooth movement.

Influence on Treatment

Periodontitis can affect different teeth to a different extent in the same mouth. As such, the orthodontist may want to alter the usual extraction pattern and remove a more compromised tooth to create the required space and leave the remaining teeth, which may have a more predictable prognosis.

3. Reduced Bone Support

Although reduced bone support may mean that there is less bone to resist orthodontic tooth movement, it also means that the teeth are more susceptible to tipping rather than bodily movement, as the centre of rotation is lower. Under these circumstances, using a force that would be suitable for a healthy periodontium may result in "hyalinisation" within the periodontal ligament. Hyalinisation describes the cellular changes that occur if an excessive force is placed on the periodontal ligament for a prolonged period. Blood supply is compromised, and areas of sterile necrosis occur within the ligament. This in turn can result in a slowing or, in extreme cases, prevention of tooth movement.

Influence on Treatment

Periodontal–orthodontic patients are usually treated with fixed, as opposed to removable, appliances, allowing greater control of the force and the direction of the force. Practically, the orthodontist applies a significantly lighter force to the teeth to avoid potential tipping problems and still achieve the desired tooth movement.

> **KEY POINT 6**
>
> Teeth with reduced bone support are more susceptible to tipping rather than bodily movement.

4. Missing Teeth and Poor Anchorage

Tooth loss due to periodontitis is relatively common, and this can cause problems for the orthodontist who requires anchorage for orthodontic appliances.

Influence on Treatment

In a stabilised periodontal patient where there may be missing teeth, anchorage can be obtained using dental implants or, more recently, temporary anchorage devices (TADs). TADs are narrow diameter mini-implants, often placed horizontally between teeth or in edentulous areas, that allow an anchor point from which forces can be applied. Conventional implants can be restored on completion of the orthodontic treatment, whereas TADs are removed when no longer needed.

5. Relapse and Retention

Post-orthodontic retention is a well-documented requirement for all patients to prevent orthodontic relapse which leads to extraction sites reopening or realigned teeth drifting. Retention can be fixed by way of bonded retainers or using removable retainers such as Essix retainers. Sometimes a combination of the two systems may be used. Studies have shown that there are biological and anatomical differences in the tissue reaction between adults and children who

have orthodontic treatment (Melsen 1991). This difference means that adult retention periods are usually significantly longer than those of children. It should be noted that fixed retainers should be inspected at every dental examination for signs of debond or damage. There are documented cases where the retainer wire appears to have been "activated", possibly by trauma to the wire, leading to unwanted orthodontic tooth movement (Figure 7.2.3).

Influence on Treatment

Adult orthodontic retention, in cases where there has been periodontal destruction, usually requires permanent retention. It is preferable that this retention is of the palatal/lingual bonded arch wire variety. The patient's consent must be obtained prior to starting treatment, and permanent retention is something that a patient will need to accept and get used to if they are to maintain a successful orthodontic outcome in the long term. These bonded retainers will have an impact on self-performed plaque control, particularly with respect to interdental cleaning.

> **KEY POINT 7**
>
> After active orthodontic appliance therapy, adult retention periods are usually significantly longer than those of children and, in adults where there has been periodontal destruction, retention may have to be permanent.

6. Gingival Biotype and Gingival Recession

Localised or generalised gingival recession is relatively common, especially in thinner periodontal biotypes where there may be bone dehiscences and thin gingival tissues with little or no attached gingiva.

Influence on Treatment

The risk of post-operative recession in orthodontics relates to the periodontal biotype and the desired tooth movement. Historically, in the UK, orthodontic treatment has centred around an extraction-based approach in crowded dentitions.

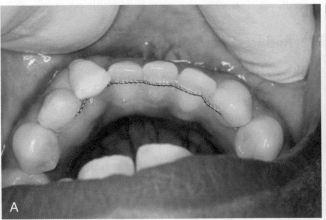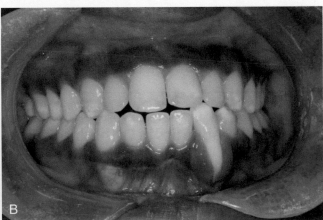

• **Figure 7.2.3** Unplanned orthodontic tooth movement in an adult at the retention stage post-orthodontics, possibly as a result of "activation" of the fixed retention wire. (A) Incisal view, (B) labial view.

Routinely, a number of premolars are removed and the remaining teeth moved around in the spaces created. More recently, there has been an increasing trend towards non-extraction, arch-expansion techniques, increasing the radius of the arch to create space for tooth movement. This results in a broader arch that is regarded by many patients as more aesthetically pleasing, but evidence suggests that this result is less stable and will require a longer period of retention. In addition, labial tooth movement may move teeth outside the alveolar bone envelope, creating a bone dehiscence or dehiscences. If the overlying soft tissue is thin, then there may well be an increased chance of developing gingival recession. Although this may not compromise the health of the dentition, it can be aesthetically displeasing in a patient undergoing an aesthetic procedure, such as orthodontics. Careful pretreatment assessment of the gingival health, periodontal biotype and desired tooth movement is essential if post-treatment recessions are to be avoided.

Interestingly, Wennström et al. (1987) have shown that it is not the apical–coronal measurement of the attached gingiva that is important in determining the chances of developing recession, but the bucco-labial "thickness" of the tissues.

Although some clinicians advocate pre-orthodontic augmentation of thin biotypes in an attempt to prevent recession, the general consensus is that this is over-treatment and the defects can be treated with free gingival grafts or coronally advanced flaps with subepithelial connective tissue grafts should they occur.

> **KEY POINT 8**
> When dental arches are expanded during orthodontic treatment, labial tooth movement may move teeth outside the alveolar bone, creating a bone dehiscence or dehiscences.

7. Minor Soft Tissue Surgery to Assist with Orthodontic Treatment

There are several simple soft tissue procedures that can complement orthodontic procedures, including pericision or fiberotomy, as discussed previously. This procedure involves severing the periodontal fibres under local anaesthetic. It needs to be repeated every 4–6 weeks and has been advocated for preventing the alveolar bone being moved down when extruding a tooth and occasionally in preventing orthodontic relapse in de-rotated teeth.

8. Frenotomy or Frenectomy

Localised gingival recession has in the past been attributed to the presence of a prominent labial frenum ("frenal pull"). There is no evidence for this attribution, and the likelihood is that the frenum may compromise adequate plaque control. Under these circumstances, a simple frenectomy can be performed to remove the unwanted tissue and aid oral hygiene.

Sometimes, a prominent labial frenum has been thought responsible for a midline diastema, especially when the maxillary labial frenum is thick and extends into the palatal tissues. In these cases, a frenotomy may be considered to remove this tissue. This is a more involved procedure compared to a frenectomy and it has been suggested that if provided towards the end of the diastema closure, the scarring and contracting of the healing tissue helps to maintain the diastema closure. However, this assertion is not evidence-based.

9. Gingival Invaginations

Occasionally, as teeth are brought together with orthodontic appliances, there is an element of soft tissue bunching inter-proximally. Whereas this usually remodels over time, occasionally, small soft tissue clefts or invaginations occur that can appear and look unsightly. Simple periodontal surgical techniques can eliminate such defects, producing a more favourable appearance.

Preparing Periodontal Patients for Orthodontic Treatment

Periodontitis is a destructive inflammatory condition that results in bone loss around affected teeth. When an orthodontic force is applied to a tooth, areas of both tension and compression are established within the periodontal ligament. On the side of the tooth under compression, osteoclasts resorb bone, and on the side of the tooth under tension, osteoblasts deposit bone, allowing a tooth to be moved within the alveolus. Orthodontic tooth movement can be thought of as primarily a periodontal ligament phenomenon that results in bone remodelling.

Studies have shown that if periodontitis is not controlled then orthodontic treatment may have an exacerbating effect on the rate of bone loss (Kessler 1976, Bollen et al. 2008) and, as such, careful preparation of a periodontal patient is essential to prevent further bone loss during the active orthodontic phase.

> **KEY POINT 9**
> If periodontal diseases are not controlled, then orthodontic treatment may have an exacerbating effect on the rate of bone loss.

Periodontal Treatment

Periodontal treatment, both non-surgical and surgical, can be very successful in controlling the destructive nature of periodontal diseases in patients who perform high levels of oral hygiene and modify their risk factors. Patients wishing to undergo orthodontic treatment should have periodontal diseases stabilised and maintained prior to embarking on active orthodontic treatment. Orthodontic treatment in the presence of active periodontal diseases is likely to result in further periodontal breakdown.

Once orthodontic treatment commences, oral hygiene may become more difficult for the patient because of the presence of orthodontic appliances, and access issues may arise. This may influence the clinician's periodontal treatment decisions towards more invasive surgical pocket reduction techniques to leave the patient with a periodontium that is easier to maintain.

Periodontally susceptible patients undergoing orthodontic treatment should have their periodontal health carefully maintained and monitored for at least 6 months prior to starting the active phase of orthodontic treatment to ensure patient compliance and stability of the treatment outcomes.

> **KEY POINT 10**
> Patients wishing to undergo orthodontic treatment should have periodontal diseases stabilised and maintained prior to embarking on active orthodontic treatment.

Monitoring and Maintenance

Patients who have successfully completed their periodontal treatment require professional maintenance or supportive care. While maintenance regimens are tailored to the individual based on a risk assessment, in practice most periodontal patients will see their dentist or dental hygienist every 3 months for non-surgical maintenance and for detailed periodontal charting at least annually.

Periodontal patients undergoing orthodontic treatment should be regarded as high-risk patients; they should be seen at least every 3 months for professional maintenance care and monitoring (Boyd et al. 1989). Anecdotally, some periodontists double the frequency of maintenance to six weekly during the active phase of orthodontics.

Any sign of lack of compliance in home care by the patient should result in orthodontic treatment being withdrawn, even if the treatment is not completed (Machen 1990).

All patients undergoing orthodontic treatment should continue with their normal dental routines by seeing their general dentist or dental hygienist at the prescribed intervals for screening of healthy dentitions or monitoring and maintenance of compromised dentitions. Referring clinicians should not abdicate their responsibility to the orthodontist and, if anything, should be especially vigilant.

> **KEY POINT 11**
> Periodontal patients undergoing orthodontic treatment should be regarded as high-risk patients.

Medico-Legal Issues

It is important to ensure that informed, valid consent is obtained when providing any treatment. This is especially important when providing orthodontic treatment for periodontally susceptible patients, for whom there may be increased risk of further loss of periodontal support.

> **KEY POINT 12**
> Informed, valid patient consent is especially important when providing orthodontic treatment for periodontally susceptible patients.

Multiple choice questions on the contents of this chapter are available online at Elsevier eBooks+.

References

Bollen AM, Cunha-Cruz J, Bakko DW, Huang GJ, Hujoel PP. The effects of orthodontic therapy on periodontal health: a systematic review of controlled evidence. *J Am Dent Assoc.* 2008;139(4):413–422.

Boyd RL, Baumrind S. Periodontal considerations in the use of bonds or bands on molars in adolescents and adults. *Angle Orthod.* 1992;62:117–126.

Boyd RL, Leggott PJ, Quinn RS, Eakle WS, Chambers D. Periodontal implications of orthodontic treatment in adults with reduced or normal periodontal tissues versus those of adolescents. *Am J Orthod Dentofacial Orthop.* 1989;96:191–199.

Corrente G, Abudo R, Re S, Cardaropoli D, Cardaropoli G. Orthodontic movement into infrabony defects in patients with advanced periodontal disease: a clinical and radiological study. *J Periodontol.* 2003;74(8):1104–1109.

Kessler M. Interrelationships between orthodontics and periodontics. *Am J Orthod.* 1976;70(2):154–172.

Machen DE. Legal aspects of orthodontic practice: risk management concepts. Periodontal evaluation and updates: don't abdicate your duty to diagnose and supervise. *Am J Orthod Dentofacial Orthop.* 1990;98(1):84–85.

Melsen B. Limitations in adult orthodontics. In: Melsen B, ed. *Current Controversies in Orthodontics.* Chicago: Quintessence; 1991:147–180.

Melsen B, Agerbaek N, Markenstam G. Intrusion of incisors in adult patients with marginal bone loss. *Am J Orthod Dentofacial Orthop.* 1989;(3):232–242.

Tarnow DP, Magner AW, Fletcher P. The effect of the distance from the contact point to the crest of bone on the presence or absence of the interproximal dental papilla. *J Periodontol.* 1992;63:995–996.

Wennström JL, Lindhe J, Sinclair F, Thilander B. Some periodontal tissue reactions to orthodontic tooth movement in monkeys. *J Clin Periodontol.* 1987;14(3):121–129.

7.3

Dental Implants – Anatomy, Complications, Management of Peri-Implant Diseases

COLIN PRIESTLAND AND NEIL MEREDITH

CHAPTER OUTLINE

OVERVIEW OF THE CHAPTER

This chapter outlines the anatomical differences between teeth and implants, the monitoring and maintenance of implants and the management of complications including peri-implant mucositis and peri-implantitis.

By the end of the chapter the reader should:

- Understand the anatomical differences, and their significance, between the supporting tissues of natural teeth and those of dental implants
- Understand the key elements of treatment planning and the use of diagnostic information including 3D imaging
- Understand the clinical stages in the routine maintenance of implants
- Understand the complications arising from dental implant treatment, their possible causes and methods of treatment.

The chapter covers the following topics:

- The anatomical architecture of natural teeth and dental implants
- Dental implant maintenance, complications and management
- Peri-implant inflammatory diseases.

There is also an online component to this chapter which covers the following:

- Development of modern dental implantology
- Treatment planning for dental implant therapy
- The insertion and restoration of dental implants
- Grafting and augmentation materials in dental implantology.

The Anatomical Architecture of Natural Teeth and Dental Implants

Macro- and Micro-Anatomy of Natural Teeth and Dental Implants

The anatomy of the interface between a natural tooth and the surrounding soft tissues, periodontal ligament and bone differs markedly from the anatomy around an implant (see Figure 7.3.1). These macro-anatomical differences are manifest in the different orientation and absence of groups of gingival connective tissue fibres, the absence of a periodontal ligament around an implant, and the direct relationship between the implant surface and bone seen in osseointegration.

The collagen fibre arrangement in the connective tissues around implants differs markedly from the arrangement seen around natural teeth. Gingival fibres are inserted into the root surface of natural teeth but not generally into an implant surface. The attachment in the implant situation exists at the most coronal point of osseointegration.

The primary orientation of connective tissue fibres around implants is similar to that of circular gingival fibres around teeth, there being a complete absence of oblique fibres, trans-septal or dentogingival fibres. This difference in the arrangement of fibres, including the absence of dentogingival fibres, in particular, and the existence of a passive soft tissue "cuff" relationship between the soft tissues and the implant surface, may play a role in the increased susceptibility of the peri-implant tissues to plaque-induced inflammation over the susceptibility of the periodontal tissue arrangement around a natural tooth.

The anatomy of the interdental or inter-implant papillae differs; dentogingival fibres associated with natural

teeth support the soft tissue architecture of the interdental papilla (Palmer 1999). Such a papilla between two adjacent implants relies on other factors including the underlying bone architecture, soft tissue thickness, restorative emergence profile and the distance from the bone crest to the contact point between the two restorations (Tarnow et al. 1992). Other factors that play a role in the stability of the soft tissues around dental implants are as follows:

- The biologic width (now referred to as the "supracrestal tissue attachment") has been investigated in a cadaver study by Gargiulo et al. (2002). The dentogingival junction was reported to have a mean width of 2.04 mm comprising supra-crestal connective tissue and junctional epithelial attachment. Encroachment to within 2 mm of the bone crest appears to result in bone loss in a similar manner at both teeth and implants leading to soft tissue recession.
- The attachment of the long junctional epithelium to the tooth surface appears to be mediated by hemi-desmosomes along the entire length of the junctional epithelium while such an attachment appears to exist only in the apical region of the peri-implant cuff epithelium to the implant surface (Stern 1981). This apparently reduced attachment at implants may also contribute to the weaker soft tissue barrier to bacterial ingress (Hermann et al. 2001). The micro-anatomical interface between tooth or implant and the surrounding tissues may play an important role in the difference in susceptibility to bacterial ingress and the degree of extension of the associated inflammatory lesion in the local soft tissue.
- Further histomorphometric analysis conducted on the attachment zones between the soft tissues, bone and the tooth or implant have been reported to demonstrate comparable ratios of collagen, blood vessels and

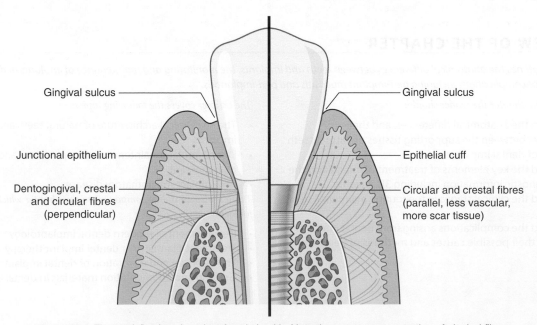

- **Figure 7.3.1** The tooth/implant–host interface in health. Note the greater concentration of gingival fibres around teeth compared to implants (Renvert & Giovannoli 2012).

plasma cells. However, analysis at implants demonstrated reduced proportions of macrophages and polymorpho-nuclear leucocytes. This was interpreted to reflect a weaker immuno-inflammatory barrier at implants than found around teeth (Ivanovski & Lee 2018).

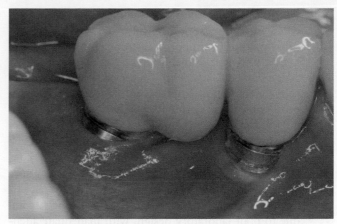

• **Figure 7.3.2** Peri-implantitis around implants with no keratinised gingival margin.

Natural teeth are generally surrounded by a band of keratinised attached gingiva, whereas the positioning of implants with respect to keratinised tissue remains under the control of the surgeon. In cases where there has been a need for significant bone augmentation and hence, an expansion of the ridge volume, the buccal tissues are often advanced coronally to achieve primary closure of the surgical wound. Where there was a pre-existing wide band of keratinised gingiva prior to placing the bone augmentation material and achieving primary closure, it is likely that after primary closure, the muco-gingival junction will remain on the labial or buccal alveolar plate, albeit positioned more coronally. This will result in the implant retaining a reduced width of keratinised gingiva.

In many cases, however, the coronal advancement of the labial or buccal flap, with a pre-existing narrow band of keratinised gingiva, results in the mucogingival junction being located on the ridge crest of the alveolar process so that the buccal aspect of the implant has a non-keratinised alveolar mucosal cuff around the buccal aspect of the implant, abutment or restoration.

It has been suggested that, at sites where the band of keratinised peri-implant tissue is less than 2 mm in width, greater plaque accumulation is found in conjunction with inflammation, but further research is required to clarify if this tissue arrangement is a significant aetiological factor in the development of peri-implant inflammation resulting in peri-implant mucositis, peri-implantitis or recession.

The need for keratinised tissue has been investigated and reported by Wennström & Derks (2012), but following review of 19 studies, they concluded that there was insufficient comparable data to draw any scientific and statistical conclusions regarding the relationship between the width of keratinised tissue around implants and the degree of plaque accumulation, peri-implant inflammation and recession around implants (see Figure 7.3.2). However, it should remain the aim in all implant surgery to achieve keratinised tissue around implants whenever possible (see Figures 7.3.3 and 7.3.4).

Soft Tissue Biotype

The soft tissue biotype refers to the thickness and contour of the gingival tissues. There is no clear definition of biotype, but it is generally believed that where a thin biotype exists, it is more difficult to achieve a stable soft tissue–implant relationship than would be the case in the presence of a thick biotype. Definitive measurements within the classification of thick versus thin biotype have yet to be universally accepted, but generally <1 mm thickness is thin biotype and >2 mm is thick biotype. The tissue between 1 mm and 2 mm may provide some confusion when attempting to interpret the literature and the effects of biotype on tissue susceptibility to peri-implant mucositis, implantitis, recession and crestal bone loss.

Implant Complications

There is a misconception that once successfully integrated, dental implants will last a lifetime. This is both inaccurate and misleading. Failures and complications may arise because of either biomechanical or biological factors, or a combination of the two.

- Biomechanical factors include:
  - *Occlusal overload* – can result in peri-implant bone loss typically with the radiographic appearance of a vertical or funnel-shaped defect. This may be due to poor occlusal design. Such situations may include the use of distal cantilever pontics and occlusal schemes with increased load application in the intercuspal position/centric occlusion (ICP/CO) or interferences during various mandibular excursions from ICP/CO. High levels of occlusal loading can be applied to implants by bruxing and other parafunction, including clenching, or by poor biomechanical prosthesis design. The consequence of excessive loads can result in bone loss and also implant, abutment screw and prosthesis fracture. Provision of an occlusal splint should be considered in patients exhibiting parafunction.
  - *Poor implant angulation* – generally occlusal forces should be applied along the long axis of an implant. This is not always achievable but should generally be the aim. Overloading or angulated loading can typically result in implant or component fracture.

Exceptions exist to this general rule, for example, when implants are joined by a bar or laser-welded sub-structure to support a fixed or removable bridge, hybrid bridge or over-denture.

- *Inappropriate components* – poor-quality components can contribute to implant failure and components must conform to nationally accepted standards.

- Biological factors:
  - *Plaque-induced inflammation* – this may be due to a lack of patient motivation to perform detailed plaque control procedures, poor manual dexterity that may arise as a patient ages or as their health deteriorates, or difficulty in achieving adequate access for plaque removal due to poor laboratory design, with inadequate attention being paid to the accessibility of cleaning aids to enable the patient to maintain plaque control beneath the prosthetic device and around the implant cuff to maintain soft and hard tissue health. Resulting peri-implant inflammation may arise, leading to the development of peri-implant mucositis or peri-implantitis.
  - *Smoking* – there is an association between those patients who smoke and peri-implant diseases. A contributing factor to oral disease in smokers is the vasoconstriction in the oral and circum-oral region, resulting from numerous chemicals present in the smoke to which the oral tissues are exposed. This reduces vascularity and blood flow to the oral and circum-oral tissues that may cause oxidative stress of the tissues, increasing their susceptibility to infection and adversely affecting the tissues' ability to heal. Smoking must therefore be considered an important risk factor in the aetiology of peri-implant mucositis and peri-implantitis, and smokers should be strongly encouraged to quit before embarking on an implant treatment plan.
  - *Past history of periodontal disease* – those patients who are susceptible to chronic inflammatory periodontal disease and suffer significant destructive changes with loss of periodontal attachment levels are generally found to be more susceptible to peri-implant inflammatory diseases, with those who have more severe periodontal diseases being the most susceptible to peri-implant complications (Sousa et al. 2016). However, past periodontal patients who have received treatment and who have continued to maintain excellent plaque control may continue to enjoy good peri-implant health after implant therapy. These patients will continue to be genetically susceptible to peri-implant inflammatory disease in the presence of reduced oral hygiene and plaque accumulation.
  - *Thin tissue biotype* – a thin biotype has been identified as a risk factor for the development of peri-implant inflammation and recession in the presence of sub-optimal hygiene. It may be prudent to alter the nature of the surrounding soft tissue by the provision of a sub-epithelial connective tissue or free gingival graft. Alternative xenogenic and allograft materials are also available to extend the keratinised zone or thicken the adjacent soft tissue.
  - *Uncontrolled or inadequately controlled diabetes* – patients suffering diabetes that remains inadequately controlled by diet, medication or both are more prone to infection. However, well-controlled diabetics who maintain good oral hygiene are not considered to have any greater susceptibility to infection than non-diabetic patients. Patients who fail to demonstrate a commitment to maintaining both good oral hygiene and effective diabetic control are therefore not ideal for implant therapy.

> **KEY POINT 3**
>
> Implants are susceptible to failures and complications due to either biomechanical or biological factors, or a combination of the two.

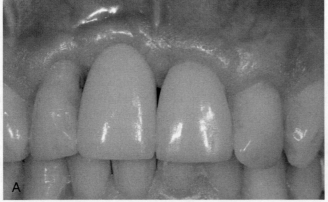 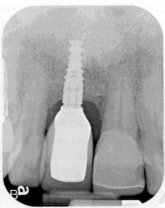

- **Figure 7.3.3** (A) An implant at UR1 with healthy gingival margins (B) Radiograph of the same implant showing good bone support

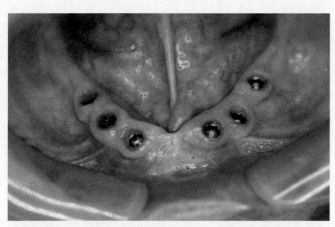

• **Figure 7.3.4** Peri-implant health in an edentulous mandible in a patient with a number of risk factors, including xerostomia, but with excellent oral hygiene. This patient had been provided with a mandibular bar and clip-retained over-denture to allow for proper self-care and professional maintenance.

Aetiology and Pathogenesis of Peri-Implant Diseases

Biofilm Formation and Maturation

There are over 700 microbial species that exist in the human mouth from which the biofilm can develop (Aas et al. 2005). Periodontitis (and by inference peri-implant diseases) is a biofilm-associated disease (Darveau et al. 1997, Marsh 2005) and many microbial interactions take place to protect the bacterial species and increase their pathogenicity and potential to induce tissue destruction (Schaudinn et al. 2009).

Specific Microbial Findings with Implants

Healthy osseo-integrated implants have been found to have relatively little biofilm and minimal inflammation associated with the peri-implant sulcus (Lekholm et al. 1986; Leonhardt et al. 1992). The flora found around healthy implant sites are similar to the flora found in gingival health around natural teeth (Mombelli & Meriscke-Stern 1990, Rams et al. 1991). It has also been demonstrated that the presence of putative periodontopathogens is more common in dentate implant patients rather than edentulous patients, suggesting that periodontal pockets present around natural teeth may serve as a reservoir for organisms from which colonisation of titanium implants may occur (Apse et al. 1989, Quiryen & Listgarten 1990, Leonhardt et al. 1999).

The microbiological studies carried out in patients who have suffered bone loss around implants indicate similar findings to those reported in periodontitis. In a study involving 51 patients with healthy implant-supporting tissues and 37 patients with one or more implants with loss of attachment of three or more threads accompanied by bleeding on probing and suppuration, subgingival plaque samples were collected using paper points. Culture studies were performed that demonstrated putative pathogens *Porphyromonas gingivalis, Prevotella intermedia, Prevotella nigrescens,* and *Aggregatibacter actinomycetemcomitans* in 60% of cases. Organisms not normally associated with periodontitis, including *Staphylococcus* spp., enteric organisms and *Candida* spp., were found in 55% of peri-implantitis sites, whereas healthy sites around implants demonstrated a microbiota associated with periodontal health around natural teeth.

In summary, Leonhardt and co-workers suggest healthy implant sulci harbour a similar flora to healthy gingival crevices around teeth. However, sites with peri-implantitis were found to be populated with organisms associated with periodontitis in almost equal proportions to additional flora, including *Staphylococci*, yeasts and enteric organisms (Leonhardt et al. 1999).

It has also been demonstrated by ligature-induced plaque formation in the dog model that, where the implant surface is exposed to microbial contamination, the degree of roughness of an implant surface influences the nature of the flora that develops on that surface (Berglundh et al. 2007). It was also found that rougher implant surfaces exhibit accelerated progression of peri-implantitis. This explains the general preference for implants with a relatively smooth collar despite the high degree of roughness of that part of the implant designed for osseointegration within the bone.

> ### KEY POINT 4
> Implants can accumulate both a health- and disease-associated biofilm in the same manner as teeth.

Incidence of Peri-Implant Inflammation

In several large-scale and international research studies, patients have received implant therapy and have then returned to the ongoing care of their general dentist. Large numbers of such patients have then been recalled for re-examination to assess the health of the soft tissues and the bone surrounding the implants. The results show that unless implant patients are given specific implant care (including professional cleaning and oral hygiene advice), a progressive reduction in peri-implant bone can be expected. The extent of inflammation and bone loss around dental osseo-integrated implants in those patients who fail to get the professional support they need is disturbing.

The results vary between studies largely because of a variation in definitions and thresholds. Zitzmann & Berglundh (2008) reported peri-implant mucositis occurred in approximately 80% of the subjects and in 50% of the implants. It has also been reported that around 50% of implant patients are found to exhibit peri-implant inflammatory changes (Koldsland et al. 2010) and around 20% of all implant patients and 10–15% of implants were found to have suffered from peri-implantitis (Mombelli et al. 2012). It is therefore imperative that the periodontal and implant communities agree to common threshold levels for peri-implant mucositis and implantitis to allow comparison of research studies on this subject.

Patients who have a history of periodontitis are susceptible to the destructive effects of periodontal inflammation around implants as well as natural teeth. These patients must receive meticulous periodontal therapy to reduce the plaque to below the threshold required to initiate inflammation in that patient. The elimination of this inflammation can then stabilise peri-implant disease. Once clinically and radiographically classified as stable, implant patients should be provided with regular ongoing periodontal supportive treatment in the presence of patient cooperation.

In a study of periodontally susceptible patients who were receiving periodontal supportive therapy, 786 implants were assessed in 239 patients. Data was analysed at both the subject and implant level. Peri-implant mucositis was diagnosed in 24.7% of subjects and 12.8% of implants whereas peri-implantitis was diagnosed in 15.1% of subjects and 9.8% of implants (Aguirre-Zorzano et al. 2015). They concluded that the level of peri-implant inflammatory disease was clinically significant with aetiologically significant factors being plaque index and implant location. However, these figures appear to be no greater than studies of patients with no history of periodontal disease (Mombelli et al. 2012, Koldsland et al. 2010) thereby demonstrating the benefits of supportive periodontal care for implant patients who remain susceptible to peri-implant inflammatory disease.

Atieh et al. (2012) carried out a meta-analysis of 9 studies with 1497 subjects and 6283 implants included in the analysis. It was found that the frequency of peri-implant mucositis was 63.4% of subjects and 30.7% of implants, and the frequency of peri-implantitis was 18.8% of subjects and 9.6% of implants. When the data for smokers were analysed separately, a frequency of peri-implantitis was found to be 36.3%. The authors therefore concluded that supportive periodontal therapy appeared to reduce the rate of occurrence of peri-implantitis. They further concluded that peri-implant diseases are not uncommon following implant therapy. Long-term maintenance care for high-risk groups is essential to reduce the risk of peri-implantitis. It was also proposed that informed consent for patients receiving implant treatment must include patient acceptance of the need for appropriate maintenance therapy.

> ### KEY POINT 5
> Peri-implant diseases are not uncommon following implant therapy, and long-term maintenance care is essential to reduce the risk of peri-implant diseases.

Histopathology of Periodontitis and Peri-Implantitis

There are histopathological differences between lesions of periodontitis around natural teeth and lesions of peri-implantitis at implant sites. Results of studies and analysis of human biopsy material have shown that peri-implantitis lesions are poorly encapsulated and are more closely associated with the adjacent bone (Berglundh et al. 2011) (see Figure 7.3.5). Inflammatory lesions are larger and extend nearer the bone crest than equivalent lesions seen in periodontitis, consistent with the reduced connective tissue fibres around implants compared to natural teeth. Lesions of peri-implantitis have been found to contain larger proportions of neutrophils and osteoclasts than would normally be seen in sites of periodontitis around natural teeth (Carcuac et al. 2013).

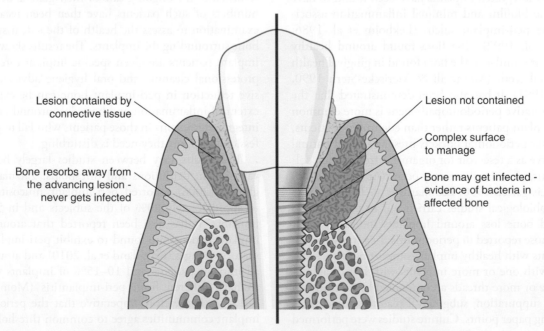

Lesion contained by connective tissue

Bone resorbs away from the advancing lesion – never gets infected

Lesion not contained

Complex surface to manage

Bone may get infected – evidence of bacteria in affected bone

• **Figure 7.3.5** The tooth/implant–host interface in disease (Renvert & Giovannoli 2012).

Comparing Periodontal Diseases and Peri-Implant Diseases

The microbiological, immunological and anatomical findings of research suggests that there are similarities between natural teeth and implants in health, and similarities between periodontitis and peri-implantitis, but differences remain that have still to be completely explained when comparing lesions of periodontitis and peri-implantitis.

Implant failure has been divided into early, late and noninfectious (overload) (Esposito et al. 1998). There are a large number of interrelated factors and cofactors that may contribute to peri-implant disease; these include cardiovascular disease, diabetes, smoking, medication and implant surface topography. The complexity of the aetiology makes isolation of single factors difficult to achieve.

It has long been established that the regular and effective biofilm control is required to prevent the development of gingivitis around natural teeth (Löe et al. 1965, Theilade et al. 1966, Löe et al. 1967) and that poor biofilm control will allow the progression from gingivitis to severe loss of periodontal support in a proportion of subjects, but not all. This indicated that periodontal disease may be a disease of a high-risk, susceptible group consisting of around 15–30% of the population. Chapter 1.3 identifies the epidemiology of periodontal diseases. It is also confirmed that the cause of this progression is multifactorial in nature with genetics, smoking exposure, systemic disease, immunological factors, local factors and oral hygiene all playing a role. This complex relationship between the causative factors, periodontal tissues and immunological defence mechanisms resulting in chronic periodontitis around natural teeth has been researched for many years. The relationship between implants and peri-implant inflammatory disease has been researched for only a fraction of that time and therefore it is not surprising that many questions remain unanswered.

The current understanding of the relationship between implants, implant restorations and peri-implant soft and hard tissue health is that peri-implant mucositis is largely equivalent to gingivitis whereas peri-implantitis is largely equivalent to periodontitis.

KEY POINT 6

Peri-implant mucositis is the equivalent of gingivitis, and peri-implantitis is the equivalent of periodontitis.

It is generally accepted that peri-implant mucositis is found where there is plaque accumulation. The quantity of plaque is difficult to assess objectively, as the aetiological flora inhabit the subgingival environment and limitations exist in objective quantitative and qualitative assessment of this primarily anaerobic ecological niche of microorganisms.

Implant Factors in Peri-Implant Disease

The association between the aetiology of peri-implant disease and implant surface design is a contentious one. Historically there has been a clear association between bone loss, implant failure and various implant surfaces and designs. Surfaces including TPS (titanium plasma sprayed) and some hydroxyapatite coatings were clearly linked to clinical failure as were hollow and basket-shaped designs. Several studies are cited that demonstrate little or no bone loss around rough-surfaced implants having a surface roughness S_a value of 1.5 or greater. However, many experienced clinicians are observing a higher level of peri-implantitis in "real-world" clinical groups where rougher surfaces have been used.

The question remains: is a conservative, moderately rough implant surface and design sufficient to achieve the early integration desired today and yet provide the long-term stability and bone level maintenance essential to long-term clinical success?

Ideal implant anatomy involves an intimate relationship between the prosthetic abutment and the peri-implant soft tissue cuff. The implant collar should be deeply placed, level with the crest of the bone allowing for close adaptation of the gingival tissue to the implant abutment. Some implant manufacturers, in order to increase the connective tissue volume around the connection between the implant and the prosthetic abutment, have adopted a platform-switch design in an attempt to maintain tissue stability. Other implants exhibit surface design features to encourage the attachment of connective tissue to the collar zone of the implant, whereas other systems employ a collar that exhibits a far smoother texture than the surface of the implant that is designed to encourage bone apposition or soft tissue desmosomal attachment.

Implants that have a relatively smooth, machined collar attract less plaque deposition and are far easier to maintain plaque free with correct hygiene techniques. Implants with a uniform rough surface throughout the body and collar of the implant encourage plaque accumulation at the collar and present a difficult surface from which to remove plaque, when exposed to the subgingival environment or when exposed to the oral cavity. When presenting for treatment, the dental hygienist, dentist or periodontist will encounter greater difficulty in achieving adequate disinfection and removal of toxins, including lipopolysaccharide endotoxin, from any implant where the rough surface has become contaminated.

As in periodontally susceptible patients, it remains the responsibility of the patient to maintain adequate biofilm control on a daily basis. There are many techniques available to access the more anatomically inaccessible sites to disrupt the biofilm. This is a fundamental requirement to avoid plaque biofilm accumulation, development of periodontal or peri-implant inflammation and associated periodontal or peri-implant attachment destruction.

KEY POINT 7

It is the responsibility of the patient to maintain adequate biofilm control around implants on a daily basis.

Routine, professional follow-up is an essential tool in order to maintain a functional and healthy implant/tissue interface to ensure long-term implant success and to identify and manage any potential complications early. Serial intraoral radiographs are a useful adjunct to clinical examination in monitoring bone levels, but to be most effective, the view should be taken in a reproducible technique; with the film parallel to the implant long axis, the central beam of the X-rays should be directed at right angles to the implant, and the film providing a clear and detailed image of the implant thread and the bone. By repeated imaging in such a reproducible manner, changes in bone level can be identified, ensuring timely periodontal support before significant peri-implant support is lost.

Classification and Diagnosis of Peri-Implant Diseases

The 2018 World Workshop on the Classification of Periodontal and Peri-implant Diseases and Conditions proposed a new classification system for both periodontal and peri-implant diseases (Caton et al. 2018) which has now been globally accepted. Peri-implant health, peri-implant mucositis and peri-implantitis were defined clinically and histologically. The clinical definitions of these various states of peri-implant health and disease are described in Table 7.3.1.

Diagnosis of Peri-Implant Mucositis

The diagnostic signs of peri-implant mucositis include an alteration in the soft tissue colour with erythema, changed soft tissue contour, bleeding on probing and/or suppuration, commonly associated with increased probing depths of up to 4 mm in the absence of radiographic loss of bone from around the implant.

The incidence reported in the literature varies widely depending on diagnostic criteria adopted. Peri-implant mucositis has been reported to affect between 25% and 80% of subjects and 13% and 50% of implants according to Roos-Jansaker et al. (2006), Zitzmann & Berglundh (2008) and Aguirre-Zorzano et al. (2015). Such wide variations in prevalence indicates the need for globally agreed diagnostic criteria.

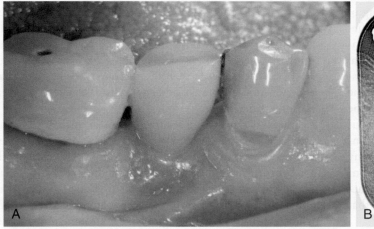
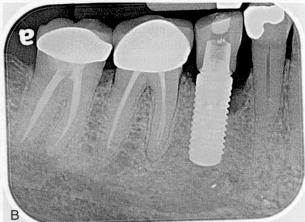

• **Figure 7.3.6** (A) Peri-implantitis around an implant with attached gingivae; (B) radiograph of the same implant.

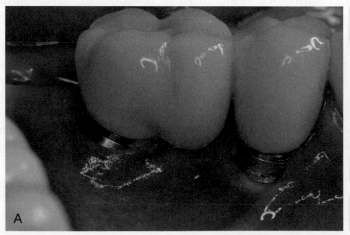
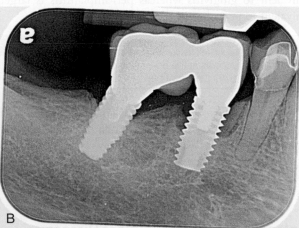

• **Figure 7.3.7** (A) Peri-implantitis around an implant with no attached gingivae; (B) radiograph of the same implant.

TABLE 7.3.1	Clinical definitions of peri-implant health and disease	
Condition	Clinical features	
Peri-implant health	• absence of signs of inflammation • absence of bleeding and/or suppuration on gentle probing • no increase in probing depth compared to previous examinations • *Note: peri-implant health can exist around implants with some pocketing* • absence of bone loss beyond crestal bone levels • *Note: peri-implant health can exist around implants with variable levels of bone support*	
Peri-implant mucositis	• presence of bleeding and/or suppuration on gentle probing with or without increased probing depth compared to previous examinations • absence of bone loss beyond crestal bone levels • *Note: visual signs of inflammation can vary and peri-implant mucositis can exist around implants with variable levels of bone support*	
Peri-implantitis (established patient)	• presence of bleeding and/or suppuration on gentle probing • increased probing depth compared to previous examinations • presence of bone loss beyond crestal bone levels	
Peri-implantitis (new patient)	• presence of bleeding and/or suppuration on gentle probing • probing depths ≥6 mm • bone levels ≥ 3 mm apical to the most coronal portion of the intraosseous part of the implant • *Note: visual signs of inflammation can vary, and recession of the mucosal margin should be considered in probing depth evaluation*	

(World Workshop on the Classification of Periodontal and Peri-implant Diseases and Conditions 2018)
Reprinted from *Journal of Clinical Periodontology* 45(S20):8, Maurizio S Tonetti et al. (2018), with permission from John Wiley & Sons.

Experimental studies of peri-implant mucositis indicate that inflammatory changes are reversible following thorough anti-infective therapy (Pontoriero et al. 1994, Salvi et al. 2012), with elimination of the biofilm from the implant, prosthetic abutment and restoration surfaces.

Left untreated, peri-implant mucositis appears to be the precursor to peri-implantitis in many cases, in the same way as gingivitis is a precursor to periodontitis. However, just as patients suffering from gingivitis may experience a stable gingivitis that does not progress to a destructive periodontitis, it appears that peri-implant mucositis does not necessarily progress to peri-implantitis. However, if peri-implant mucositis is found to be present, treatment should be directed at its elimination and future prevention to avoid the potential for the development of peri-implantitis.

Diagnosis of Peri-Implantitis

In addition to peri-implant inflammation, with or without suppuration, peri-implantitis presents with bone loss that may be detectable either clinically or radiographically (see Figures 7.3.6 and 7.3.7). Early detection of bone loss relies on accurate and reproducible radiography with a film parallel to the long axis of the implant. The bone crest may then be related to the thread of the implant, providing accurate interpretation when judging if the crest has remained stable or has reduced. Periodontal probing is also a useful examination to determine whether the implant thread can be detected. The incidence of peri-implantitis varies between studies, but when the criteria for radiographic bone loss is set at 2 mm or greater, then incidence is generally reported around 20% of subjects and 10% of implants (Atieh et al. 2012, Aguirre-Zorzano et al. 2015). Globally accepted diagnostic criteria need to be adopted to ensure comparability of peri-implantitis studies, thereby increasing the number of studies that may be accepted for systematic reviews.

Management of Peri-Implant Diseases

Patient Prophylaxis

Daily biofilm disruption around all implants and teeth should be achieved using an accepted technique. Brushing with a conventional manual toothbrush is often ineffective for a number of reasons that include:
• incorrect size of the brush head,
• use of a scrubbing motion,
• use of hard bristles,
• use of excessive force,
• inadequate frequency of brushing,
• inadequate brushing time,
• missing areas because of a lack of a standardised sequence of brushing.

A systematic review of 59 studies revealed an average plaque removal of 42% (range 30–53%) depending on the particular plaque index chosen. Differences in bristle tuft design were found to influence the outcome with angled designs being more effective, achieving a plaque reduction of 62%. Brushing duration was also important in plaque removal.

Systematic reviews of studies investigating the effectiveness of powered brushes versus manual brushes have been published. These have demonstrated more effective plaque removal with powered brushes than manual brushes (Niedermann 2003, Deery et al. 2004). More recently the incorporation of accelerometer sensors into powered brushes altering the brushing mode depending on brush position further improves the effectiveness of plaque removal.

• A high frequency electric vibration brush can be effective in maintaining a high standard of plaque control; however, this technique should be supplemented with floss and proximal brushes of various designs between teeth/implants to obtain the best plaque control possible.

- For manual brushing a single-tufted interproximal brush may also be effective used at an angle of 45 degrees to the restoration or tooth surface, the bristles should be splayed apart, and then advanced subgingivally before initiating a very small vibratory movement. This requires a fair degree of manual dexterity that not all patients possess.
- Antimicrobial agents may be used on the brush, though the length of time the active ingredient remains in the crevice/cuff is likely to be short and will therefore have a limited antimicrobial effect.

Professional Support

Regular and thorough professional debridement of the implant/abutment/restoration surfaces exposed to contamination must take place. This can be achieved using several techniques, all of which have a place in the prevention and treatment of periodontal and peri-implant disease.

- Ultrasonic or piezo-electric scalers with non-damaging tips for implant surfaces including Teflon, plastic or titanium inserts. The inserts must be very narrow to gain access to the relatively inaccessible sites where debridement or biofilm disruption is required, particularly in the interdental areas and within the peri-implant cuff.
- Hand instrumentation is best limited to removing calculus that remains despite piezo-electric or ultrasonic scaling.
- Following mechanical biofilm disruption, adjunctive methods may be employed to achieve as near as possible to complete elimination of the microbial plaque if there is a periodontal or peri-implant inflammatory response to established plaque. These adjunctive techniques may include the following:
  - Lasers may be beneficial using light energy of a wavelength that is absorbed by particular pigments produced by many anaerobic, pathogenic bacteria. The application of laser light energy that is preferentially absorbed by those particular pigments will result in the destruction of the pigment-containing bacteria. Furthermore, if there is an associated inflammatory response to the presence of those pathogenic bacteria, and the laser light energy is preferentially absorbed by haemoglobin in the expanded vasculature, then this inflamed tissue will also be destroyed. This will have the effect of reducing the extent of the inflammatory lesion.
  - The use of air polishing (a pressurised air jet with abrasive particles) can be effective in removing particles from the supra- and subgingival environments and from tooth or implant surfaces.
  - Submucosal application of chlorhexidine may also have a beneficial effect on microbial control. The literature is equivocal on the benefits of antimicrobials and antiseptics to enhance plaque control and control periodontal inflammation. There appears to be inadequate scientific evidence and guidance on the use of sub-mucosal application of antibiotic and antiseptic preparations to achieve effective control of flora in peri-implant disease.

Management of Peri-Implant Mucositis

The successful management of this early stage of peri-implant inflammatory disease is dependent on clear communication of suitable home plaque control measures and motivation of the patient to achieve improved biofilm disruption in order to resolve inflammation and maintain improved peri-implant health. Once the patient is able and willing to perform the necessary hygiene measures, then the peri-implant environment should be professionally cleaned in a thorough manner using ultrasonic or piezo-electric scaling tips suitable for use against the implant surface. Hand instrumentation is relatively ineffective, particularly when the biofilm is attached to the microscopically rough surface of the implant.

Adjunctive use of antimicrobials, air polishing or suitable laser therapy may be applied at the clinician's discretion to improve antimicrobial activity. Review of the site is essential to ensure healing is taking place, and a longer-term maintenance regime should be agreed upon with the patient to ensure the improvement in peri-implant health is maintained. Once a patient has been identified as being susceptible to peri-implant mucositis, their susceptibility remains, and they should therefore be considered a higher-risk patient and provided with an enhanced professionally supported maintenance care plan.

> ### KEY POINT 8
> Both daily home care and professional support are essential to ensure long-term peri-implant health.

Management of Peri-Implantitis

Heitz-Mayfield & Mombelli (2014) conducted a systematic review and concluded that generally treatment of peri-implantitis results in an improvement in the clinical condition. However, peri-implantitis in some patients appears to present a degree of resistance to therapy. In these patients there was a recurrence or progression of peri-implantitis that required re-treatment or removal of the implant. The effectiveness of therapy appears to relate to the thoroughness of anti-infective treatment with elimination of the biofilm from the surfaces of the implant/abutment/restoration being the aim. The most appropriate treatment protocol will be individually driven by patient and site-specific factors.

Increasing concern has been expressed for sites with peri-implantitis resulting from the incomplete removal of cement left in the subgingival space around dental implants following cementation of the implant restoration (Wilson 2009). The cementation of crowns on implants is still a common practice, though screw retention is preferable for retrievability in case of restorative fractures or peri-implant inflammatory disease. Several commonly used luting cements are undetectable on radiographs (Wadhwani et al. 2010) and therefore can only be found by careful periodontal probing with an appropriate instrument. The cement surface topography is likely to provide a suitable plaque-retentive surface for the development of a biofilm with resulting inflammation. Complete removal of all cement deposits is required to prevent progressive loss of attachment and the development of a severe peri-implantitis.

A detailed assessment of the extent and degree of peri-implantitis should be undertaken combining visual, radiographic and probing examinations to achieve a clear picture of the underlying bone contour and possible implant surface exposure due to bone dehiscence. An assessment should also be made of the degree of biofilm accumulation and the patient educated on the correct performance of biofilm control. It is very often helpful to remove the prosthesis and replace with healing abutments to facilitate easier access for home care throughout the period of treatment for the peri-implantitis.

Once the patient is able to carry out home care to the necessary standard, professional cleaning should be performed and the patient reviewed over time to confirm their continued cooperation and healing. It is likely that the peri-implant sulcus depth will be deeper where peri-implantitis has been present, and biofilm control techniques may have to be modified to achieve this more challenging biofilm disruption and more frequent professional support in a less accessible location. More adjunctive therapeutic techniques may be applied from the outset in order to achieve control of the destructive lesion. The use of a diode laser has been found to be extremely effective in conjunction with thorough debridement, and air-polishing use can also provide an effective means of debridement of the rough implant surface, the peri-implant sulcus and the soft tissue outer wall of the sulcus, such as the EMS AirFlow, PerioFlow and Piezon approach to guided biofilm therapy. However, lesions of peri-implantitis do not always respond adequately to an entirely non-surgical approach to treatment.

Where several threads of the implant are no longer covered by bone and there has been an aggressive inflammatory response seen clinically in the adjacent soft tissues, accompanied by recession, open debridement of the site may have to follow the non-surgical approach adopted initially. Thorough debridement of the implant surface is fundamental to achieving a good clinical outcome.

Several authors advocate the use of various chemicals to assist in this implant surface preparation (Salvi et al. 2007, Kotsovilis et al. 2006). The use of citric acid in combination with mechanical debridement is reported to have been successful in achieving a satisfactory outcome when treating peri-implantitis. Some authors have also suggested using tetracycline, ethylene-diamine-tetra-acetic acid (EDTA) and various antimicrobials.

Ultimately after healing is established, the site must be assessed for its stability and its anatomical susceptibility to further damage including recession, leading to further implant thread exposure, creating a greater hygiene challenge for the patient. In these cases the application of a sub-epithelial connective tissue graft may thicken the tissues significantly and provide a more robust barrier to the development of peri-implantitis in the future, where formerly the implant was surrounded by non-keratinised alveolar mucosa. Modification of the implant surface may also provide additional benefits by removing supra-gingival threads and rough implant surface and achieving a polished surface more conducive to plaque removal by the patient. However, such surface modification of the titanium implant surface may be challenging because of poor access proximally.

Appropriate treatment depends on correct diagnosis, identification of relevant contributing factors and assessment of the level of bone destruction taking place. While management of peri-implant mucositis is within the scope of practice of a general dentist with implant training, the identification of such a lesion from one where peri-implantitis is becoming established can be challenging. For that reason, the referral of such patients for specialist assessment and management should be considered at an early stage in the disease process, rather than providing incomplete therapy that allows further deterioration and loss of supporting bone that may endanger the longevity of the implant and restoration. Early referral is far preferable to late referral and will both maintain the patient's confidence in their general dental practitioner and provide the practitioner with a measure of medico-legal defence should peri-implantitis endanger the implant and the patient wish to enter into litigation.

> ### KEY POINT 9
> If peri-implantitis is diagnosed or suspected, early referral to a periodontal specialist is indicated.

Individualised Implant Maintenance

All patients who receive implant therapy should be assessed for their future risk of plaque-associated periodontal and peri-implant inflammation. Once their degree of risk has been identified, an individualised supportive protocol should be developed with the patient's involvement to ensure the oral environment presents the lowest risk possible to the establishment of periodontal or peri-implant inflammatory diseases.

Patients with very few risk factors would include patients who have suffered no previous periodontitis, have no detectable family history of periodontal disease or premature tooth loss, are systemically healthy, do not smoke and maintain excellent plaque control with gingival crevices around natural teeth of no more than 3 mm at any site. These patients should be seen by a dental hygienist to monitor their plaque control, check the health of the oral soft tissues and help to re-motivate the patient to continue their commitment to maintaining good plaque control. The frequency of review may depend on dental and non-dental factors, including the oral findings and the patient's ability to afford regular care and support. Frequency of review may vary between six-monthly and annually.

Patients who are considered to have an increased risk of periodontal or peri-implant inflammatory diseases include patients with a history of some of the following risk factors, including previous periodontitis, a family history of periodontal disease and/or premature tooth loss, systemic disease including sub-optimally controlled diabetes (Heitz-Mayfield 2008, Kotsovilis et al. 2006) or an indication of a compromised immunological response, a recent history of smoking or continued smoking (Lang & Berglundh 2011, Ong et al. 2008), the presence of sites exhibiting periodontal inflammation with sub-optimal plaque control (Serino & Ström 2009) and the presence of periodontal pockets of more than 3 mm in depth with bleeding on blunt probing and/or suppuration. The deeper pockets provide a suitable ecological niche in which a reservoir of flora can thrive to initiate recolonisation of implant and restorative surfaces with putative pathogens (Papaioannou et al. 1996, Gouvoussis et al. 1997), especially in patients with a history of aggressive periodontitis (DeBoever & DeBoever 2006). High-risk patients require a different approach, incorporating a greater frequency of professional support and a higher level of profession intervention (Karoussis et al. 2007, Lindhe & Meyle 2008, Lang & Berglundh 2011, Ong et al. 2008).

High-risk patients should not normally receive implant therapy, but should such therapy have been provided, then they would normally be reviewed and supported by a dental hygienist at a frequency of 2–4 monthly, and additional review with the implant dentist or periodontist would normally take place every 6–12 months. At each review an assessment of plaque accumulation should take place with plaque disclosure preceding observation of the patient's own efforts to maintain plaque control. Correction of plaque control measures would take place where necessary, and further observation of the patients corrected techniques should follow. A full-mouth debridement should take place around the implants and natural teeth to minimise the reservoir of bacteria available to repopulate the oral environment, and in particular, the periodontal and peri-implant sulci and pockets. Following debridement the use of an air-polishing system can be useful to remove any residual flora or debris.

It is accepted that patients who have active chronic or aggressive periodontitis should not receive implant therapy due to the higher risk of implant failure and the raised likelihood of their implants being affected by peri-implantitis. However, patients who have a past history of chronic or aggressive periodontitis and who have subsequently received periodontal treatment and have co-operated fully with the requirement for meticulous plaque control, and have received periodontal debridement resulting in the elimination of active disease with resolution of periodontal inflammation, may receive implant therapy but should be carefully monitored for ongoing compliance and absence of periodontal inflammation. Their innate susceptibility to periodontal and peri-implant disease remains because of their genetic profile. Therefore they must be prepared to maintain an absolute commitment to their periodontal and peri-implant plaque control on a life-long basis. Failure to keep up this high standard of home care will certainly lead to a reinfection of the subgingival sites with a pathogenic flora and resulting destructive inflammation with the re-development of periodontitis and peri-implantitis. This can present a problem for elderly patients whose manual dexterity, cognitive function and self-care can become compromised.

Follow-Up and Support

With implant treatment being so widely available, many implant patients are returning to their own general dentist for their ongoing dental and implant care and supervision. It is therefore extremely important that all dentists and their oral healthcare teams provide the necessary high standard of clinical and radiological monitoring and regular professional periodontal debridement of implants and natural teeth in conjunction with support of the patients in their home care and plaque removal. This is a task that can be performed most effectively by dental hygienists, and these regular maintenance visits are the best support an implant patient can receive.

Summary

Dental implants represent a successful and long-term therapy for the replacement of missing teeth and, in many cases, they are the treatment of choice in providing anchorage for single-tooth, partial and full prostheses. Several fundamental principles remain essential in achieving success in implant therapy, including the early identification of risk factors and any predisposition to periodontal disease, as well as appropriate patient follow-up and management to minimise the risk of plaque-induced peri-implant inflammatory disease.

Multiple choice questions on the contents of this chapter are available online at Elsevier eBooks+.

References

Aas JA, Paster BJ, Stokes LN, Olsen I, Dewhirst FE. Defining the normal bacterial flora of the oral cavity. *J Clin Microbiol.* 2005;43:5721–5732.

Aguirre-Zorzano LA, Estefania-Fresco R, Telletxea O, Bravo M. Prevalence of peri-implant inflammatory disease in patients with a history of periodontal disease who receive supportive periodontal therapy. *Clin Oral Impl Res.* 2015;26:1338–1344.

Apse P, Ellen RP, Overall CM, Zarb GA. Microbiota and crevicular fluid collagenase activity in the osseointegrated dental implant sulcus: a comparison of sites in edentulous and partially edentulous patients. *J Perio Res.* 1989;24:96–105.

Atieh MA, Zadeh H, Stanford CM, Cooper LF. Survival of short dental implants for treatment of posterior partial edentulism: a systematic review. *Int J Oral & Maxillofacial Impl.* 2012;1:27.

Berglundh T, Gotfredsen K, Zitzmann NU, Lang NP, Lindhe J. Spontaneous progression of ligature induced peri–implantitis at implants with different surface roughness: an experimental study in dogs. *Clin Oral Impl Res*. 2007;18:655–661.

Berglundh T, Zitzmann NU, Donati M. Are peri–implantitis lesions different from periodontitis lesions? *J Clin Perio*. 2011;38(suppl 11):188–202.

Carcuac O, Abrahamsson I, Albouy JP, Linder E, Larsson L, Berglundh T. Experimental periodontitis and peri–implantitis in dogs. *Clin Oral Impl Research*. 2013;24:363–371.

Caton JG, Armitage G, Berglundh T, Chapple ILC, Jepson S, Kornman KS, Mealey BL, Papapanou PN, Sanz M, Tonetti MS. A new classification scheme for periodontal and peri-implant diseases and conditions - introduction and key changes from the 1999 classification. *J Periodontol*. 2018;89(suppl 1):S1–S8.

Darveau RP, Tanner A, Page RC. The microbial challenge in periodontitis. *Periodontol 2000*. 1997;14:12–32.

DeBoever AL, DeBoever JA. Early colonization of non-submerged dental implants in patients with a history of advanced aggressive periodontitis. *Clin Oral Impl Res*. 2006;17:8–17.

Deery C, Heanue M, Deacon S, Robinson PG, Walmsley AD, Worthington H, Shaw W, Glenny AM. The effectiveness of manual versus powered toothbrushes for dental health: a systematic review. *J Dent*. 2004;32:197–211.

Eriksson RA, Albrektsson T, Gran B, McQueen D. Thermal injury to bone. A vital microscopic description of heat effects. *Int J Oral Surg*. 1982;11:115–121.

Esposito M, Hirsch JM, Lekholm U, Thomsen P. Biological factors contributing to failures of osseointegrated oral implants,(II). Etiopathogenesis. *Eur J Oral Sci*. 1998;106:721–764.

Gargiulo AW, Yoon J, Misch CE, Wang HL. The cause of early implant bone loss: myth or science? *J Periodontol*. 2002;73:322–333.

Gouvoussis J, Sindhusake D, Yeung S. Cross-infection from periodontitis sites to failing implant sites in the same mouth. *Int J Oral & Maxillofac Impls*. 1997;12:666–673.

Heitz–Mayfield LJ. Peri–implant diseases: diagnosis and risk indicators. *J Clin Perio*. 2008;35(suppl 8):292–304.

Heitz-Mayfield LJ, Mombelli A. The therapy of peri-implantitis: a systematic review. *Int J Oral Maxillofac Impls*. 2014;29(suppl 1):325–345.

Hermann JS, Buser D, Schenk RK, Schoolfield JD, Cochran DL. Biologic width around one- and two-piece titanium implants. *Clin Oral Impls Res*. 2001;12:559–571.

Ivanovski S, Lee R. Comparison of peri-implant and periodontal marginal soft tissues in health and disease. *Periodontol 2000*. 2018;76:116-130.

Karoussis IK, Kotsovilis S, Fourmousis I. A comprehensive and critical review of dental implant prognosis in periodontally compromised partially edentulous patients. *Clinl Oral Impls Res*. 2007;18:669–679.

Koldsland OC, Scheie AA, Aass AM. Prevalence of peri-implantitis related to severity of the disease with different degrees of bone loss. *J Perio*. 2010;81:231–238.

Kotsovilis S, Karoussis IK, Fourmousis I. A comprehensive and critical review of dental implant placement in diabetic animals and patients. *Clin Oral Impls Res*. 2006;17:587–599.

Lang NP, Berglundh T. Periimplant diseases: where are we now?– Consensus of the Seventh European Workshop on Periodontology. *J Clin Perio*. 2011;38(suppl 11):178–181.

Lekholm U, Ericsson I, Adell R, Slots J. The condition of the soft tissues at tooth and fixture abutments supporting fixed bridges A microbiological and histological study. *J Clin Perio*. 1986;13:558–562.

Leonhardt Å, Berglundh T, Ericsson I, Dahlén G. Putative periodontal and teeth in pathogens on titanium implants and teeth in experimental gingivitis and periodontitis in beagle dogs. *Clinl Oral Impls Res*. 1992;3:112–119.

Leonhardt Å, Renvert S, Dahlén G. Microbial findings at failing implants. *Clin Oral Impls Res*. 1999;10:339–345.

Lindhe J, Meyle J. Peri–implant diseases: Consensus Report of the Sixth European Workshop on Periodontology. *J Clin Perio*. 2008;35(suppl 8):282–285.

Löe H, Theilade E, Jensen SB. Experimental gingivitis in man. *J Period*. 1965;36:177–187.

Löe H, Theilade E, Jensen SB, Schiøtt CR. Experimental gingivitis in man. *J Perio Res*. 1967;2:282–289.

Marsh PD. Dental plaque: biological significance of a biofilm and community life–style. *J Clin Perio*. 2005;32(suppl 6):7–15.

Mombelli A, Meriscke-Stern R. Microbiological features of stable osseointegrated implants used as abutments for overdentures. *Clin Oral Impls Res*. 1990;1:1–7.

Mombelli A, Müller N, Cionca N. The epidemiology of peri–implantitis. *Clinl Oral Impls Res*. 2012;23(suppl 6):67–76.

Niederman, R1. Manual versus powered toothbrushes: the Cochrane review. *J Am Dent Assoc*. 2003;134:1240–1244.

Ong CTT, Ivanovski S, Needleman IG, Retzepi M, Moles DR, Tonetti MS, Donos N. Systematic review of implant outcomes in treated periodontitis subjects. *J Clin Perio*. 2008;35:438–462.

Palmer R. Teeth and implants. *Br Dent J*. 1999;187:183–188.

Papaioannou W, Quirynen M, Van Steenberghe D. The influence of periodontitis on the subgingival flora around implants in partially edentulous patients. *Clin Oral Impls Res*. 1996;7:405–409.

Pontoriero R, Tonelli MP, Carnevale G, Mombelli A, Nyman SR, Lang NP. Experimentally induced peri–implant mucositis. A clinical study in humans. *Clin Oral Impls Res*. 1994;5:254–259.

Quiryen M, Listgarten MA. The distribution of bacterial morphotypes around natural teeth and titanium implants ad modum Brånemark. *Clin Oral Impls Res*. 1990;1:8–12.

Rams TE, Roberts TW, Feik D, MoIzan AK, Slots J. Clinical and microbiological findings on newly inserted hydroxyapatite–coated and pure–titanium human dental implants. *Clin Oral Impls Res*. 1991;2:121–127.

Roos–Jansåker AM, Renvert H, Lindahl C, Renvert S. Nine–to fourteen–year follow–up of implant treatment. Part III: factors associated with peri–implant lesions. *J Clin Perio*. 2006;33:296–301.

Salvi GE, Persson GR, Heitz-Mayfield LJ, Frei M, Lang NP. Adjunctive local antibiotic therapy in the treatment of peri-implantitis II: clinical and radiographic outcomes. *Clin Oral Impls Res*. 2007;18:281–285.

Salvi GE, Aglietta M, Eick S, Sculean A, Lang NP, Ramseier CA. Reversibility of experimental peri–implant mucositis compared with experimental gingivitis in humans. *Clin Oral Impls Res*. 2012;23:182–190.

Schaudinn C, Gorur A, Keller D, Sedghizadeh PP, Costerton JW. Periodontitis: an archetypical biofilm disease. *JAMA*. 2009;140:978–986.

Serino G, Ström C. Peri–implantitis in partially edentulous patients: association with inadequate plaque control. *Clin Oral Impls Res*. 2009;20:169–174.

Sousa V, Mardas N, Farias B, Petrie A, et al. A systematic review of implant outcomes in treated periodontitis patients. *Clin Oral Implants Res*. 27(7):787–844.

Stern IB. Current concepts of the dento-gingival junction: the epithelial and connective tissue attachments to the tooth. *J Periodontol*. 1981;52:465–476.

Tarnow DP, Magner AW, Fletcher P. The effect of the distance from contact point to the crest of bone on the presence or absence of the interproximal dental papilla. *J Periodontol*. 1992;63:995–996.

Theilade E, Wright WH, Jensen SB, Löe H. Experimental gingivitis in man. *J Perio Res*. 1966;1:1–3.

Wadhwani C, Hess T, Faber T, Piñeyro A, Chen CS. A descriptive study of the radiographic density of implant restorative cements. *J Pros Dent*. 2010;103:295–302.

Wennström JL, Derks J. Is there a need for keratinized mucosa around implants to maintain health and tissue stability? *Clin Oral Impls Res*. 2012;23(suppl 6):136–146.

Wilson Jr TG. The positive relationship between excess cement and peri-implant disease: a prospective clinical endoscopic study. *J Perio*. 2009;80:1388–1392.

Zitzmann NU, Berglundh T. Definition and prevalence of peri-implant diseases. *J Clin Perio*. 2008;55(suppl 8):286–291.

World Workshop on Classification of Periodontal and Peri-implant Diseases and Conditions 2017 - Staging and Grading of Periodontitis

Staging

Periodontitis stage		Stage I	Stage II	Stage III	Stage IV
Severity	Interdental CAL at site of greatest loss	1 to 2 mm	3 to 4 mm	≥5 mm	≥5 mm
	Radiographic bone loss	Coronal third (<15%)	Coronal third (15%–33%)	Extending to mid-third of root and beyond	Extending to mid-third of root and beyond
	Tooth loss	No tooth loss due to periodontitis		Tooth loss due to periodontitis of ≤4 teeth	Tooth loss due to periodontitis of ≥5 teeth
Complexity	Local	Maximum probing depth ≤4 mm Mostly horizontal bone loss	Maximum probing depth ≤5 mm Mostly horizontal bone loss	In addition to stage II complexity: Probing depth ≥6 mm Vertical bone loss ≥3 mm Furcation involvement class II or III Moderate ridge defect	In addition to stage III complexity: Need for complex rehabilitation due to: Masticatory dysfunction Secondary occlusal trauma (tooth mobility degree ≥2) Severe ridge defect Bite collapse, drifting, flaring Less than 20 remaining teeth (10 opposing pairs)
Extent and distribution	Add to stage as descriptor	For each stage, describe extent as localized (<30% of teeth involved), generalized, or molar/incisor pattern			

CAL: Clinical attachment loss.

Grading

Periodontitis grade			Grade A: Slow rate of progression	Grade B: Moderate rate of progression	Grade C: Rapid rate of progression
Primary criteria	Direct evidence of progression	Longitudinal data (radiographic bone loss or CAL)	Evidence of no loss over 5 years	<2 mm over 5 years	≥2 mm over 5 years
	Indirect evidence of progression	% bone loss/age	<0.25	0.25 to 1.0	>1.0
		Case phenotype	Heavy biofilm deposits with low levels of destruction	Destruction commensurate with biofilm deposits	Destruction exceeds expectation given biofilm deposits; specific clinical patterns suggestive of periods of rapid progression and/or early onset disease (e.g., molar/incisor pattern; lack of expected response to standard bacterial control therapies)
Grade modifiers	Risk factors	Smoking	Non-smoker	Smoker <10 cigarettes/day	Smoker ≥10 cigarettes/day
		Diabetes	Normoglycemic/no diagnosis of diabetes	HbA1c <7.0% in patients with diabetes	HbA1c ≥7.0% in patients with diabetes

CAL: Clinical attachment loss; I IbA1c: glycated haemoglobin.

(Reprinted from Tonetti, M., Greenwell, H., Kornman, K. J. Staging and grading of periodontitis: Framework and proposal of a new classification and case definition. J Periodontol. 2018 Jun;89 Suppl 1:S159-S172. doi: 10.1002/JPER.18-0006., with permission from Wiley.)

Appendix 2

Implementing the 2017 Classification of Periodontal Diseases to Reach a Diagnosis in Clinical Practice

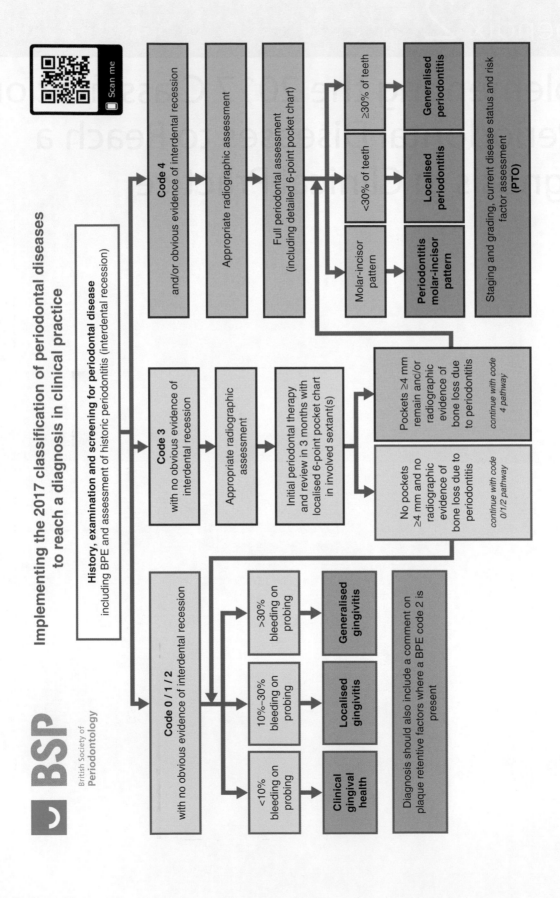

Implementing the 2017 classification of periodontal diseases to reach a diagnosis in clinical practice

British Society of Periodontology

History, examination and screening for periodontal disease
including BPE and assessment of historic periodontitis (interdental recession)

Code 0 / 1 / 2 with no obvious evidence of interdental recession
- <10% bleeding on probing → **Clinical gingival health**
- 10%–30% bleeding on probing → **Localised gingivitis**
- >30% bleeding on probing → **Generalised gingivitis**

Diagnosis should also include a comment on plaque retentive factors where a BPE code 2 is present

Code 3 with no obvious evidence of interdental recession
→ Appropriate radiographic assessment
→ Initial periodontal therapy and review in 3 months with localised 6-point pocket chart in involved sextant(s)
- No pockets ≥4 mm and no radiographic evidence of bone loss due to periodontitis — *continue with code 0/1/2 pathway*
- Pockets ≥4 mm remain and/or radiographic evidence of bone loss due to periodontitis — *continue with code 4 pathway*

Code 4 and/or obvious evidence of interdental recession
→ Appropriate radiographic assessment
→ Full periodontal assessment (including detailed 6-point pocket chart)
- Molar-incisor pattern → **Periodontitis molar-incisor pattern**
- <30% of teeth → **Localised periodontitis**
- ≥30% of teeth → **Generalised periodontitis**

Staging and grading, current disease status and risk factor assessment **(PTO)**

Scan me

BSP
British Society of Periodontology

Staging

Radiographic assessment
(periapicals or OPG/DPT)
if not clinically justified or if bitewings only available use CAL or bone loss from CEJ

Interproximal bone loss
(use worst site of bone loss due to periodontitis)

<15% (or <2 mm attachment loss from CEJ)	Coronal third of root	Mid-third of root	Apical third of root
Stage I (early/mild)	Stage II (moderate)	Stage III (severe)	Stage IV (very severe)

Grading

% bone loss ÷ patient age
(use worst site of bone loss due to periodontitis)

<0.5	0.5–1.0	>1.0
Grade A (slow rate of progression)	Grade B (moderate rate of progression)	Grade C (rapid rate of progression)

Assessment of current periodontitis status

Currently stable
BoP <10%
PPD ≤4 mm
No BoP at 4 mm sites

Currently in remission
BoP ≥10%
PPD ≤4 mm
No BoP at 4 mm sites

Currently unstable
PPD ≥5 mm or
PPD ≥4 mm & BoP

Risk factor assessment

For example:
• Smoking, including cigarettes/day
• Sub-optimally controlled diabetes

Diagnosis statement: Extent - periodontitis - stage - grade - stability - risk factors
e.g.: Generalised periodontitis stage 3 grade B - currently unstable - risk(s): Smoker 15/day

Reproduced with the kind permission of the British Society of Periodontology and Implant Dentistry: www.bsperio.org.uk

European Federation of Periodontology S3-Level Clinical Treatment Guidelines - Stepwise Approach

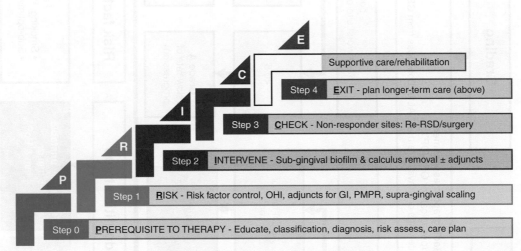

(Reprinted with permission from Springer Nature: Br. Dent. J. Evidence-based, personalised and minimally invasive treatment for periodontitis patients - the new EFP S3-level clinical treatment guidelines, Kebschull, M., Chapple, I., copyright 2020.)

Appendix 4

BSP UK Clinical Practice Guidelines for the Treatment of Periodontal Diseases

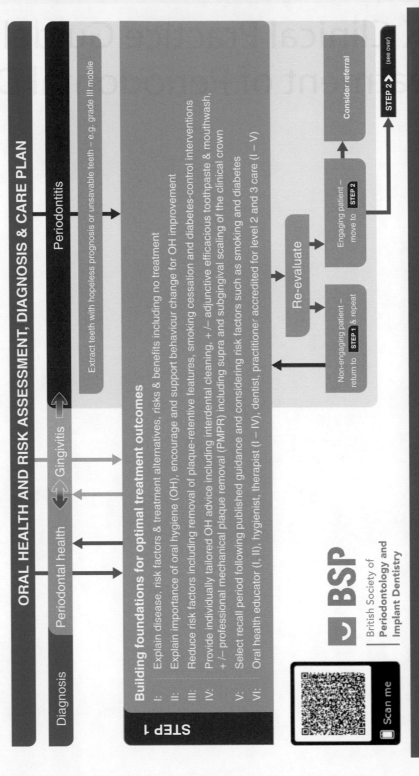

BSP UK clinical practice guidelines for the treatment of periodontal diseases

Supported by
gsk

ORAL HEALTH AND RISK ASSESSMENT, DIAGNOSIS & CARE PLAN

Diagnosis

Periodontal health | Gingivitis | Periodontitis

Extract teeth with hopeless prognosis or unsavable teeth – e.g. grade III mobile

STEP 1

Building foundations for optimal treatment outcomes

I: Explain disease, risk factors & treatment alternatives, risks & benefits including no treatment

II: Explain importance of oral hygiene (OH), encourage and support behaviour change for OH improvement

III: Reduce risk factors including removal of plaque-retentive features, smoking cessation and diabetes-control interventions

IV: Provide individually tailored OH advice including interdental cleaning, +/– adjunctive efficacious toothpaste & mouthwash, +/– professional mechanical plaque removal (PMPR) including supra and subgingival scaling of the clinical crown

V: Select recall period following published guidance and considering risk factors such as smoking and diabetes

VI: Oral health educator (I, II), hygienist, therapist (I – IV), dentist, practitioner: accredited for level 2 and 3 care (I – V)

Re-evaluate

Non-engaging patient – return to STEP 1 & repeat

Engaging patient – move to STEP 2

Consider referral

STEP 2 ❯ (see over)

BSP
British Society of
**Periodontology and
Implant Dentistry**

Scan me

www.bsperio.org.uk

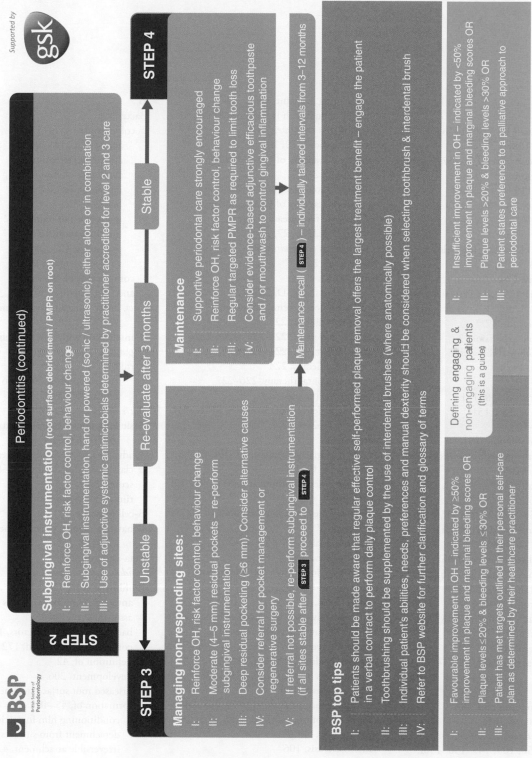

Supported by
gsk

BSP
British Society of
Periodontology

Periodontitis (continued)

STEP 2

Subgingival instrumentation (root surface debridement / PMPR on root)

- I: Reinforce OH, risk factor control, behaviour change
- II: Subgingival instrumentation, hand or powered (sonic / ultrasonic), either alone or in combination
- III: Use of adjunctive systemic antimicrobials determined by practitioner accredited for level 2 and 3 care

Re-evaluate after 3 months

Unstable → STEP 3

Stable → STEP 4

STEP 3

Managing non-responding sites:

- I: Reinforce OH, risk factor control, behaviour change
- II: Moderate (4–5 mm) residual pockets – re-perform subgingival instrumentation
- III: Deep residual pocketing (≥6 mm). Consider alternative causes
- IV: Consider referral for pocket management or regenerative surgery
- V: If referral not possible, re-perform subgingival instrumentation (if all sites stable after STEP 3) proceed to STEP 4

STEP 4

Maintenance

- I: Supportive periodontal care strongly encouraged
- II: Reinforce OH, risk factor control, behaviour change
- III: Regular targeted PMPR as required to limit tooth loss
- IV: Consider evidence-based adjunctive efficacious toothpaste and / or mouthwash to control gingival inflammation

Maintenance recall (STEP 4) – individually tailored intervals from 3–12 months

BSP top tips

- I: Patients should be made aware that regular effective self-performed plaque removal offers the largest treatment benefit – engage the patient in a verbal contract to perform daily plaque control
- II: Toothbrushing should be supplemented by the use of interdental brushes (where anatomically possible)
- III: Individual patient's abilities, needs, preferences and manual dexterity should be considered when selecting toothbrush & interdental brush
- IV: Refer to BSP website for further clarification and glossary of terms

Defining engaging & non-engaging patients (this is a guide)

- I: Favourable improvement in OH – indicated by ≥50% improvement in plaque and marginal bleeding scores OR
- II: Plaque levels ≤20% & bleeding levels ≤30% OR
- III: Patient has met targets outlined in their personal self-care plan as determined by their healthcare practitioner

- I: Insufficient improvement in OH – indicated by <50% improvement in plaque and marginal bleeding scores OR
- II: Plaque levels >20% & bleeding levels >30% OR
- III: Patient states preference to a palliative approach to periodontal care

Reproduced with the kind permission of the British Society of Periodontology and Implant Dentistry: www.bsperio.org.uk

Index

Page numbers followed by '*f*' indicate figures those followed by '*t*' indicate tables and '*b*' indicate boxes.